D1442271

Atlas of Palpatory Anatomy of Limbs and Trunk

Atlas of Palpatory Anatomy of Limbs and Trunk

Serge Tixa

Instructor of Anatomy
and Palpatory Anatomy
Swiss School of Osteopathy
of Lausanne

Including illustrations by Frank H. Netter

Icon Learning Systems · Teterboro, New Jersey

Published by Icon Learning Systems, LLC, a subsidiary of MediMedia USA, Inc.
Copyright © 2003 MediMedia, Inc.

FIRST EDITION

ISBN 1-929007-24-8
Library of Congress Catalog No. 2003110692

NOTICE

Executive Editor: Paul Kelly
Editorial Director: Greg Otis
Managing Editor: Jennifer Surich
Production Editor: Stephanie Klein
Art Director: Colleen Quinn
Print Production Manager: Mary Ellen Curry

TRANSLATION

Sections I to VII translated by Icon Learning Systems. Sections VIII to XII translated by Normand Miller, MD, FRCSC

10   9   8   7   6   5   4   3   2   1

Printed and bound by Banta Book Group

This book presents a method of palpatory anatomy based on the manual inspection of surface forms, or MISF. This method can be used to learn and become familiar with anatomic structures including bones, ligaments, tendons, muscle bodies, nerves, and the vasculature. It is a highly visual approach that relies on photographs showing the structure under investigation with accompanying text that instructs the reader how to apply the proper techniques.

For Whom Is It Intended?

The author conceived this book as a helpful reference for physicians, physical therapists, exercise physiologists, sports trainers, and other professionals who require a method of applied anatomy.

How Is the Book Organized?

This book includes more than 700 photographs of the neck, trunk, sacrum and upper and lower extremities. It is divided into 12 sections corresponding to body regions; each section is in turn subdivided into chapters covering osteology, myology (or musculotendinous structures), arthrology (joints and ligaments), and nerves and vessels.

Each section of the book is introduced with anatomic illustrations by the highly regarded medical illustrator Frank H. Netter, MD, the author of the *Atlas of Human Anatomy,* the most widely-used anatomy atlas in the world.

Within each section, there are two types of photographs.

• Photographs of presentation

— General presentation, introducing a region of the body.

— Topographic presentation, showing a comprehensive view of a region with structures accessible to palpation (e.g., the lateral inguinofemoral region or the lateral border of the foot).

— Structural presentation, illustrating, when possible, the anatomic structure and its relationships with the adjacent structures. These are mainly presentations of muscles or muscular groups (e.g., the quadriceps extensor muscle).

• MISF photographs

— The essential part of this work, demonstrating the investigated structure and describing the technique of approach.

How should it be used?

There are two possible methods:

• To study a region (e.g., the knee) or part of a region (e.g., the lateral border of the foot) thoroughly, refer to the part or chapter of interest in the Table of Contents.

• To study a specific structure from all possible angles, refer to the Index, which lists all photographs related to the subject (e.g., the sartorius muscle is dealt with in Part II, "The Thigh," as well as Parts I and III, "The Hip" and "The Knee").

Note

• The delimitation of the regions studied in each part should not be interpreted too strictly, since some muscles, for example, extend beyond the areas of emphasis. This is justified by the fact that each muscle is studied not only in a transverse approach, in relation to the adjacent structures, but also longitudinally in terms of its origin, body, and site of insertion (e.g., the iliopsoas muscle, which extends far beyond the medial inguinofemoral region, found also in the abdominal region).

• In the text, the hand or grip of the examiner is often labeled "proximal" or "distal," depending on whether it is moving closer to or further away from the origin of the limb being examined.

TABLE OF CONTENTS

PART I: UPPER EXTREMITIES

SECTION I: THE NECK

Gross Anatomy

Chapter 1: Osteology

Chapter 2: Myology

Chapter 3: Nerves and Vessels

SECTION II: THE TRUNK AND THE SACRUM

Gross Anatomy

Chapter 4: Osteology

Chapter 5: Myology

Chapter 6: Nerves and Vessels

SECTION III: THE SHOULDER

Gross Anatomy

Chapter 7: Osteology

TABLE OF CONTENTS

TABLE OF CONTENTS

TABLE OF CONTENTS

TABLE OF CONTENTS

UPPER EXTREMITIES

THE NECK

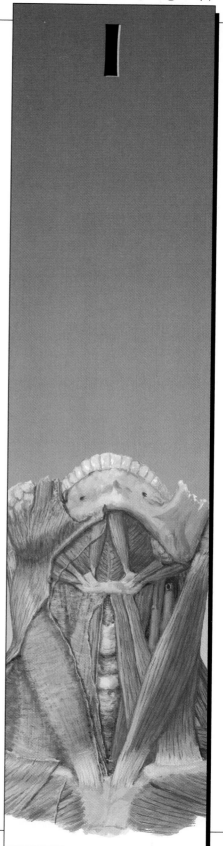

MUSCLES OF THE NECK: ANTERIOR VIEW

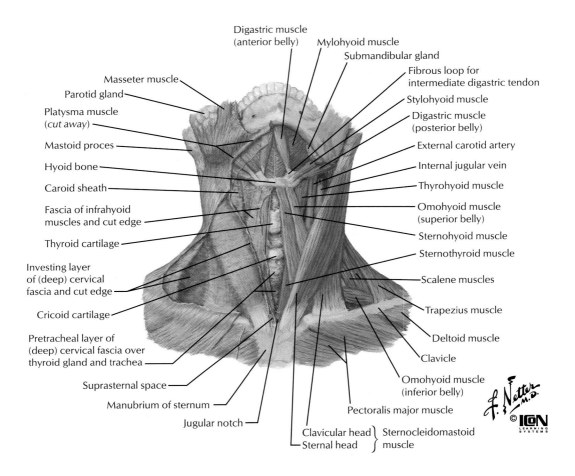

Digastric muscle (anterior belly)

Mylohyoid muscle

Submandibular gland

Masseter muscle

Parotid gland

Platysma muscle (*cut away*)

Mastoid proces

Hyoid bone

Caroid sheath

Fascia of infrahyoid muscles and cut edge

Thyroid cartilage

Investing layer of (deep) cervical fascia and cut edge

Cricoid cartilage

Pretracheal layer of (deep) cervical fascia over thyroid gland and trachea

Suprasternal space

Manubrium of sternum

Jugular notch

Fibrous loop for intermediate digastric tendon

Stylohyoid muscle

Digastric muscle (posterior belly)

External carotid artery

Internal jugular vein

Thyrohyoid muscle

Omohyoid muscle (superior belly)

Sternohyoid muscle

Sternothyroid muscle

Scalene muscles

Trapezius muscle

Deltoid muscle

Clavicle

Omohyoid muscle (inferior belly)

Pectoralis major muscle

Clavicular head } Sternocleidomastoid
Sternal head   } muscle

MUSCLES OF THE NECK: LATERAL VIEW

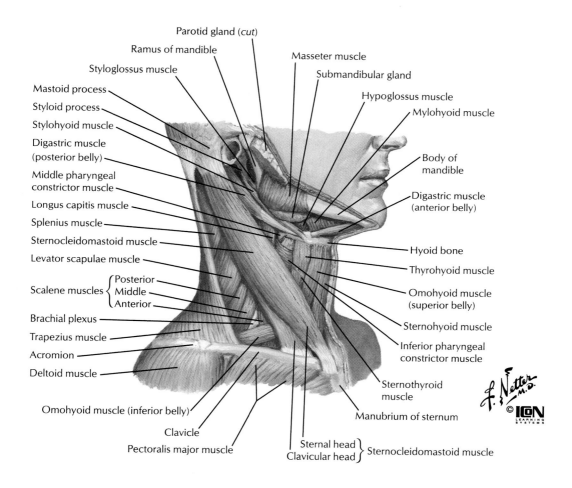

Parotid gland (*cut*)

Ramus of mandible

Masseter muscle

Styloglossus muscle

Submandibular gland

Mastoid process

Hypoglossus muscle

Styloid process

Mylohyoid muscle

Stylohyoid muscle

Digastric muscle
(posterior belly)

Body of
mandible

Middle pharyngeal
constrictor muscle

Digastric muscle
(anterior belly)

Longus capitis muscle

Splenius muscle

Sternocleidomastoid muscle

Hyoid bone

Levator scapulae muscle

Thyrohyoid muscle

Scalene muscles { Posterior
Middle
Anterior

Omohyoid muscle
(superior belly)

Brachial plexus

Sternohyoid muscle

Trapezius muscle

Inferior pharyngeal
constrictor muscle

Acromion

Deltoid muscle

Sternothyroid
muscle

Omohyoid muscle (inferior belly)

Manubrium of sternum

Clavicle

Pectoralis major muscle

Sternal head }
Clavicular head } Sternocleidomastoid muscle

SUBOCCIPITAL TRIANGLE

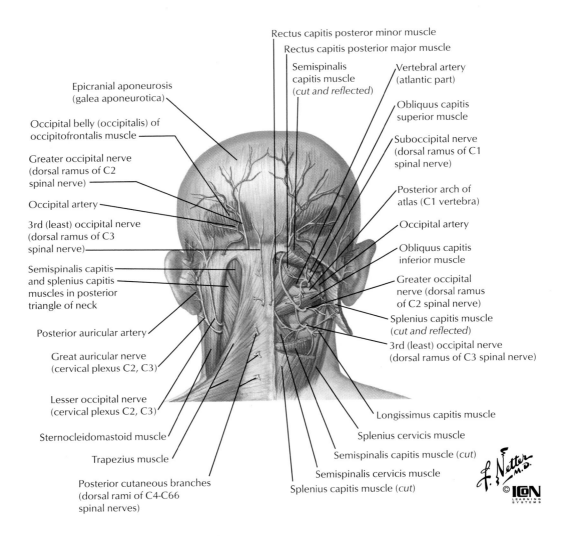

Rectus capitis posteror minor muscle

Rectus capitis posterior major muscle

Semispinalis capitis muscle (*cut and reflected*)

Vertebral artery (atlantic part)

Epicranial aponeurosis (galea aponeurotica)

Obliquus capitis superior muscle

Occipital belly (occipitalis) of occipitofrontalis muscle

Suboccipital nerve (dorsal ramus of C1 spinal nerve)

Greater occipital nerve (dorsal ramus of C2 spinal nerve)

Posterior arch of atlas (C1 vertebra)

Occipital artery

Occipital artery

3rd (least) occipital nerve (dorsal ramus of C3 spinal nerve)

Obliquus capitis inferior muscle

Semispinalis capitis and splenius capitis muscles in posterior triangle of neck

Greater occipital nerve (dorsal ramus of C2 spinal nerve)

Splenius capitis muscle (*cut and reflected*)

3rd (least) occipital nerve (dorsal ramus of C3 spinal nerve)

Posterior auricular artery

Great auricular nerve (cervical plexus C2, C3)

Lesser occipital nerve (cervical plexus C2, C3)

Longissimus capitis muscle

Sternocleidomastoid muscle

Splenius cervicis muscle

Semispinalis capitis muscle (*cut*)

Trapezius muscle

Semispinalis cervicis muscle

Posterior cutaneous branches (dorsal rami of C4-C66 spinal nerves)

Splenius capitis muscle (*cut*)

f. Netter
m.d.

© IꞒN
LEARNING
SYSTEMS

TOPOGRAPHIC PRESENTATION OF THE NECK

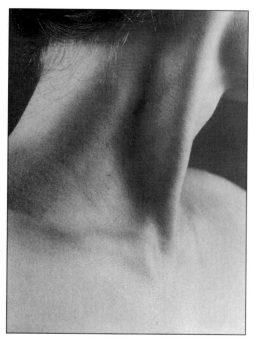

FIGURE 1-1
PRESENTATION OF THE NECK REGION

CHAPTER One

OSTEOLOGY

The notable structures accessible by palpation are

- The cervical region (Fig. 1-3)
- The spinous process of the seventh cervical vertebra (vertebra prominens, C7) (Fig. 1-4)
- The spinous process of the sixth cervical vertebra (C6) (Fig. 1-5)
- The posterior tubercle of the atlas (C1) (Fig. 1-6)
- The spinous process of the axis (C2) (Fig. 1-7)
- The transverse process of the atlas (C1) (Fig. 1-8)
- The transverse process of the axis (C2) (Fig. 1-9)
- The transverse processes of the third to the seventh cervical vertebrae (Fig. 1-10)
- The articular process of the cervical vertebrae — global approach (Figs. 1-11 and 1-12)

- The thyroid cartilage (Fig. 1-13)
- The thyroid cartilage and the laryngeal prominence (Adam's apple) — lateral view (Fig. 1-14)
- The thyroid cartilage and the laryngeal prominence (Adam's apple) — anterior view (Fig. 1-15)
- The cricoid cartilage (Fig. 1-16)
- The body of the hyoid bone — step 1 (Fig. 1-17)
- The body of the hyoid bone — step 2 and the median hyoid tubercle (Fig. 1-18)
- The body of the hyoid bone — the lesser cornu (horn) (Fig. 1-19)
- The body of the hyoid bone — the greater cornu (horn) and its posterior tubercle (Fig. 1-20)

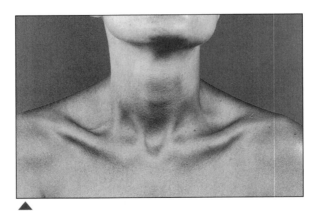

▲

FIGURE 1-2
ANTERIOR VIEW OF THE NECK REGION

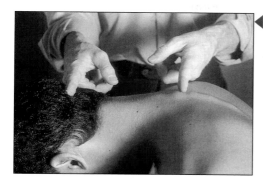

FIGURE 1-3

THE CERVICAL REGION

The general topographic location of the cervical region, which is situated between the occipital bone and the first thoracic vertebra, is indicated by the two index fingers. The seven cervical vertebrae are positioned one under the other, each separated from the one below by an articulation.

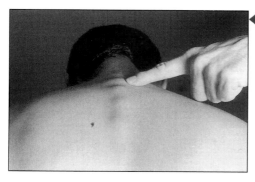

FIGURE 1-4

THE SPINOUS PROCESS OF THE SEVENTH CERVICAL VERTEBRA (VERTEBRA PROMINENS, C7)

This long and prominent process presents only a single tubercle at its extremity. To avoid confusing this process with that of the first thoracic vertebra, see Figures 4-33 and 4-34.

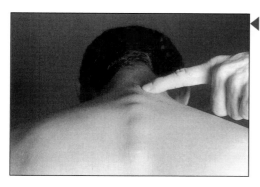

FIGURE 1-5

THE SPINOUS PROCESS OF THE SIXTH CERVICAL VERTEBRA (C6)

Once you have clearly identified the spinous process of the seventh cervical vertebra (see Fig. 1-4, above, and Figs. 4-33 and 4-34), it is easy to find the spinous process of the sixth, which is located immediately above. Repeated right and left rotations of the subject's head help confirm its identification (the spinous process of C6 is clearly felt moving in relation to the spinous process of C7).

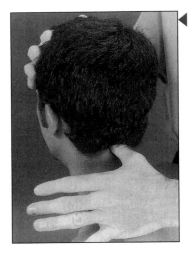

◀ FIGURE 1-6
THE POSTERIOR TUBERCLE OF THE ATLAS (C1)

This structure is found in the extension of the external occipital crest, on the external surface of the occipital bone. Under your fingers, you will feel the posterior border of the foramen magnum and, just below this border (caudally), a small depression, where your thumb comes in contact with the posterior tubercle of the atlas.

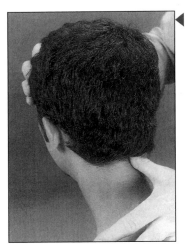

◀ FIGURE 1-7
THE SPINOUS PROCESS OF THE AXIS (C2)

Below the small depression referred to in Figure1-6 (at the bottom of which the posterior tubercle of the atlas is located), under your fingers you can feel a bony structure, which is the spinous process of the axis. This very prominent process will be obvious if you place your other hand on the subject's forehead and perform light flexion and extension movements of the subject's head.

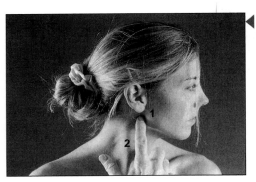

◀ FIGURE 1-8
THE TRANSVERSE PROCESS OF THE ATLAS (C1)

The index finger indicates the space between the ramus of the mandible (1) and the sternocleidomastoid muscle (2), where the single tubercle of the transverse process of the atlas may be palpated.

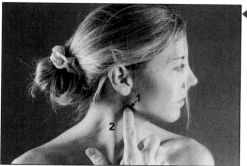

◀ **FIGURE 1-9**

THE TRANSVERSE PROCESS OF THE AXIS (C2)

The landmark for locating this structure is the angle of the mandible (1). This process can be palpated either in front of or behind the sternocleidomastoid muscle (2). Unlike the transverse process of the atlas, the transverse process of the axis is not very pronounced.

Comment: As with all the structures in the neck region, approach this structure very carefully.

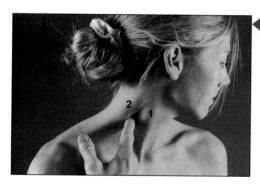

◀ **FIGURE 1-10**

THE TRANSVERSE PROCESSES OF THE THIRD TO THE SEVENTH CERVICAL VERTEBRAE

In this figure the index finger indicates the region between the sternocleidomastoid muscle (1) and the trapezius muscle (2), where you need to slide your grip in order to come into contact with the transverse processes.

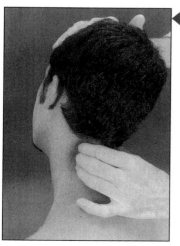

◀ **FIGURE 1-11**

THE ARTICULAR PROCESSES OF THE CERVICAL VERTEBRAE — GLOBAL APPROACH

This is a global grip. Place your thumb and fingers just anterior to the cervical part of the trapezius muscle (Fig. 1-20), in contact with the articular processes of the cervical vertebrae. With your other hand placed on the subject's forehead, direct alternating movements of lateral flexion. You will feel these processes under your fingers.

Comment: After you locate the lateral border of the cervical aspect of the trapezius muscle as described above, be certain that this muscle is totally relaxed before you palpate the articular processes.

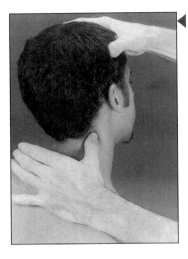

FIGURE 1-12
THE ARTICULAR PROCESS OF THE CERVICAL VERTEBRAE — GLOBAL APPROACH

This grip is identical to the one described in Figure 1-11. This picture shows the precise location of the thumb.

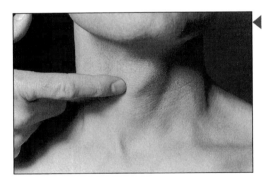

FIGURE 1-13
THE THYROID CARTILAGE

Place the subject's head in hyperextension for better visualization. This structure is located between the hyoid bone (Figs. 1-17 through 1-20) superiorly and the cricoid cartilage (Fig. 1-16) inferiorly. The thyroid cartilage, indicated by the index finger, is the largest of all the laryngeal cartilages. It owes its name to its form, which resembles a shield (thyroid means "shield-shaped" in Greek), and its position, in that it covers the other elements of the larynx anteriorly.

Comment: This unpaired and median cartilage tends to ossify in adults and elderly people.

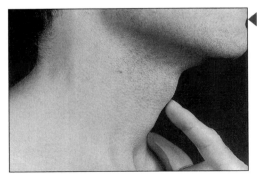

FIGURE 1-14
THE THYROID CARTILAGE AND THE LARYNGEAL PROMINENCE (ADAM'S APPLE) — LATERAL VIEW

The anterior surface of this cartilage, strongly convex anteriorly, presents along its median line an angular projection—the Adam's apple (much more pronounced in men than in women), indicated by the index finger.

Comment: Three of the eleven laryngeal cartilages are unpaired and median: the thyroid cartilage, the cricoid cartilage, and the epiglottis.

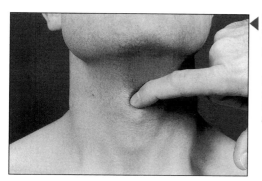

FIGURE 1-15
THE THYROID CARTILAGE AND THE LARYNGEAL PROMINENCE (ADAM'S APPLE) — ANTERIOR VIEW

In this figure, the index finger is placed on the median notch, located on the superior border of the thyroid cartilage, at the level of the Adam's apple (see also Figs. 1-13 and 1-14).

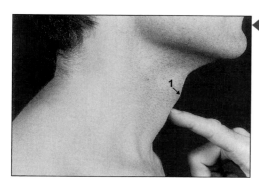

FIGURE 1-16
THE CRICOID CARTILAGE

This is the lowest cartilage of the larynx. Indicated by the index finger, this structure is located two fingerbreadths below the laryngeal prominence (1) (Fig. 1-14). The cricoid cartilage constitutes the base of the laryngeal pyramid and ensures the transition between the larynx and the first tracheal ring.

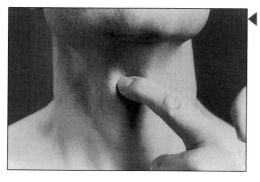

FIGURE 1-17
THE BODY OF THE HYOID BONE — STEP 1

Place the index finger on the superior border of the thyroid cartilage (Fig. 1-15). This is the first step in locating the body of the hyoid bone, which is situated above.

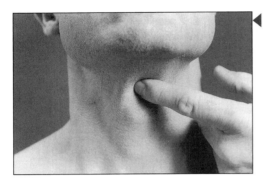

◀ FIGURE 1-18
THE BODY OF THE HYOID BONE —
STEP 2 AND THE HYOID MEDIAN TUBERCLE

After completing Step 1, place the subject's neck in slight extension and move your index finger upward to make contact with the body of the hyoid bone, which is located one fingerbreadth toward the mandible. The hyoid median tubercle forms a bony projection directly perceptible under the skin.

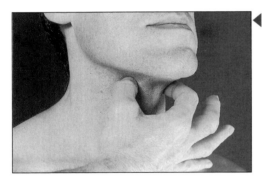

◀ FIGURE 1-19
THE HYOID BONE — THE LESSER CORNU (HORN)

After locating the superior border of the thyroid cartilage (Fig. 1-15) and the hyoid body with its median tubercle (Figs. 1-17 and 1-18), move your thumb–index finger grip slightly laterally, staying in the plane of the hyoid body, to come in contact with two little bony projections that resemble little horns pointing upward.

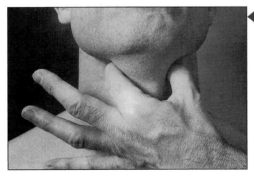

◀ FIGURE 1-20
THE HYOID BONE — THE GREATER CORNU (HORN) AND ITS POSTERIOR TUBERCLE

After locating the body of the hyoid bone (Figs. 1-17 and 1-18) and the lesser cornua (horns) (Fig. 1-19), and using the same grip as above, press gently laterally to make contact with the greater cornua, which extend the body of the hyoid bone superiorly, posteriorly, and laterally. The greater cornua end posteriorly with a tubercle, also perceptible under your fingers. Position the subject's head in extension to better perceive these structures.

C H A P T E R
T w o

MYOLOGY

THE STERNOCLEIDOMASTOID REGION

The notable structures accessible by palpation are

- The distal insertion of the sternal portion of the sternocleidomastoid muscle (Fig. 2-2)
- The two parts of the sternal portion of the sternocleidomastoid muscle (Fig. 2-3)
- The belly of the sternal portion of the sternocleidomastoid muscle (Fig. 2-4)

- The clavicular portion of the sternocleidomastoid muscle (Fig. 2-5)
- The mastoid insertion of the sternocleidomastoid muscle (Fig. 2-6)

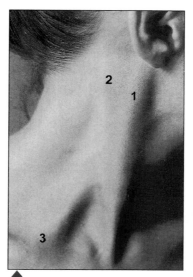

▲
FIGURE 2-1
LATERAL VIEW OF THE
STERNOCLEIDOMASTOID MUSCLE

(1) Sternal portion of the sternocleidomastoid muscle
(2) Occipital portion of the sternocleidomastoid muscle
(3) Clavicular portion of the sternocleidomastoid muscle

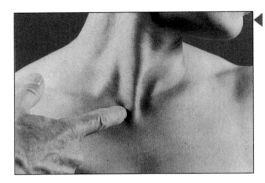

FIGURE 2-2

THE DISTAL INSERTION OF THE STERNAL PORTION OF THE STERNOCLEIDOMASTOID MUSCLE

The index finger indicates the insertion of this portion of the muscle into the sternal manubrium, medial to the stern-oclavicular interspace, with its strong tendon. To make this muscle protrude, ask the subject to perform a contralateral rotation of the head with a slight ipsilateral lateral flexion.

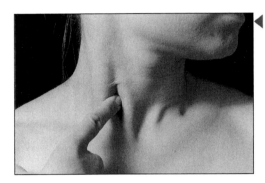

FIGURE 2-3

THE TWO PARTS OF THE STERNAL PORTION OF THE STERN-OCLEIDOMASTOID MUSCLE

The sternal portion is sometimes divided into two bundles: sternomastoid and sternooccipital. These two fasciculi insert into the sternum through two distinct tendons: the tendon of the sternooccipital portion is located lateral to the tendon of the sternomastoid portion. Ask the subject for the same action as described in Fig. 2-2. You can slide your index finger between the two portions (if they exist), as shown in this figure.

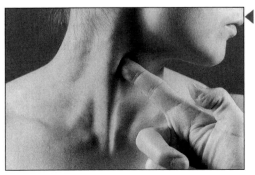

FIGURE 2-4

THE BELLY OF THE STERNAL PORTION OF THE STERNOCLEI-DOMASTOID MUSCLE

The muscle belly appears above the sternoclavicular joint and is directed upward, backward, and outward. Ask the subject to perform the same movements as described in Fig. 2-2.

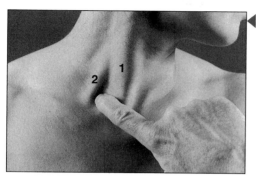

FIGURE 2-5
THE CLAVICULAR PORTION OF THE STERNOCLEIDOMASTOID MUSCLE

The index finger indicates the cleidooccipital portion of the muscle, which is a superficial and oblique portion that arises from the medial third of the superior surface of the clavicle. It covers the cleidomastoid portion, which has a vertical orientation. Ask the subject to perform the same muscular action as described in Figure 2-2 but with a more pronounced ipsilateral lateral flexion, as well as a slight flexion of the neck.

Comment: In this figure, the index finger is placed in the triangular space with an inferior base that separates the two heads of the sternocleidomastoid muscle: sternal (1) and clavicular (2).

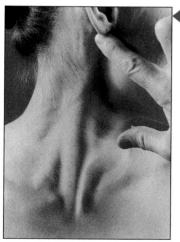

FIGURE 2-6
THE MASTOID INSERTION OF THE STERNOCLEIDOMASTOID MUSCLE

The sternocleidomastoid muscle inserts into the skull through four portions: two occipital portions, which insert into the lateral aspect of the superior nuchal line (not shown in this figure), and two mastoid portions, which insert into the mastoid process of the temporal bone (this structure is indicated by the index finger). The cleidomastoid portion inserts into the lateral surface of this process, and the sternomastoid portion inserts into the apex.

THE LATERAL REGION OF THE NECK

The notable structures accessible by palpation are

• The bellies of the posterior scalene muscle and the middle scalene muscle (Fig. 2-8)

• The belly of the anterior scalene muscle (Fig. 2-9)

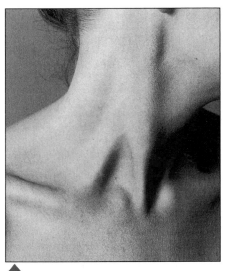

▲
FIGURE 2-7
ANTEROLATERAL VIEW OF THE NECK

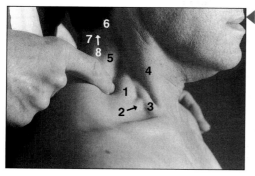

(1) Muscular mass representing the bellies of the middle and posterior scalene muscles

(2) Inferior belly of the omohyoid muscle

(3) Sternocleidomastoid muscle (clavicular portion)

(4) Sternocleidomastoid muscle (sternal portion)

(5) Levator scapulae muscle

(6) Sternocleidomastoid muscle (cleidooccipital portion)

(7) Trapezius muscle (cervical portion)

(8) Splenius cervicis muscle

FIGURE 2-8
THE BELLIES OF THE POSTERIOR SCALENE MUSCLE AND THE MIDDLE SCALENE MUSCLE

The scalenes, classically described as three muscles, can also be considered a single muscular mass at the level of their proximal attachments. The muscular mass (1) indicated by the index finger represents the bellies of the middle and posterior scalenes; the most posterior aspect can be considered the posterior scalene muscle. In order to make this mass protrude, ask the subject to perform brief, repeated inspirations with the upper part of the thorax (this action of accessory inhaling is one of the actions of the scalenes if you consider the cervical vertebrae fixed).

Comment: The distal attachment of the posterior scalene is on the superolateral surface of the second rib. The distal attachment of the middle scalene is on the superior surface of the first rib, behind the tubercle for the anterior scalene (scalene tubercle of Lisfranc) and behind the groove for the subclavian artery.

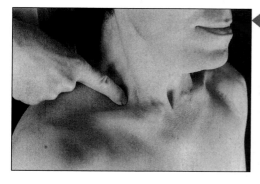

FIGURE 2-9
THE BELLY OF THE ANTERIOR SCALENE MUSCLE

After locating the clavicular portion of the sternocleidomastoid muscle (Fig. 2-5), place one or two fingertips on the muscular portion, slightly set back from the clavicle, to come in contact with the anterior scalene muscle. (This muscle is perceptible through the clavicular portion.) Then ask the subject to perform brief, repeated inspirations to move the upper part of the rib cage; this is one of the muscular actions of the anterior scalene if the cervical vertebrae are considered fixed.

Comment: This muscle inserts into the superior surface of the first rib, on the tubercle for the anterior scalene (scalene tubercle of Lisfranc), between the groove for the subclavian artery posteriorly and the groove for the subclavian vein anteriorly.

THE ANTERIOR REGION OF THE NECK

The notable structures accessible by palpation are

- The platysma (Fig. 2-11)
- The mylohyoid muscle (Fig. 2-12)
- The anterior belly of the digastric muscle (Fig. 2-13)
- The sternohyoid muscle — topographic visualization (Fig. 2-14)
- The belly of the sternohyoid muscle (Fig. 2-15)
- The superior belly of the omohyoid muscle (Fig. 2-16)
- The sternothyroid muscle (Fig. 2-17)

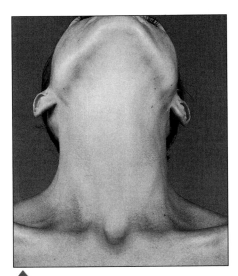

▲
FIGURE 2-10
**PRESENTATION OF THE ANTERIOR
REGION OF THE NECK**

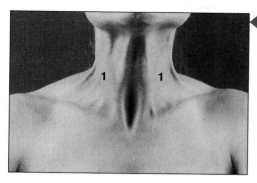

◄ **FIGURE 2-11**
THE PLATYSMA

Ask the subject to "pull" the corners of the mouth downward, backward, and outward (laterally) in order to demonstrate this structure (1), which extends from the lip commissures and the inferior border of the mandible to the skin of the pectoral and deltoid regions. The platysma is attached to the deep surface of the skin.

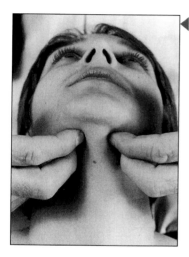

◄ **FIGURE 2-12**
THE MYLOHYOID MUSCLE

The mylohyoid muscle is the principal muscle of the floor of mouth. Its inferior surface is covered by the anterior belly of the digastric muscle (Fig. 2-13); its superior surface, by the geniohyoid muscle. Ask the subject to lower the mandible, open the mouth, or swallow (this action lifts the hyoid bone if the mandible is considered fixed) to allow you to feel the contraction below and medial to the free inferior border of the mandible.

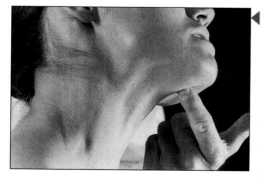

◄ **FIGURE 2-13**
THE ANTERIOR BELLY OF THE DIGASTRIC MUSCLE

This muscle is located superior to the hyoid bone (Figs. 1-17 to 1-20), and it and the mylohyoid muscle (Fig. 2-12) together constitute the muscles of the floor of the mouth. Place your index finger in the interspace between the two anterior digastric muscle bellies, in contact with the raphe where the two mylohyoid muscles meet. The digastric muscles cover the inferior surface of the mylohyoid muscles. To feel the contraction, ask the subject to lower the jaw.

Comment: Because of its two bellies (anterior and posterior), the digastric muscle belongs to two different muscular groups, the posterior belly belonging to the lateropharyngeal muscles.

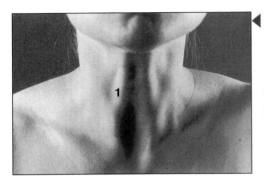

FIGURE 2-14
THE STERNOHYOID MUSCLE — TOPOGRAPHIC
VISUALIZATION

The sternohyoid muscle (1) inserts distally into the dorsal surface of the sternoclavicular joint and covers the adjacent aspects of the clavicle and the manubrium. Proximally, it inserts into the inferior border of the body of the hyoid bone, near the median line. These two muscles project obliquely upward and slightly inward (medially).

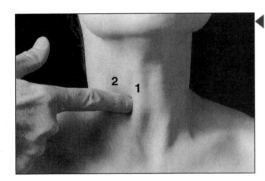

FIGURE 2-15
THE BELLY OF THE STERNOHYOID MUSCLE

In this figure, the index finger separates the sternohyoid muscle (1) from the sternocleidomastoid muscle (2).

Comment: Not all subjects present muscle bellies that are easy to identify.

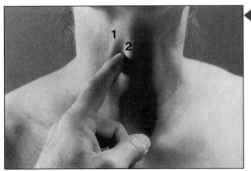

FIGURE 2-16
THE SUPERIOR BELLY OF THE OMOHYOID MUSCLE

This muscle (1), which projects slightly obliquely downward and laterally, follows the lateral border of the sternohyoid muscle (2) (see also Fig. 2-15) and then continues with the inferior belly (see Fig. 2-8) through an intermediate tendon. This tendon marks the change of direction of the muscle; the internal jugular vein is slightly deeper than the muscle at this point. The inferior belly ends at the anterior surface of the scapular body, near the superior border, medial to the scapular notch.

Comment: The contraction of the omohyoid muscle may influence the flow of blood in the internal jugular vein.

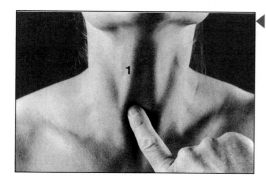

FIGURE 2-17
THE STERNOTHYROID MUSCLE

Push the sternohyoid muscle (1) (Figs. 2-14 and 2-15) later-ally with your index finger to gain access to the sternothy-roid muscle, which is not perceptible under the fingers as such.

THE NUCHAL REGION

The notable structures accessible by palpation are

- The muscular boundaries of the lateral region of the neck (Fig. 2-19)
- The cervical portion (or superior fasciculus) of the trapezius muscle (Fig. 2-20)
- The levator scapulae muscle — anterior view (Fig. 2-21)
- The levator scapulae muscle — lateral view (Fig. 2-22)
- The splenius muscle (Fig. 2-23)

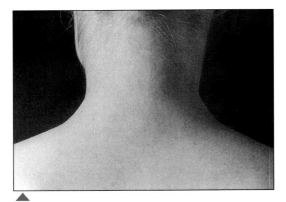

▲
FIGURE 2-18
PRESENTATION OF THE NUCHAL REGION

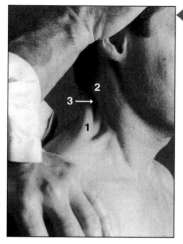

◀ **FIGURE 2-19**
THE MUSCULAR BOUNDARIES OF THE LATERAL REGION OF THE NECK

This figure shows the muscular boundaries of the lateral region of the neck, including the cervical aspect of the trapezius muscle (1) posteriorly (dorsally) and the occipital portion of the sternocleidomastoid muscle (2) anteriorly (ventrally). To make these boundaries protrude, ask the subject to resist pressure applied to the lateral aspect of the head while you press down on the subject's shoulder. These muscles are approached in the posterior aspect of this region (3).

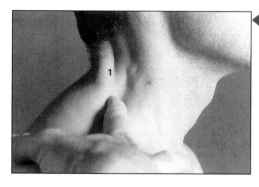

◀ **FIGURE 2-20**
THE CERVICAL PORTION (OR SUPERIOR FASCICULUS) OF THE TRAPEZIUS MUSCLE

The index finger indicates the cervical portion of the trapezius muscle (1) (see also Fig. 2-8).

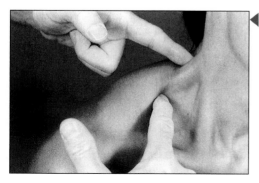

◀ **FIGURE 2-21**
THE LEVATOR SCAPULAE MUSCLE — ANTERIOR VIEW

In this figure, the levator scapulae muscle is grasped between the two index fingers. To make the muscle protrude more, ask the subject to perform a retropulsion of the shoulder and to lift the scapula, so that the superior angle of the scapula reaches its highest point. The inferior fibers of the levator scapulae muscle are attached to this superior angle.

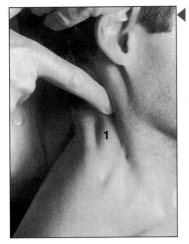

FIGURE 2-22
THE LEVATOR SCAPULAE MUSCLE — LATERAL VIEW

This figure presents a lateral view of the belly of the levator scapulae muscle (1). It can also be demonstrated with a double muscular action applied against resistance (see Figs. 2-19 and 2-21), i.e., lateral flexion of the head and lifting of the shoulder.

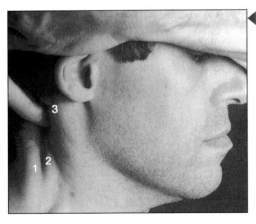

FIGURE 2-23
THE SPLENIUS MUSCLE

This muscle is palpated in the triangular space located between the trapezius muscle (1) posteriorly, the levator scapulae muscle (2) inferiorly, and the cleidooccipital portion (3) of the sternocleidomastoid muscle anteriorly. The muscular actions requested of the subject and the resistance applied are the same as those described in Figure 2-19.

CHAPTER
Three

NERVES
AND VESSELS

The notable structures accessible by palpation are

• The subclavian artery (Fig. 3-2)
• The brachial plexus (Fig. 3-3)

• The internal carotid artery — taking the pulse (Fig. 3-4)

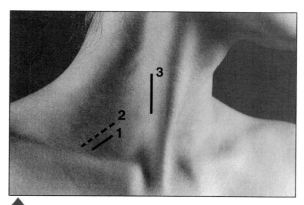

▲
FIGURE 3-1
PRESENTATION OF THE NERVES AND VESSELS OF THE NECK

(1) Subclavian artery
(2) Brachial plexus
(3) Internal carotid artery

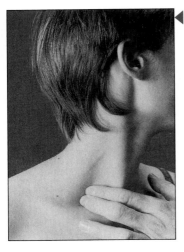

◄ FIGURE 3-2
THE SUBCLAVIAN ARTERY

Locate the clavicular portion of the sternocleidomastoid muscle (see Fig. 2-5) by asking the subject to perform a contralateral rotation of the head (rotation away from the sternocleidomastoid muscle). Place a large digital grip on the medial third of the clavicle on the sternocleidomastoid muscle; you will feel the pulse of this artery under your fingers.

Comment: The subclavian artery runs just deep to the anterior scalene muscle (Fig. 2-9).

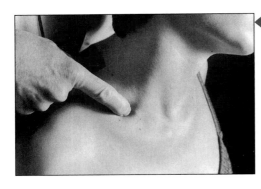

◄ FIGURE 3-3
THE BRACHIAL PLEXUS

The approach is identical to that described in Figure 3-2. This structure can be felt through the sternocleidomastoid muscle as a full cylindrical cord. To tighten this structure and thus make it more perceptible, ask the subject to perform a contralateral rotation and a contralateral lateral flexion of the head and place the upper limb of the subject in external rotation and extension.

Comment: The brachial plexus and the subclavian artery pass between the anterior scalene muscle (Fig. 2-9) and the middle scalene muscle (Fig. 2-8).

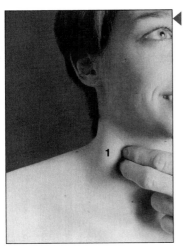

◄ FIGURE 3-4
THE INTERNAL CAROTID ARTERY — TAKING THE PULSE

The carotid pulse can be felt either anterior and medial to the sternal portion of the sternocleidomastoid muscle (1), as shown in this figure, or posterior and lateral to this same muscle.

Comment: The carotid pulse must be taken on only one side at a time, so that the cerebral circulation is not completely blocked. Pressure should be applied very carefully on this artery as atheromatous plaques can detach and cause a cerebral embolism. Taking the carotid pulse is very useful in an emergency because it allows you to feel a pulse with a very weak pressure —around 60 mmHg— a pressure just high enough to prevent the brain from becoming hypoxic.

THE TRUNK AND THE SACRUM

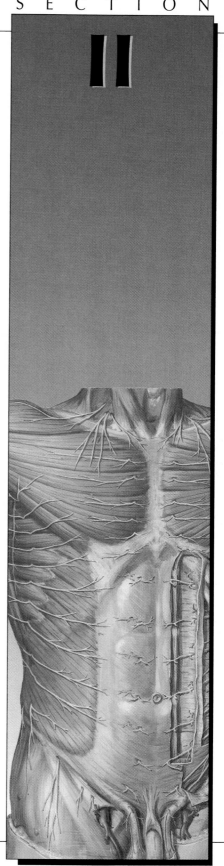

MUSCLES OF THE BACK: SUPERFICIAL LAYERS

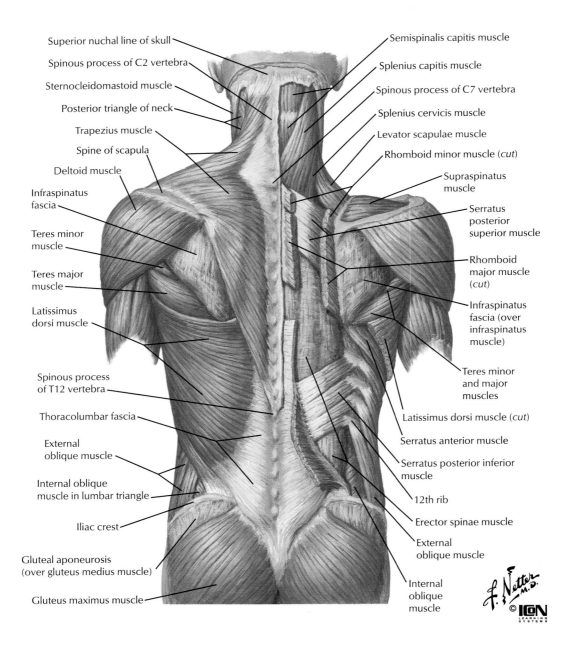

Superior nuchal line of skull

Spinous process of C2 vertebra

Sternocleidomastoid muscle

Posterior triangle of neck

Trapezius muscle

Spine of scapula

Deltoid muscle

Infraspinatus fascia

Teres minor muscle

Teres major muscle

Latissimus dorsi muscle

Spinous process of T12 vertebra

Thoracolumbar fascia

External oblique muscle

Internal oblique muscle in lumbar triangle

Iliac crest

Gluteal aponeurosis (over gluteus medius muscle)

Gluteus maximus muscle

Semispinalis capitis muscle

Splenius capitis muscle

Spinous process of C7 vertebra

Splenius cervicis muscle

Levator scapulae muscle

Rhomboid minor muscle (cut)

Supraspinatus muscle

Serratus posterior superior muscle

Rhomboid major muscle (cut)

Infraspinatus fascia (over infraspinatus muscle)

Teres minor and major muscles

Latissimus dorsi muscle (cut)

Serratus anterior muscle

Serratus posterior inferior muscle

12th rib

Erector spinae muscle

External oblique muscle

Internal oblique muscle

ANTERIOR THORACIC WALL

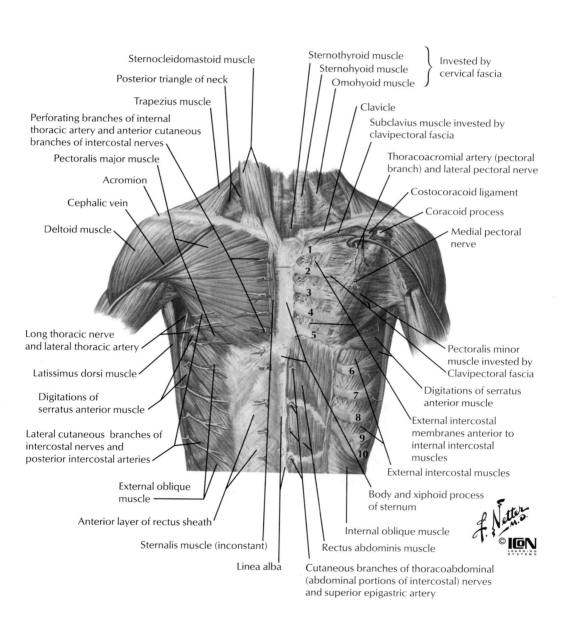

Sternocleidomastoid muscle

Posterior triangle of neck

Trapezius muscle

Perforating branches of internal thoracic artery and anterior cutaneous branches of intercostal nerves

Pectoralis major muscle

Acromion

Cephalic vein

Deltoid muscle

Long thoracic nerve and lateral thoracic artery

Latissimus dorsi muscle

Digitations of serratus anterior muscle

Lateral cutaneous branches of intercostal nerves and posterior intercostal arteries

External oblique muscle

Anterior layer of rectus sheath

Sternalis muscle (inconstant)

Linea alba

Sternothyroid muscle
Sternohyoid muscle
Omohyoid muscle
} Invested by cervical fascia

Clavicle

Subclavius muscle invested by clavipectoral fascia

Thoracoacromial artery (pectoral branch) and lateral pectoral nerve

Costocoracoid ligament

Coracoid process

Medial pectoral nerve

Pectoralis minor muscle invested by Clavipectoral fascia

Digitations of serratus anterior muscle

External intercostal membranes anterior to internal intercostal muscles

External intercostal muscles

Body and xiphoid process of sternum

Internal oblique muscle

Rectus abdominis muscle

Cutaneous branches of thoracoabdominal (abdominal portions of intercostal) nerves and superior epigastric artery

F. Netter M.D.

© ICON LEARNING SYSTEMS

NERVES OF THE ANTERIOR ABDOMINAL WALL

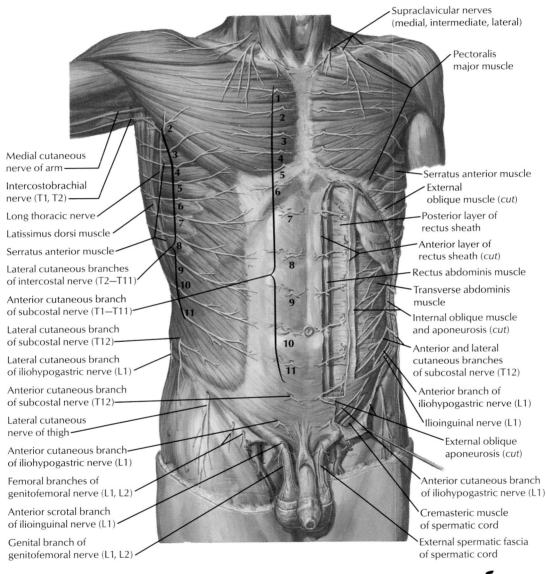

Medial cutaneous nerve of arm

Intercostobrachial nerve (T1, T2)

Long thoracic nerve

Latissimus dorsi muscle

Serratus anterior muscle

Lateral cutaneous branches of intercostal nerve (T2–T11)

Anterior cutaneous branch of subcostal nerve (T1–T11)

Lateral cutaneous branch of subcostal nerve (T12)

Lateral cutaneous branch of iliohypogastric nerve (L1)

Anterior cutaneous branch of subcostal nerve (T12)

Lateral cutaneous nerve of thigh

Anterior cutaneous branch of iliohypogastric nerve (L1)

Femoral branches of genitofemoral nerve (L1, L2)

Anterior scrotal branch of ilioinguinal nerve (L1)

Genital branch of genitofemoral nerve (L1, L2)

Supraclavicular nerves (medial, intermediate, lateral)

Pectoralis major muscle

Serratus anterior muscle

External oblique muscle (cut)

Posterior layer of rectus sheath

Anterior layer of rectus sheath (cut)

Rectus abdominis muscle

Transverse abdominis muscle

Internal oblique muscle and aponeurosis (cut)

Anterior and lateral cutaneous branches of subcostal nerve (T12)

Anterior branch of iliohypogastric nerve (L1)

Ilioinguinal nerve (L1)

External oblique aponeurosis (cut)

Anterior cutaneous branch of iliohypogastric nerve (L1)

Cremasteric muscle of spermatic cord

External spermatic fascia of spermatic cord

TOPOGRAPHIC PRESENTATION
OF THE TRUNK AND SACRUM

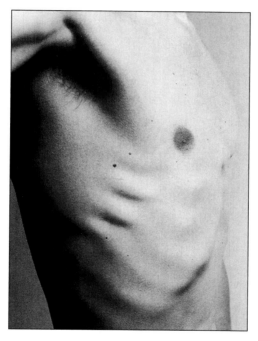

FIGURE 4-1
ANTEROLATERAL VIEW OF THE TRUNK

CHAPTER
Four

OSTEOLOGY

THE THORAX

The notable structures accessible by palpation are

- The sternum—general presentation (Fig. 4-3)
- The sternal manubrium (Fig. 4-4)
- The jugular (or suprasternal) notch (Fig. 4-5)
- The sternal angle (angle of locus) (Fig. 4-6)
- The body of the sternum (Fig. 4-7)
- The xiphoid process (Fig. 4-8)
- The thoracic inlet (superior thoracic aperture) (Fig. 4-9)
- The first costal cartilage (Fig. 4-10)
- The first rib—the body above the clavicle (Fig. 4-11)
- The posterior (or dorsal) extremity of the body of the first rib (Fig. 4-12)
- Close-up of the posterior (or dorsal) extremity of the body of the first rib (Fig. 4-13)
- The tubercle for the anterior scalene muscle (Fig. 4-14)
- The anterior (or ventral) extremity of the body of the second rib (Fig. 4-15)
- The body of the second rib at the anterior (or ventral) aspect of the thorax (Fig. 4-16)
- The second rib in the lateral region of the neck (Fig. 4-17)

- The posterior (or dorsal) extremity of the body of the second rib (Fig. 4-18)
- The true ribs (Fig. 4-19)
- The false ribs (Fig. 4-20)
- The thoracic outlet (inferior thoracic aperture) (Fig. 4-21)
- The notches of the costal arch (seventh, eighth, ninth, and tenth costal cartilages) (Fig. 4-22)
- The eleventh rib (Fig. 4-23)
- The eleventh rib—the anterior (or ventral) extremity (Fig. 4-24)
- The twelfth rib (Fig. 4-25)
- The twelfth rib: the anterior (or ventral) extremity—lateral view (Fig. 4-26)
- The twelfth rib: the anterior (or ventral) extremity—anterolateral view (Fig. 4-27)
- The tenth rib (Fig. 4-28)
- The costal angle (Fig. 4-29)

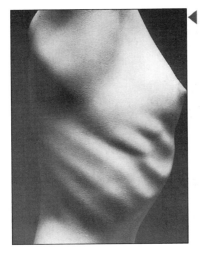

◀ **FIGURE 4-2**
LATERAL VIEW OF THE THORAX

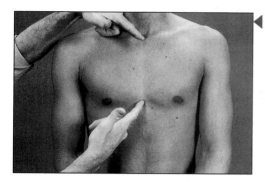

FIGURE 4-3
THE STERNUM — GENERAL PRESENTATION

This flat and unpaired bone occupies the ventral and median aspect of the thorax, indicated between the two index fingers. The sternum has three parts: a superior portion, the manubrium (Fig. 4-4); a middle portion, the body (Fig. 4-7); and an inferior portion, the xiphoid process (Fig. 4-8).

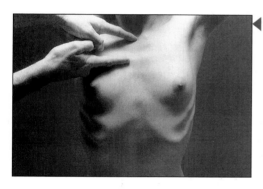

FIGURE 4-4
THE STERNAL MANUBRIUM

This structure, shown between the two index fingers, occupies the superior third of the sternum. It joins the body of the sternum at the level of the second rib.

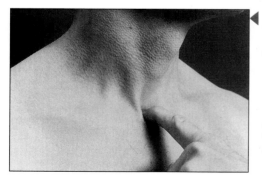

FIGURE 4-5
THE JUGULAR (OR SUPRASTERNAL) NOTCH

The jugular notch is located at the base (superior border) of the sternum. You will feel it under your index finger as a superior concavity.

Comment: The other two notches of this segment of the sternum are the clavicular notches, which articulate with the clavicle. They are concave transversely, flattened front to back, and directed upward and laterally.

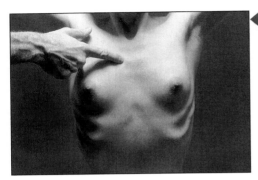

◀ **FIGURE 4-6**
THE STERNAL ANGLE (ANGLE OF LOUIS)

This structure, indicated by the index finger, represents the line where the manubrium (Fig. 4-4) and the body of the sternum (Fig. 4-7) join. It is situated at the level of the second rib, and it forms the edge of a bony ridge projecting forward.

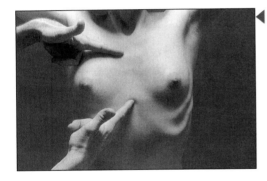

◀ **FIGURE 4-7**
THE BODY OF THE STERNUM

The two index fingers show globally the position of this portion of the sternum, located between the sternal angle (Fig. 4-6) and the xiphoid process (Fig. 4-8). Palpation of the anterior aspect of this structure reveals three or four transverse crests (vestiges of the welding of the sternebrae), as well as rough vertical patches where the sternochondral fasciculi of the pectoralis major muscle are attached (see also Fig. 8-3).

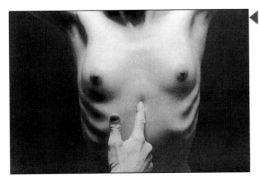

◀ **FIGURE 4-8**
THE XIPHOID PROCESS

This structure is located at the inferior extremity of the body of the sternum (Fig. 4-7), in the extension of the posterior (or dorsal) surface. Consequently, it is slightly set back for palpation. Also, the xiphoid process ends with an apex that is sometimes bifid and that may be deviated forward, backward, or to the side; it is therefore not always very accessible.

Comment: This structure ossifies with age.

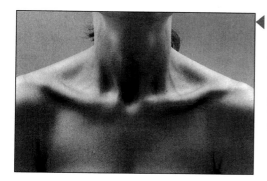

FIGURE 4-9

THE THORACIC INLET (SUPERIOR THORACIC APERTURE)

This elliptical opening, which is wider than it is deep, is inclined downward and forward. It is limited anteriorly by the jugular notch (Fig. 4-5), which projects over the inferior border of the second thoracic vertebra, laterally by the first rib, and posteriorly by the superior border of the first thoracic vertebra.

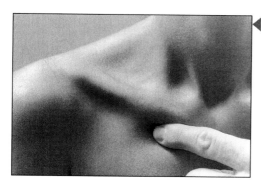

FIGURE 4-10

THE FIRST COSTAL CARTILAGE

To find this structure, place your index finger immediately below the clavicle and in contact with the lateral border of the manubrium. If necessary, ask the subject to perform rapid, repeated high costal inspirations to make it easier for you to feel the structure under your index finger.

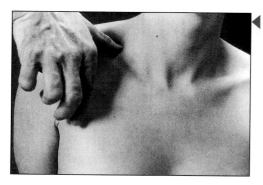

FIGURE 4-11

THE FIRST RIB — THE BODY ABOVE THE CLAVICLE

This structure can be felt as a density behind and above the clavicle. Nearly the whole structure is accessible.

Comment: The first rib is a true rib, that is, a rib joined to the sternum by means of a costal cartilage.

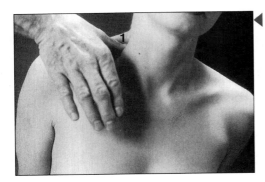

FIGURE 4-12
THE POSTERIOR (OR DORSAL) EXTREMITY OF THE BODY OF THE FIRST RIB

The first rib is easily accessible at this level after you push back the superior fibers of the trapezius muscle (1).

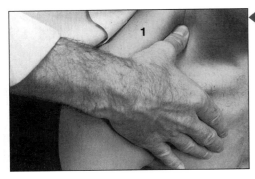

FIGURE 4-13
CLOSE-UP OF THE POSTERIOR (OR DORSAL) EXTREMITY OF THE BODY OF THE FIRST RIB

As shown in the figure, push back the superior fibers of the trapezius muscle (1) with your thumb to reach the most posterior (or dorsal) aspect of the superior surface of the first rib.

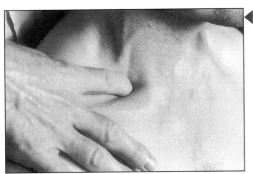

FIGURE 4-14
THE TUBERCLE FOR THE ANTERIOR SCALENE MUSCLE

To feel the structure of interest, place your index finger above and behind the clavicle and then relax all the muscles of the region (by asking the subject to perform an ipsilateral rotation and deviation of the head). In some subjects, the tubercle is felt through the thickness of the two clavicular portions of the sternocleidomastoid muscle.

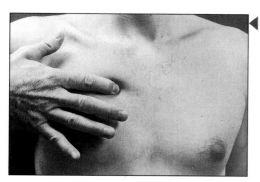

◀ **FIGURE 4-15**

THE ANTERIOR (OR VENTRAL) EXTREMITY OF THE BODY OF THE SECOND RIB

This structure is located between the first rib and the middle ribs, in the extension of the sternal angle (Fig. 4-6). In this figure, the index finger is placed in the second intercostal space and is in contact with the inferior aspect of the second rib.

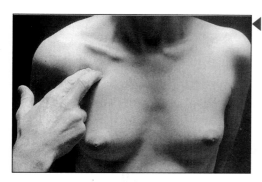

◀ **FIGURE 4-16**

THE BODY OF THE SECOND RIB AT THE ANTERIOR (OR VENTRAL) ASPECT OF THE THORAX

As shown in this figure, it is possible to follow the second rib right up to its passage under the clavicle.

Comment: The second rib is a true rib (see comment Fig. 4-11).

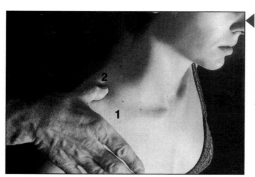

◀ **FIGURE 4-17**

THE SECOND RIB IN THE LATERAL REGION OF THE NECK

You can feel this structure as a density under your fingers behind the lateral extremity of the clavicle (1) while you push back the trapezius muscle (2). To feel it better, direct your grip downward and ask the subject to perform brief, repeated inspirations to mobilize the upper aspect of the rib cage and consequently the second rib.

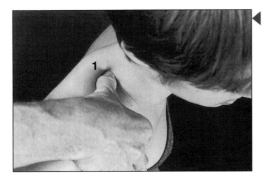

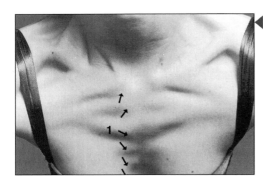

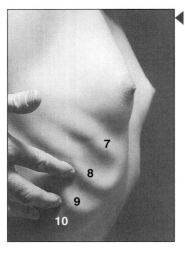

FIGURE 4-18
THE POSTERIOR (OR DORSAL) EXTREMITY
OF THE BODY OF THE SECOND RIB

This figure shows palpation of the vertebral extremity of the second rib. Push back the trapezius muscle (1) and place your grip behind and below the first rib (see Fig. 4-12).

FIGURE 4-19
THE TRUE RIBS

This figure shows the sternal extremity of the first six true ribs (1) (the seventh is visible in Fig. 4-20). It is easy to count the true ribs, starting from the sternal angle (see Fig. 4-6), which corresponds to the second rib. There are seven true ribs.

See comment Figure 4-11.

FIGURE 4-20
THE FALSE RIBS

Each of the three false ribs (eighth, ninth, and tenth) (8, 9, 10) joins the costal cartilage of the rib above through the cartilage that extends from its anterior (or ventral) extremity. Together with the cartilage of the seventh rib, the cartilages of the false ribs form the costal arch (7).

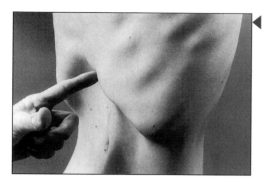

FIGURE 4-21
THE THORACIC OUTLET (INFERIOR THORACIC APERTURE)

This elliptical opening, which is wider than it is deep, is nearly three times as big as the thoracic inlet (Fig. 4-9). It is inclined downward and backward. It is limited anteriorly by the xiphoid process (Fig. 4-8), which projects over the tenth thoracic vertebra, and posteriorly by the body of the twelfth thoracic vertebra. It is bounded laterally by the costal arch (seventh, eighth, ninth, and tenth costal cartilages) and the floating ribs (see Figs. 4-23 through 4-27).

Comment: This opening is covered by the diaphragm.

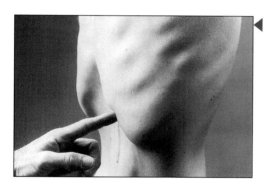

FIGURE 4-22
THE NOTCHES OF THE COSTAL ARCH (SEVENTH, EIGHTH, NINTH, AND TENTH COSTAL CARTILAGES)

Starting from the xiphoid process and following the inferior border of the costal arch, you will feel two notches. The first notch (indicated by the index finger in Fig. 4-21) corresponds to the union of the eighth and the seventh costal cartilages; the second notch corresponds to the union of the tenth and the ninth costal cartilages (indicated by the index finger in this figure).

Comment: These two notches are not always very pronounced.

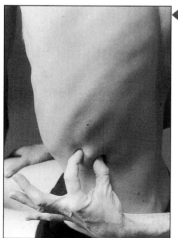

FIGURE 4-23
THE ELEVENTH RIB

This figure shows the eleventh rib grasped between the thumb and the index finger. For a better approach to this structure, stand behind the subject and place both hands on the inferior border of the costal arch (Fig. 4-20), that is, at the inferior border of the tenth rib. After locating the tenth rib, move your grip to the level of the anterolateral side of the abdomen toward the iliac crest to find a rib that is situated immediately below the inferior border of the costal arch and that has a free anterior (or ventral) extremity.

Comment: The iliac crest is shown in Fig. 17-4.

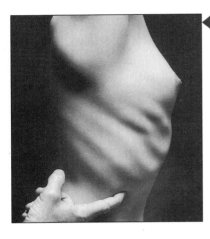

FIGURE 4-24
THE ELEVENTH RIB — THE ANTERIOR (OR VENTRAL) EXTREMITY

In this figure, the index finger is placed at the anterior (or ventral) extremity of the eleventh rib, which is unattached and covered with cartilage. This is called a floating rib.

Comment: The anterior (or ventral) extremity of the eleventh rib, which is about 20 cm (8 inches) long, is usually at a distance from the inferior border of the tenth rib, but it can be very close to or even merge with the tenth rib.

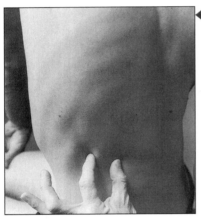

FIGURE 4-25
THE TWELFTH RIB

This figure shows the eleventh rib grasped between the thumb and the index finger. After locating the eleventh rib (Figs. 2-23 and 2-24), move your grip downward and backward toward the iliac crest to find the twelfth rib, which is shorter than the eleventh.

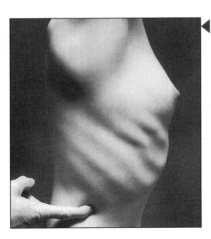

FIGURE 4-26
THE TWELFTH RIB: THE ANTERIOR (OR VENTRAL) EXTREMITY — LATERAL VIEW

In this figure, the index finger is placed on the anterior (or ventral) extremity of the twelfth rib, which is unattached and covered with cartilage.

Comment: The twelfth rib is also a floating rib. It usually measures 10 cm to 14 cm (4–6 inches), but it can also be very short (3–6 cm or 1–2 inches), in which case it may be mistaken for a transverse process of a lumbar vertebra.

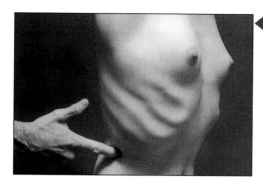

◀ FIGURE 4-27
THE TWELFTH RIB: THE ANTERIOR (OR VENTRAL)
EXTREMITY — ANTEROLATERAL VIEW

In this figure, the index finger is placed on the anterior (or ventral) extremity of the twelfth rib. This anterolateral view allows the visualization of the position of the twelfth rib in relation to the position of the eleventh rib and the positions of the seventh, eighth, ninth, and tenth ribs, which form the costal arch (Fig. 4-20).

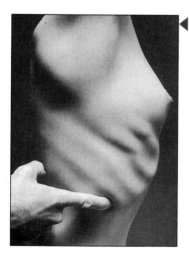

◀ FIGURE 4-28
THE TENTH RIB

The anterior (or ventral) extremity of the tenth rib may not be attached to the cartilage of the ninth rib. In this case, its anterior extremity remains free. In this figure, the thumb–index finger grip moves this extremity.

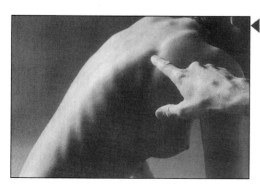

◀ FIGURE 4-29
THE COSTAL ANGLE

This angle corresponds to the first change of direction of the rib at the dorsal aspect of the thorax, from which point the rib is directed anteriorly and downward.

THE THORACIC AND LUMBAR VERTEBRAE

The notable structures accessible by palpation are

- The thoracic vertebrae T1 to T12 (Fig. 4-31)
- The cervicothoracic joint C7-T1 (Fig. 4-32)
- Location of C7 and T1 — test with rotation of the head (Fig. 4-33)
- Location of C7 and T1 — test with extension of the head (Fig. 4-34)
- Visualization of the relationship between the scapula and the spinous processes (Fig. 4-35)
- Location of the spinous process of T1 (Fig. 4-36)
- Location of the spinous process of T3 (Fig. 4-37)
- Location of the spinous process of T7 (Fig. 4-38)
- The costal processes of the thoracic vertebrae (Fig. 4-39)
- The lumbar vertebrae L1 to L5 (Fig. 4-40)
- Location of the fourth (L4) and fifth (L5) lumbar vertebrae (Fig. 4-41)
- Location of the fifth lumbar vertebra (L5) (Fig. 4-42)
- The transverse processes of the lumbar vertebrae (Fig. 4-43)

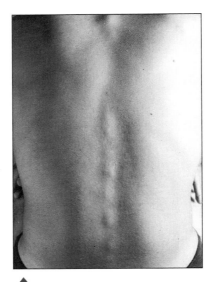

▲
FIGURE 4-30
POSTERIOR (OR DORSAL) VIEW
OF THE THORACIC AND LUMBAR
VERTEBRAE

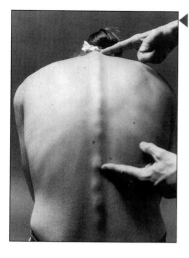

FIGURE 4-31
THE THORACIC VERTEBRAE T1 TO T12

In this figure, the two index fingers indicate the thoracic vertebrae from T1 to T12.

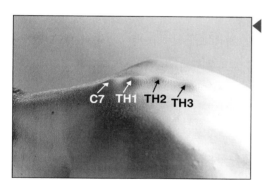

FIGURE 4-32
THE CERVICOTHORACIC JOINT C7-T1

In this figure, you can clearly see the spinous processes of the last cervical vertebra C7 and of the first thoracic vertebrae T1, T2, and T3.

Comment: The subject is seated, with the head bent forward.

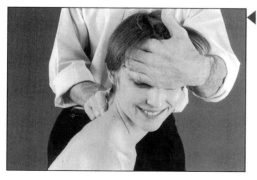

FIGURE 4-33
LOCATION OF C7 AND T1 — TEST WITH ROTATION OF THE HEAD

The subject is seated, with the head in a neutral position (not flexed, not extended). Stand next to the subject and place your index and middle fingers on the spinous processes of the seventh cervical vertebra C7 (Fig. 4-32) and the first thoracic vertebra T1 (Fig. 4-32). Starting from this position, with the other hand, rotate the subject's head to the right, then to the left, several times if necessary. You will feel a slight movement at the level of C7; there is no movement at the level of T1.

Comment: The slight movement felt may be more pronounced while turning the head to one side than while turning it to the other; therefore, it is of interest to perform the test on both sides.

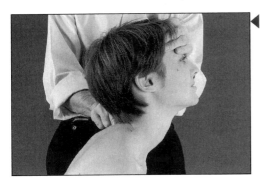

FIGURE 4-34
LOCATION OF C7 AND T1 — TEST WITH
EXTENSION OF THE HEAD

The subject is seated, with the head in a neutral position (not flexed, not extended). Stand next to the subject and place your index and middle fingers on the spinous processes of the seventh cervical vertebra C7 and the first thoracic vertebra T1 (Fig. 4-32). Place the palm of your other hand across the subject's forehead and hyperextend the subject's head: the spinous process of C7 disappears in the physiological cervical lordosis, while the spinous process of T1 does not move under your fingers.

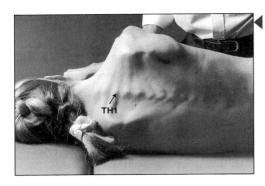

FIGURE 4-35
VISUALIZATION OF THE RELATIONSHIP BETWEEN
THE SCAPULA AND THE SPINOUS PROCESSES

In this figure, notice that the superior angle of the scapula is at the level of the first thoracic vertebra T1. The medial extremity of the scapular spine is facing the spinous process of T3. The inferior angle of the scapula is facing the spinous process of T7.

Comment: This approach is a technique for rapidly locating the spinous processes — location must be completed by "counting" from C7 (see Figs. 4-32, 4-33, and 4-34) or from L5 (see Figs. 4-41 and 4-42). The landmarks mentioned above are only indicators. The position of the scapula on the rib cage, the position of the subject on the table, and various dysmorphisms that may exist at the level of the spine (kyphosis, flat back, scoliosis) noticeably modify the topographic relationships between the scapula and the spine.

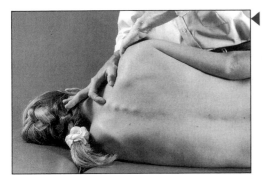

FIGURE 4-36
LOCATION OF THE SPINOUS PROCESS OF T1

This figure highlights the relationship (see Fig. 4-35) between the superior angle of the scapula, indicated by the thumb, and the spinous process of the first thoracic vertebra T1, indicated by the index finger.

See comment Fig. 4-35.

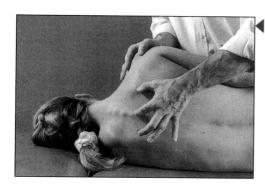

FIGURE 4-37
LOCATION OF THE SPINOUS PROCESS OF T3

This figure highlights the relationship (see also Fig. 4-35) between the medial extremity of the scapular spine, indicated by the thumb, and the spinous process of the third thoracic vertebra T3, indicated by the index finger.

See comment Fig. 4-35.

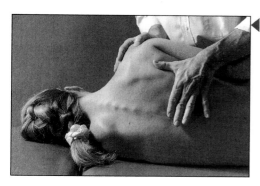

FIGURE 4-38
LOCATION OF THE SPINOUS PROCESS OF T7

This figure highlights the relationship (see also Fig. 4-35) between the inferior angle of the scapula, indicated by the thumb, and the spinous process of the seventh thoracic vertebra T7, indicated by the index finger.

See comment Fig. 4-35.

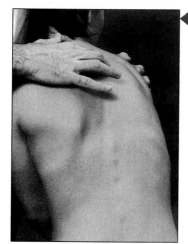

FIGURE 4-39
THE COSTAL PROCESSES OF THE THORACIC VERTEBRAE

With the subject seated, stand next to the subject and cradle the anterior aspect of the subject's shoulders with your palms. Search for a density medial to the costal angle, about two fingerbreadths lateral to the spinous processes. The cradle grip allows you to rotate the subject's trunk so you can better feel this structure, which is difficult to access in most subjects because of the presence of the spinal muscles.

Comment: The purpose of this figure is to show the technique of approach, not the bony structure itself.

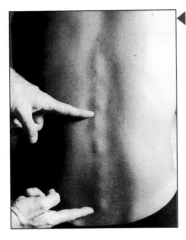

◄ **FIGURE 4-40**
THE LUMBAR VERTEBRAE L1 TO L5

In this figure, the two index fingers indicate the lumbar spine (the set of lumbar vertebrae from L1 to L5).

Comment: The lumbar column, made up of five vertebrae, can have its number increased by lumbarization of the first sacral vertebra S1 or decreased by sacralization of the last lumbar vertebra L5.

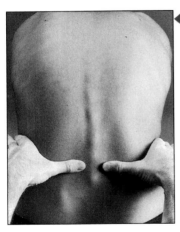

◄ **FIGURE 4-41**
LOCATION OF THE FOURTH (L4) AND FIFTH (L5) LUMBAR VERTEBRAE

As shown in this figure, place your hands on the iliac crest, with your thumbs pointing toward the lumbar vertebrae. If you place your thumbs naturally, they are at the level of the intervertebral disc L4–L5; if you keep your thumbs at the same level as your palm, they point to the spinous process of the fourth lumbar vertebra L4.

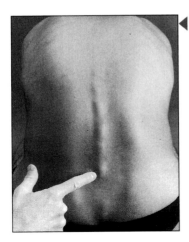

◄ **FIGURE 4-42**
LOCATION OF THE FIFTH LUMBAR VERTEBRA (L5)

After you locate L4 (see Fig. 4-41), it is easy to locate the spinous process of the vertebra below, indicated by the index finger.

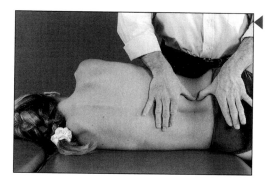

◄ **FIGURE 4-43**
THE TRANSVERSE PROCESSES OF THE LUMBAR VERTEBRAE

With the subject lying on his or her side, facing you, place your thumbs lateral to the erector spinae muscles and move your grip toward the lumbar vertebrae until you come in contact with a density, which is the structure of interest.

Comments:

·In very muscular subjects, look for this structure posteriorly through the muscular mass of the erector spinae muscles.

·The transverse process of the first lumbar vertebra is shorter than the transverse processes of the other lumbar vertebrae. The transverse process of the fifth lumbar vertebra is longer than the transverse processes of the other lumbar vertebrae. Its overdevelopment can fuse L5 with the iliac bone, which is called sacralization (see also comment Fig. 4-40).

THE SACRUM

The notable structures accessible by palpation are

- Posterolateral visualization of the sacrum (Fig. 4-45)
- The posterior (or dorsal) and lateral aspect of the first sacral vertebra (S1) (Fig. 4-46)
- The spinous process of the first sacral vertebra (S1) (Fig. 4-47)
- The spinous process of the second sacral vertebra (S2)—step 1 (Fig. 4-48)
- The spinous process of the second sacral vertebra (S2)—step 1 (other approach) (Fig. 4-49)

- The spinous process of the second sacral vertebra (S2)—step 2 (Fig. 4-50)
- The median sacral crest (Fig. 4-51)
- The sacral cornua (horns) (Fig. 4-52)
- The sacral hiatus (Fig. 4-53)
- The lateral border of the sacrum—posterolateral view (Fig. 4-54)
- The lateral border of the sacrum—posterior (or dorsal) view (Fig. 4-55)

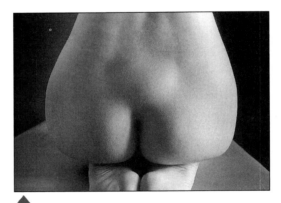

▲
FIGURE 4-44
POSTERIOR VIEW OF THE PELVIS AND THE SACRUM

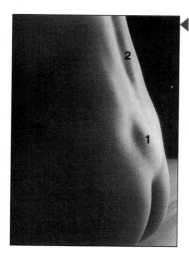

FIGURE 4-45
POSTEROLATERAL VISUALIZATION OF THE SACRUM

In this figure, the sacrum (1) appears "positive" (in relief) inferior to the lumbar vertebrae (2).

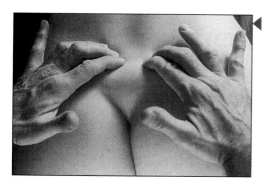

FIGURE 4-46
THE POSTERIOR (OR DORSAL) AND LATERAL ASPECT OF THE FIRST SACRAL VERTEBRA (S1)

With the subject in a prone position, stand at the level of the greater trochanter and place your hands on both sides of the lumbar vertebrae. With a slight pressure, slide your hands down along these vertebrae until you feel a "stop" inferior to L5; this stop is the structure of interest.

Comment: When sliding past L5, the hands naturally land on the sacrum, because its posterior (or dorsal) surface is facing dorsally and superiorly (backward and upward).

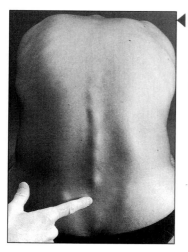

FIGURE 4-47
THE SPINOUS PROCESS OF THE FIRST SACRAL VERTEBRA (S1)

After you locate the spinous process of L5 (Figs. 4-41 and 4-42), move your grip downward to feel the structure of interest, which is the first tubercle sitting along the median sacral crest.

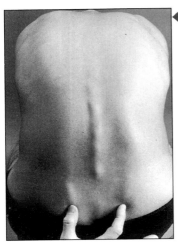

◀ FIGURE 4-48
THE SPINOUS PROCESS OF THE SECOND SACRAL VERTEBRA (S2)—STEP 1

With the subject seated and leaning forward, place your thumb and your index finger on the posterior superior iliac spines of the iliac bones.

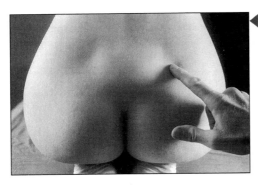

◀ FIGURE 4-49
THE SPINOUS PROCESS OF THE SECOND SACRAL VERTEBRA (S2)—STEP 1 (OTHER APPROACH)

In this figure, the index finger indicates the dimple at the level of the sacroiliac joint, which is more or less pronounced depending on the subject. This cutaneous landmark corresponds approximately to the posterior superior iliac spine.

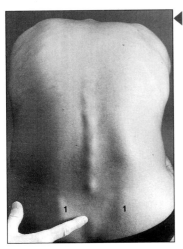

◀ FIGURE 4-50
THE SPINOUS PROCESS OF THE SECOND SACRAL VERTEBRA (S2)—STEP 2

After you locate the posterior superior iliac spines (1), whether they are clearly visible (Fig. 4-48) or not (Fig. 4-49), draw an imaginary horizontal line from one structure to the other. The middle of this line corresponds to the second tubercle of the median sacral crest, the structure of interest.

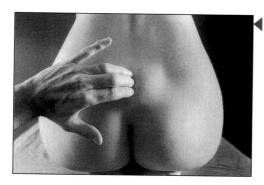

FIGURE 4-51
THE MEDIAN SACRAL CREST

Place several fingers in the middle of the posterior (or dorsal) surface of the sacrum, in line with the spinous processes of the lumbar vertebrae. With this grip, rub transversely on this crest to better feel this structure.

Comment: The median sacral crest consists of three or four tubercles remaining from the fusion of the spinous processes of the five sacral vertebrae. The spinous processes are separated from each other by slight depressions.

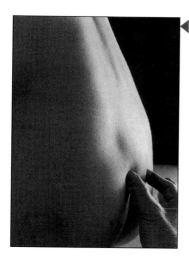

FIGURE 4-52
THE SACRAL CORNUA (HORNS)

Immediately above the intergluteal (natal) cleft, surrounding the depression of the sacral hiatus (Fig. 4-53), you can feel two small bony columns slightly lateral to the median sacral crest (Fig. 4-51).

Comment: The sacral crest splits into two bony columns at the level of the third and fourth dorsal sacral foramina. These two columns constitute the sacral cornua (horns).

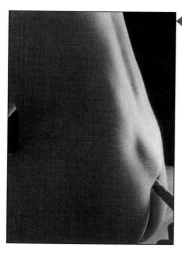

FIGURE 4-53
THE SACRAL HIATUS

Immediately above the intergluteal (natal) cleft, you can feel a depression in the extension of the median sacral crest (Fig. 4-51), as shown in this figure. This depression is formed by the divergence (downward and outward) of the sacral cornua (horns) (Fig. 4-52). The sacral canal ends in the apex of the structure of interest, which is bordered by the sacral cornua.

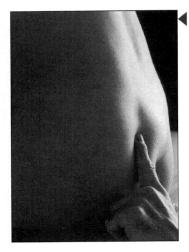

◄ FIGURE 4-54
THE LATERAL BORDER OF THE SACRUM — POSTEROLATERAL VIEW

As shown in this figure, place your index finger on the lateral border of the sacrum, which feels like a thick, blunt border.

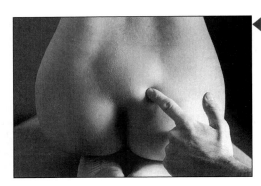

◄ FIGURE 4-55
THE LATERAL BORDER OF THE SACRUM — POSTERIOR (OR DORSAL) VIEW

This view demonstrates the position of this border between the posterior superior iliac spine (Figs. 4-48 and 4-49) and the sacral cornua (horns) (Fig. 4-52).

CHAPTER
Five

MYOLOGY

THE POSTERIOR MUSCULAR GROUP

The notable structures accessible by palpation are

- The trapezius muscle—global visualization (Fig. 5-2)
- The trapezius muscle—the superior fibers (Fig. 5-3)
- The trapezius muscle—the middle fibers (Fig. 5-4)
- The trapezius muscle—the inferior fibers (Fig. 5-5)
- The latissimus dorsi muscle—global visualization and topographic situation (Fig. 5-6)
- The latissimus dorsi muscle. (Fig. 5-7)
- The latissimus dorsi muscle—the upper or cranial aspect at the level of the thoracic vertebrae (Fig. 5-8)
- The rhomboid major muscle (Fig. 5-9)
- The plane of the serratus posterior muscles (Fig. 5-10)
- The intermediate aponeurosis of the serratus posterior muscles (Fig. 5-11)

- The erector spinae muscles—topographic situation (Fig. 5-12)
- The inferior aspect of the erector spinae muscles (Fig. 5-13)
- The iliocostalis lumborum muscle and the longissimus thoracis muscle (Fig. 5-14)
- The iliocostalis thoracis muscle and the longissimus thoracis muscle—topographic situation (Fig. 5-15)
- The iliocostalis thoracis muscle and the longissimus thoracis muscle (Fig. 5-16)
- The quadratus lumborum muscle in the lumbar quadrangle (Fig. 5-17)

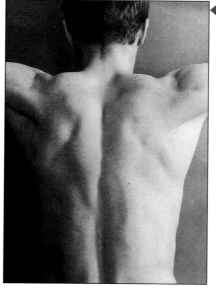

◀ FIGURE 5-1
GLOBAL VIEW OF THE POSTERIOR
MUSCLES OF THE TRUNK

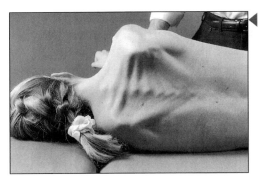

FIGURE 5-2
THE TRAPEZIUS MUSCLE — GLOBAL VISUALIZATION

This figure shows the topographic situation of the trapezius, which, together with the latissimus dorsi muscle (Figs. 5-6, 5-7, and 5-8) constitutes the most superficial plane of the muscles of the back. The middle and inferior fibers belong to the back region. This muscle inserts medially into the outer occipital plane, on the superior nuchal line, on the posterior border of the nuchal ligament, and on the spinous processes of C7 to T11 (see also Figs. 5-3, 5-4, and 5-5)

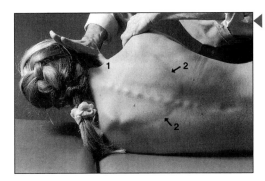

FIGURE 5-3
THE TRAPEZIUS MUSCLE — THE SUPERIOR FIBERS

With the subject is lying on his or her side, face the subject and place the palm of your hand on the lateral aspect of the subject's head and your other hand on the subject's shoulder. Ask the subject to lift the shoulder and to perform an ipsilateral lateral flexion of the head while you resist these two simultaneous actions. The muscle of interest appears at the lateral aspect of the neck (1).

Comment: The superior fibers are oblique downward and outward and insert into the lateral third of the inferior border of the clavicle and into the adjacent part of its superior surface.

The arrows (2) point to the inferolateral borders of the trapezius muscle.

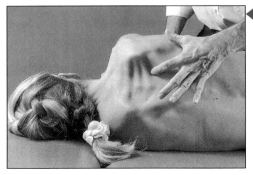

FIGURE 5-4
THE TRAPEZIUS MUSCLE — THE MIDDLE FIBERS

With the subject lying on his or her side, with both arms flexed at 90° in relation to the shoulders, apply resistance at the lateral aspect of the subject's arm, above the elbow, and ask the subject to abduct the arm horizontally while you resist this movement. The index finger indicates the middle fibers.

Comment: The transverse middle fibers insert into the acromion and the superior aspect of the posterior border of the scapular spine, with a particularly extended insertion on the tubercle for the trapezius muscle (see Fig. 7-22).

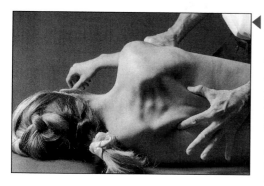

◀ FIGURE 5-5
THE TRAPEZIUS MUSCLE — THE INFERIOR FIBERS

With the subject lying on his or her side with the shoulder and the elbow flexed at 90°, apply resistance at the lateral aspect of the subject's arm, above the elbow. Ask the subject to abduct the arm horizontally. With your other hand, grasp both muscles between your thumb and your index finger.

Comment: These fibers, which are oblique upward and outward, are attached to a flattened aponeurotic lamina that inserts into the medial extremity of the scapular spine.

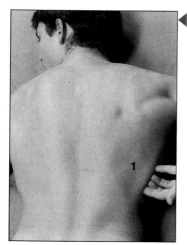

◀ FIGURE 5-6
THE LATISSIMUS DORSI MUSCLE — GLOBAL VISUALIZATION
AND TOPOGRAPHIC SITUATION

This muscle, together with the trapezius muscle (Figs. 5-2 through 5-5), forms the most superficial plane of the muscles of the back. This muscle (1) is large, flat, and triangular, with a large lateral base. It inserts into the spinous processes of T6 to T12 and L1 to L5, into the corresponding interspinal ligaments, and into the iliac crest with an aponeurotic lamina (see Figs. 5-7 and 5-8, below, and Fig. 8-17).

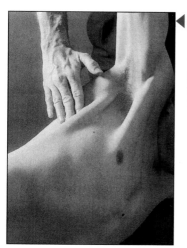

◀ FIGURE 5-7
THE LATISSIMUS DORSI MUSCLE

This figure shows an anterolateral view of the muscle of interest. The subject is lying on his or her side, and the arm is abducted at 90°. Apply resistance above the subject's elbow on the medial surface of the arm and resist the adduction of the upper limb.

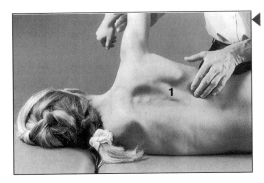

FIGURE 5-8

THE LATISSIMUS DORSI MUSCLE — THE UPPER OR CRANIAL ASPECT AT THE LEVEL OF THE THORACIC VERTEBRAE

The technique for making the inferior fibers of the trapezius muscle (1) protrude is described in Figure 5-5. After you locate this muscle, grip below the most inferior aspect of these inferior fibers in order to be in contact with the most superior aspect of the latissimus dorsi muscle at the level of the thoracic vertebrae.

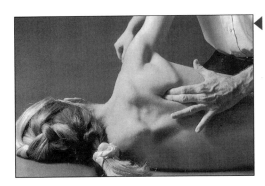

FIGURE 5-9

THE RHOMBOID MAJOR MUSCLE

First, locate the inferior fibers of the trapezius muscle (Fig. 5-5). Then, bring the scapula in external rotation, far enough to expose the rhomboid major muscle, which at this level is located directly deep to the trapezius muscle. Palpate this muscle between the thoracic vertebrae and the medial border of the scapula.

Comment: This muscle detaches from the first five thoracic vertebrae and ends on the medial border of the scapular spine.

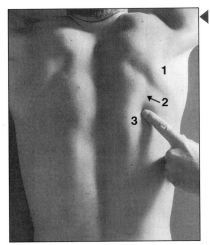

FIGURE 5-10

THE PLANE OF THE SERRATUS POSTERIOR MUSCLES

These two muscles, one superior and one inferior, are flat and quadrilateral. They are joined by an intermediate aponeurosis. They extend from the line of the spinous processes of C7 to L3 to the costal angle of all the ribs (see Fig. 5-29), slightly laterally to these angles. In this figure, the scapula (1) is drawn aside and the index finger indicates the "penetration point" (medial to the posterior angle of the ribs (2)) where you approach the plane of the serratus posterior muscles. Palpate the structure of interest through the fibers of the latissimus dorsi muscle by sliding your grip under the trapezius muscle (3).

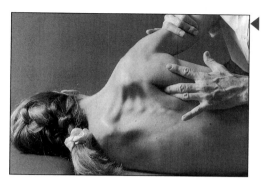

FIGURE 5-11
THE INTERMEDIATE APONEUROSIS OF THE
| SERRATUS POSTERIOR MUSCLES

In the zone between the serratus posterior superior muscle and the serratus posterior inferior muscle, the plane of the serratus posterior muscles consists of a fine intermediate aponeurotic lamina that extends between the vertebral spines and the fourth to the ninth ribs.

Comment: This figure completes the approach technique described in Fig. 5-10. The subject is lying on her side.

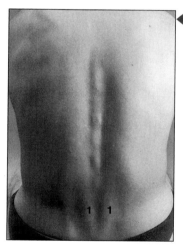

FIGURE 5-12
THE ERECTOR SPINAE MUSCLES — TOPOGRAPHIC SITUATION

These muscles (1) constitute the deep plane of the posterior muscles of the trunk. They are located on both sides of the spinous processes posterior to the lamina and the transverse processes. They extend from the cervical region to the sacrum, and they are made up of closely interlinked muscle slips (see Fig. 5-13), which fill in the vertebral grooves completely.

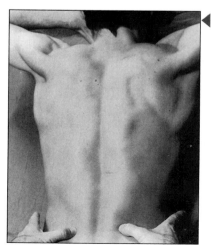

FIGURE 5-13
THE INFERIOR ASPECT OF THE ERECTOR SPINAE MUSCLES

The subject is in a prone position and is asked to extend the trunk. A muscular mass appears at the level of the vertebral grooves in the lumbar region.

Comment: These muscles include the spinalis, longissimus, and ilio-costalis muscles. They form an undivided mass.

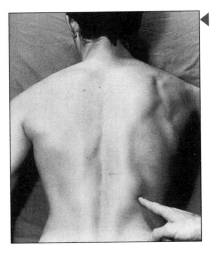

FIGURE 5-14
THE ILIOCOSTALIS LUMBORUM MUSCLE
AND THE LONGISSIMUS THORACIS MUSCLE

These two closely interlinked muscles share a common distal origin or attachment (iliac crest, iliac tubercle, and sacral crest). Ask the subject to extend the trunk in order to make the muscular mass protrude, as indicated by the index finger. The demonstration technique is the same as the one described in Figure 5-13.

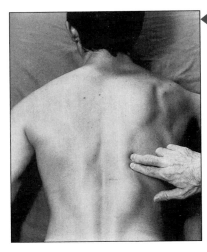

FIGURE 5-15
THE ILIOCOSTALIS THORACIS MUSCLE AND THE
LONGISSIMUS THORACIS MUSCLE — TOPOGRAPHIC SITUATION

This figure shows the topographic situation of these muscles at the level of the vertebral grooves, covered (from deep to superficial) by the plane of the serratus posterior muscles (Figs. 5-10 and 5-11), by the plane of the rhomboid major muscle (Fig. 5-9) facing the scapula, and finally by the trapezius muscle superiorly and the latissimus dorsi muscle inferiorly.

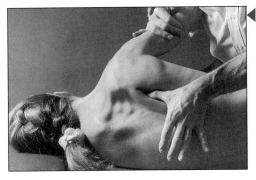

FIGURE 5-16
THE ILIOCOSTALIS THORACIS MUSCLE
AND THE LONGISSIMUS THORACIS MUSCLE

After locating the inferior fibers of the trapezius muscle (Fig. 5-5), slide a bidigital grip (the thumb may be placed as shown in this figure) under the trapezius muscle toward the thoracic vertebrae. It is possible to feel bundles of fleshy fibers under the fingers, which belong to the iliocostalis thoracis muscle laterally and to the longissimus thoracis muscle medially (see also Fig. 5-15).

Comment: Perception of these muscles is highly variable in different subjects.

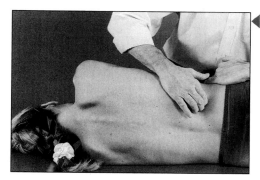

FIGURE 5-17
THE QUADRATUS LUMBORUM MUSCLE
IN THE LUMBAR QUADRANGLE

With the subject lying on his or her side, place one hand on the twelfth rib (see Figs. 4-25, 4-26, and 4-27) in the lumbar quadrangle (see comment); the other hand lies on the iliac crest. Ask the subject to move the iliac crest toward the twelfth rib while you resist this movement: you will feel the contraction of the muscle of interest under your cranial hand.

Comment: The lumbar quadrangle is an aponeurotic plane limited
· medially by the common muscular mass of the erector spinae muscles,
· inferiorly and laterally by the posterior border of the internal abdominal oblique muscle,
· superiorly and medially by the serratus posterior
· inferior muscle,
· superiorly and laterally by the inferior border of the twelfth rib.

This muscular plane is covered posteriorly by a plane where the lumbar triangle (of Jean-Louis Petit) is located. This triangle is limited by the posterior aspect of the iliac crest inferiorly, the posterior border of the external abdominal oblique muscle laterally and anteriorly, and the lateral border of the latissimus dorsi muscle medially.

These two areas (lumbar quadrangle and lumbar triangle) are the two weak points of the posterior abdominal wall.

THE MUSCLES OF THE ANTEROLATERAL SIDE OF THE THORAX AND THE ABDOMEN

The notable structures accessible by palpation are

- The external intercostal muscles (Fig. 5-19)
- The external abdominal oblique muscle: costal insertions—visualization (Fig. 5-20)
- The external abdominal oblique muscle—costal insertions (Fig. 5-21)
- The external abdominal oblique muscle: costal insertions—relationship with the serratus anterior muscle (Fig. 5-22)
- The external abdominal oblique muscle: costal insertions—relationship with the latissimus dorsi muscle (Fig. 5-23)
- The anterolateral muscles of the abdomen (Fig. 5-24)
- The psoas major muscle: technique of approach—step 1 (Fig. 5-25)
- The psoas major muscle: technique of approach—step 2 (Fig. 5-26)
- The psoas major muscle: technique of approach—step 3 (Fig. 5-27)

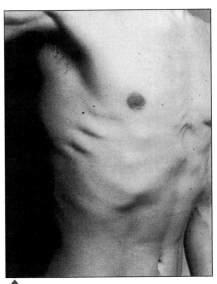

▲
FIGURE 5-18
ANTEROLATERAL VIEW OF THE THORAX
AND THE ABDOMEN

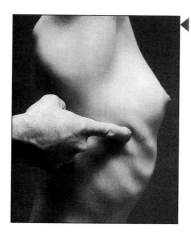

◀ FIGURE 5-19
THE EXTERNAL INTERCOSTAL MUSCLES

These muscles occupy the dorsal three quarters of the intercostal space, from the costotransverse joint to the costochondral joint. It is the topographic situation described here and shown in this figure more than the perception by palpation that should be taken in here.

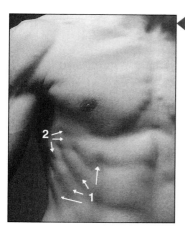

◀ FIGURE 5-20
THE EXTERNAL ABDOMINAL OBLIQUE MUSCLE: COSTAL
INSERTIONS — VISUALIZATION

This figure shows the fleshy bundles of the external abdominal oblique muscle (1), which are directed obliquely toward the last seven or eight ribs (where they insert into the external surface). This figure also shows the interdigitation of this muscle with the serratus anterior muscle (2) (see Fig. 5-22; see also Fig. 8-8).

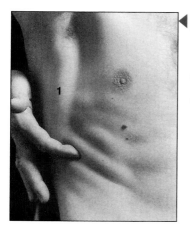

◀ FIGURE 5-21
THE EXTERNAL ABDOMINAL OBLIQUE MUSCLE — COSTAL INSERTIONS

In this figure, the index finger points to one of the digitations of the external abdominal oblique muscle (see also Figs. 5-22 and 5-23).

(1) Latissimus dorsi muscle

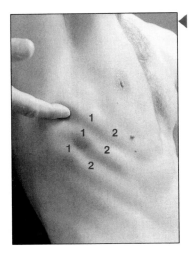

◀ **FIGURE 5-22**

THE EXTERNAL ABDOMINAL OBLIQUE MUSCLE: COSTAL
INSERTIONS — RELATIONSHIP WITH THE SERRATUS ANTERIOR MUSCLE

In this figure, the index finger points to the digitations of the serratus anterior muscle (1) and the close relationship between this muscle and the external abdominal oblique muscle (2) (see Fig. 8-8).

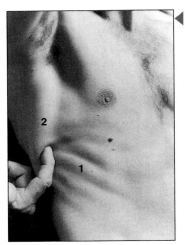

◀ **FIGURE 5-23**

THE EXTERNAL ABDOMINAL OBLIQUE MUSCLE: COSTAL
INSERTIONS — RELATIONSHIP WITH THE LATISSIMUS DORSI MUSCLE

In this figure, the index finger is placed at the same time on a digitation of the external abdominal oblique muscle (1) and on the latissimus dorsi muscle (2). This emphasizes the relationship between these two muscles — they are closely related on the lateral surface of the last three or four ribs.

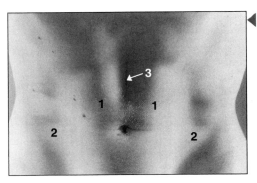

◀ **FIGURE 5-24**

THE ANTEROLATERAL MUSCLES OF THE ABDOMEN

This figure shows the two rectus abdominis muscles (1) separated by the linea alba (3). The bellies (2) of the external oblique muscles, the internal oblique muscle, and the transversus abdominis muscle are positioned in that order (from superficial to deep) on both sides of the rectus abdominis muscles.

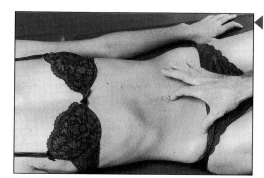

◄ **FIGURE 5-25**

THE PSOAS MAJOR MUSCLE: TECHNIQUE OF APPROACH— STEP 1

With the subject in a supine position, place your thumb on the anterior superior iliac spine and your index finger on the umbilicus.

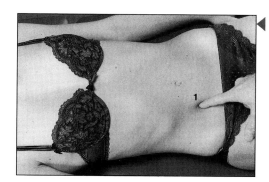

◄ **FIGURE 5-26**

THE PSOAS MAJOR MUSCLE: TECHNIQUE OF APPROACH— STEP 2

Position your thumb and your index finger as described in Figure 5-25 and imagine a line drawn between them. Place your index finger in the middle of this line, at the lateral border of the rectus abdominis muscle (1) (see also Fig. 5-24).

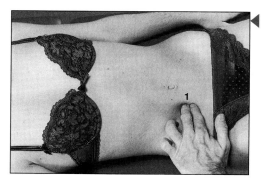

◄ **FIGURE 5-27**

THE PSOAS MAJOR MUSCLE: TECHNIQUE OF APPROACH— STEP 3

After completing the preceding two steps (Figs. 5-26 and 5-27), gently palpate the muscle of interest from the abdominal wall at the lateral border of the rectus abdominis muscle (1). You will feel a relatively large muscle belly under your fingers (an active flexion of the subject's thigh on the pelvis can help you feel this structure).

CHAPTER
Six

NERVES AND VESSELS

The notable structures accessible by palpation are

• The axillary artery (Fig. 6-2)

• The abdominal aorta (Fig. 6-3)

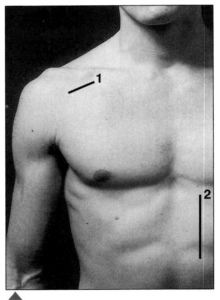

▲
FIGURE 6-1
**VISUALIZATION OF THE ROUTE
OF THE AXILLARY ARTERY AND
OF THE ABDOMINAL AORTA**

(1) Axillary artery
(2) Abdominal aorta

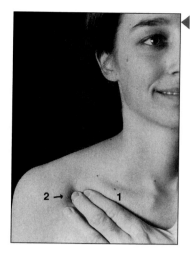

◀ FIGURE 6-2
THE AXILLARY ARTERY

Place your hand flat on the anterior surface of the pectoralis major muscle: the index finger is placed at the inferior border of the clavicle (1); the tips of the fingers are touching the medial surface of the coracoid process (2) (see Fig. 7-28). You can feel the pulse under your fingers.

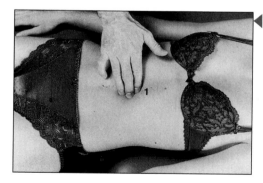

◀ FIGURE 6-3
THE ABDOMINAL AORTA

The abdominal aorta continues the thoracic aorta below the diaphragm. It descends in front and to the left of the spine before it divides into two terminal branches at the level of the L4–L5 disc. To feel the pulse of this artery, place the subject in a supine position, with the knees flexed to relax the abdominal wall. Stand at the right of the subject and place your fingers above the umbilicus, one finger-breadth to the left of the linea alba (1) (see Fig. 5-24). Press on the abdominal wall very carefully.

THE

SHOULDER

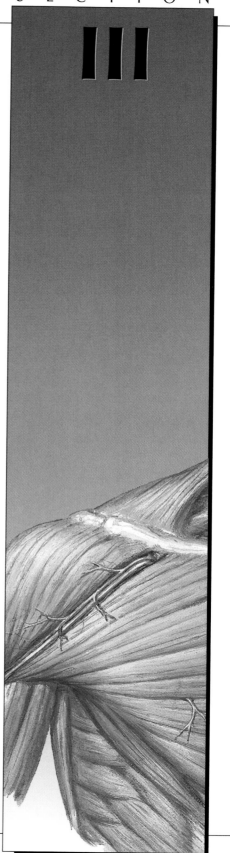

MUSCLES OF SHOULDER

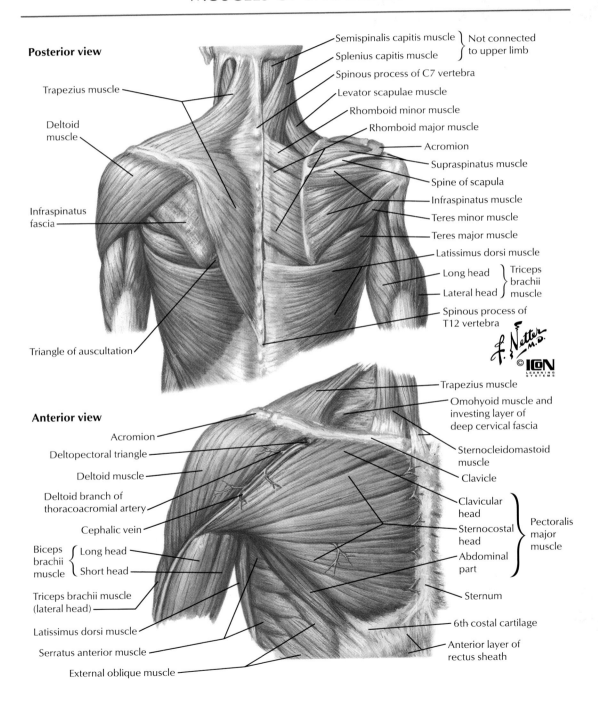

Posterior view

Semispinalis capitis muscle ⎫ Not connected
Splenius capitis muscle ⎰ to upper limb

Trapezius muscle

Spinous process of C7 vertebra

Levator scapulae muscle

Rhomboid minor muscle

Deltoid muscle

Rhomboid major muscle

Acromion

Supraspinatus muscle

Spine of scapula

Infraspinatus muscle

Teres minor muscle

Infraspinatus fascia

Teres major muscle

Latissimus dorsi muscle

Long head ⎫ Triceps
Lateral head ⎰ brachii muscle

Spinous process of T12 vertebra

Triangle of auscultation

Trapezius muscle

Omohyoid muscle and investing layer of deep cervical fascia

Anterior view

Acromion

Sternocleidomastoid muscle

Deltopectoral triangle

Clavicle

Deltoid muscle

Clavicular head ⎫
Sternocostal head ⎬ Pectoralis major muscle
Abdominal part ⎰

Deltoid branch of thoracoacromial artery

Cephalic vein

Biceps brachii muscle ⎰ Long head
⎱ Short head

Triceps brachii muscle (lateral head)

Sternum

Latissimus dorsi muscle

6th costal cartilage

Serratus anterior muscle

Anterior layer of rectus sheath

External oblique muscle

PECTORAL, CLAVIPECTORAL AND AXILLARY FASCIAE

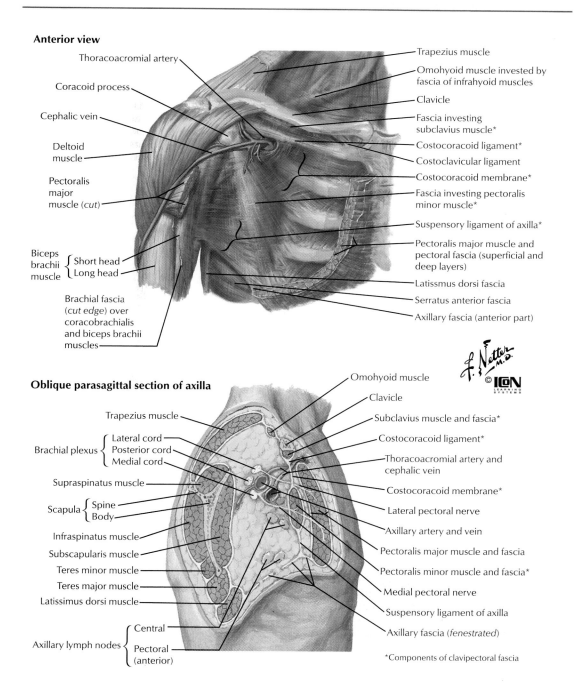

Anterior view

Thoracoacromial artery

Coracoid process

Cephalic vein

Deltoid muscle

Pectoralis major muscle (*cut*)

Biceps brachii muscle { Short head / Long head

Brachial fascia (*cut edge*) over coracobrachialis and biceps brachii muscles

Trapezius muscle

Omohyoid muscle invested by fascia of infrahyoid muscles

Clavicle

Fascia investing subclavius muscle*

Costocoracoid ligament*

Costoclavicular ligament

Costocoracoid membrane*

Fascia investing pectoralis minor muscle*

Suspensory ligament of axilla*

Pectoralis major muscle and pectoral fascia (superficial and deep layers)

Latissimus dorsi fascia

Serratus anterior fascia

Axillary fascia (anterior part)

Oblique parasagittal section of axilla

Trapezius muscle

Brachial plexus { Lateral cord / Posterior cord / Medial cord

Supraspinatus muscle

Scapula { Spine / Body

Infraspinatus muscle

Subscapularis muscle

Teres minor muscle

Teres major muscle

Latissimus dorsi muscle

Axillary lymph nodes { Central / Pectoral (anterior)

Omohyoid muscle

Clavicle

Subclavius muscle and fascia*

Costocoracoid ligament*

Thoracoacromial artery and cephalic vein

Costocoracoid membrane*

Lateral pectoral nerve

Axillary artery and vein

Pectoralis major muscle and fascia

Pectoralis minor muscle and fascia*

Medial pectoral nerve

Suspensory ligament of axilla

Axillary fascia (*fenestrated*)

*Components of clavipectoral fascia

71

TOPOGRAPHIC PRESENTATION OF THE SHOULDER

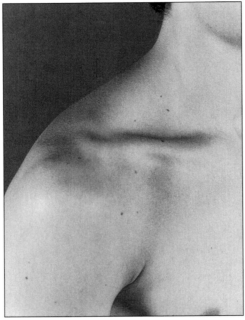

FIGURE 7-1
ANTEROLATERAL VIEW OF THE SHOULDER

| C H A P T E R | **OSTEOLOGY** |
| Seven | |

THE CLAVICLE

The notable structures accessible by palpation are

- The anterolateral concavity of the clavicle (Fig. 7-3)
- The posterolateral convexity of the clavicle (Fig. 7-4)
- The anteromedial convexity of the clavicle (Fig. 7-5)
- The posterolateral concavity of the clavicle (Fig. 7-6)
- The sternal extremity of the clavicle (Fig. 7-7)
- The acromial extremity of the clavicle (Fig. 7-8)

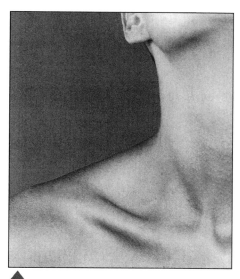

▲
FIGURE 7-2
GENERAL PRESENTATION OF THE CLAVICLE

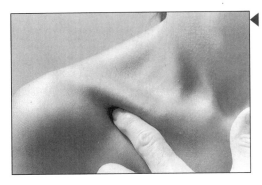

◀ FIGURE 7-3
THE ANTEROLATERAL CONCAVITY OF THE CLAVICLE

The clavicle, a long bone in the shape of an italic S, is located transversely between the scapula and the sternum. It is a key element of the shoulder girdle. The structure of interest is the site of origin or proximal attachment of the anterior fasciculus of the deltoid muscle.

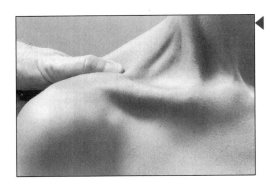

◀ FIGURE 7-4
THE POSTEROLATERAL CONVEXITY OF THE CLAVICLE

This part of the clavicle belongs to the posterior border. Convex and rough, it is the site of insertion of the clavicular fibers of the trapezius muscle (this insertion occupies the lateral third of the posterior border).

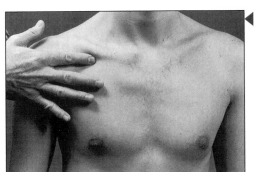

◀ FIGURE 7-5
THE ANTEROMEDIAL CONVEXITY OF THE CLAVICLE

This convexity occupies the medial two thirds of the anterior border. It is the site of origin or proximal attachment of the pectoralis major muscle.

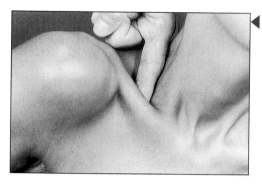

◀ **FIGURE 7-6**
THE POSTEROLATERAL CONCAVITY OF THE CLAVICLE

This concavity occupies the medial two thirds of the posterior border of the clavicle.

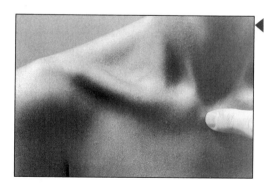

◀ **FIGURE 7-7**
THE STERNAL EXTREMITY OF THE CLAVICLE

This bulbous structure has a saddle-shaped articular surface that articulates with the sternum and the first costal cartilage.

Comment: These three structures contribute to the sternoclavicular joint.

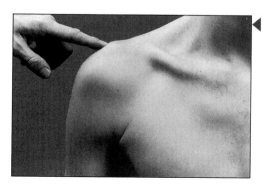

◀ **FIGURE 7-8**
THE ACROMIAL EXTREMITY OF THE CLAVICLE

This structure, flattened at the top, articulates with the acromion by means of an oval articular surface directed downward, forward, and outward.

Comment: These two structures, the acromion and the acromial extremity of the clavicle, contribute to the acromioclavicular joint.

THE SCAPULA

The notable structures accessible by palpation are

- The scapula—general approach (Fig. 7-10)
- The anterior surface of the scapula—spinal or medial approach (Fig. 7-11)
- The anterior surface of the scapula—lateral approach (Fig. 7-12)
- Visualization of the scapular spine and the acromion (Fig. 7-13)
- The scapular spine and its lateral extension—the acromion (Fig. 7-14)
- The acromial angle (Fig. 7-15)
- The posterior inferior border of the acromion medial to the acromial angle (Fig. 7-16)
- The lateral border of the acromion (Fig. 7-17)
- The apex of the acromion (Fig. 7-18)
- The medial border of the acromion (Fig. 7-19)
- The scapular spine (Fig. 7-20)
- The medial extremity of the scapular spine (Fig. 7-21)
- The tubercle for the trapezius muscle (Fig. 7-22)
- The supraspinous fossa (Fig. 7-23)
- The infraspinous fossa (Fig. 7-24)
- The medial margin of the scapula (Fig. 7-25)
- The lateral margin of the scapula (Fig. 7-26)
- The neck of the scapula (Fig. 7-27)
- The coracoid process (Fig. 7-28)
- The superior margin of the scapula (Fig. 7-29)
- The inferior angle of the scapula (Fig. 7-30)
- The superior angle of the scapula—posterior (or dorsal) approach (Fig. 7-31)
- The superior angle of the scapula—anterior approach (Fig. 7-32)

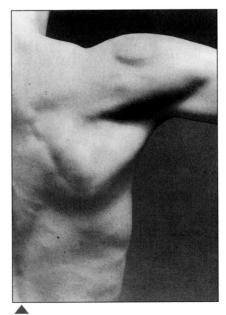

▲
FIGURE 7-9
GENERAL PRESENTATION
OF THE SCAPULA

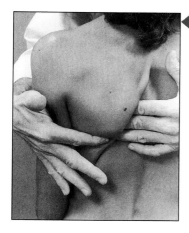

FIGURE 7-10
THE SCAPULA — GENERAL APPROACH

The scapula is a flat bone attached to the posterior surface of the rib cage, between the second and the seventh ribs. It articulates with the clavicle and the humerus.

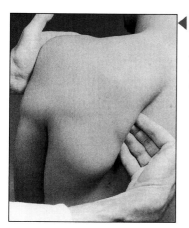

FIGURE 7-11
THE ANTERIOR SURFACE OF THE SCAPULA — MEDIAL APPROACH

The medial approach to the scapula allows contact with the insertions of the serratus anterior muscle, which is attached to the medial margin of the scapula.

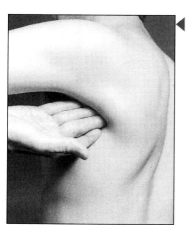

FIGURE 7-12
THE ANTERIOR SURFACE OF THE SCAPULA — LATERAL APPROACH

This approach allows contact with the fibers of the subscapularis muscle that arise from the anterior surface of the scapula.

Comment: Along the lateral margin, there is a crest that connects the neck of the scapula with the inferior angle. This bony structure is called the pillar of the scapula.

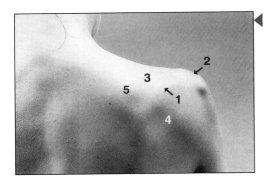

FIGURE 7-13

VISUALIZATION OF THE SCAPULAR SPINE AND THE ACROMION

The scapular spine (1), which is triangular with a medial apex, is located at the union of the superior quarter and the inferior three quarters of the scapula. It is perpendicular to the plane of the scapula: the anterior border of the scapular spine is in contact with the posterior surface of the scapula, separating the latter into two parts — the supraspinous fossa (3) (Fig. 7-23) and the infraspinous fossa (4) (Fig. 7-24). The lateral and posterior borders of the spine widen laterally to form the acromion (2).

Comment: The superior angle of the scapula (5) (see Fig. 7-31) is also visible in this figure.

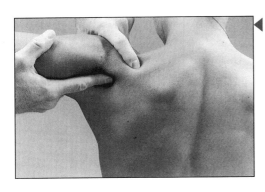

FIGURE 7-14

THE SCAPULAR SPINE AND ITS LATERAL EXTENSION — THE ACROMION

In this figure, the two index fingers indicate the lateral extremity of the scapular spine, which widens laterally to form the acromion. Flattened perpendicularly to the scapular spine, it is quadrangular and presents a superior surface, an inferior surface, a medial edge (Fig. 7-25), a lateral edge (Fig. 7-26), an apex (Fig. 7-18), and the acromial angle (Fig. 7-15).

Comment: The superior surface seems to result from a widening of the posterior border of the spine. The inferior surface seems to result from a widening of the lateral border of the spine.

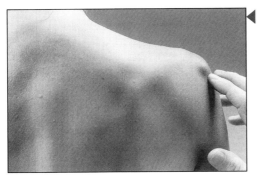

FIGURE 7-15

THE ACROMIAL ANGLE

This anatomic landmark represents the change of direction of the posterior inferior border of the acromion. It is a site of origin of the deltoid muscle.

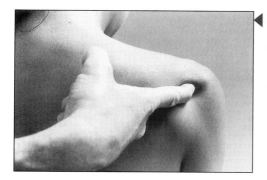

FIGURE 7-16
THE POSTERIOR INFERIOR BORDER
OF THE ACROMION MEDIAL TO THE ACROMIAL ANGLE

This border, indicated by the index finger, is a site of origin or attachment of the deltoid muscle.

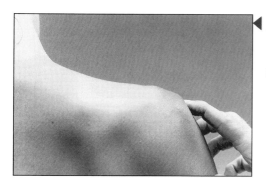

FIGURE 7-17
THE LATERAL BORDER OF THE ACROMION

In this figure, the index finger indicates the structure of interest, a site of origin of the deltoid muscle.

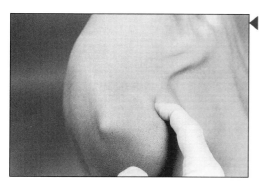

FIGURE 7-18
THE APEX OF THE ACROMION

This structure is located lateral to and in front of the lateral (or acromial) extremity of the clavicle (Fig. 7-8). It is a site of origin of the deltoid muscle.

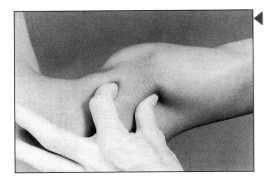

◀ **FIGURE 7-19**
THE MEDIAL BORDER OF THE ACROMION

The lateral two thirds of this border is characterized by an oval articular surface that is directed upward and medially and that articulates with the lateral extremity of the clavicle. Examine this structure with your index finger, with your thumb in contact with the posterior inferior border of the acromion, as shown in this figure.

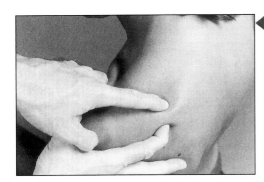

◀ **FIGURE 7-20**
THE SCAPULAR SPINE

This triangular bony structure is located transversely on the posterior surface of the scapula where its superior quarter and its inferior three quarters meet (see also Figs. 7-13 and 7-14).

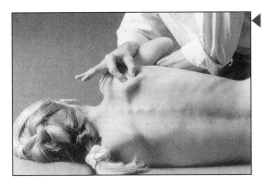

◀ **FIGURE 7-21**
THE MEDIAL EXTREMITY OF THE SCAPULAR SPINE

The scapular spine presents at its medial extremity a triangular widening, which is clearly visible in this figure (beneath the thumb–index finger grip). It ends on the medial border of the scapula.

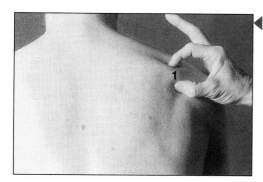

FIGURE 7-22
THE TUBERCLE FOR THE TRAPEZIUS MUSCLE

The posterior border of the scapular spine, which is directly subcutaneous, presents at its middle region a thickening. This thickening, which you can feel under your fingers as a bulge, is the tubercle for the trapezius muscle (1).

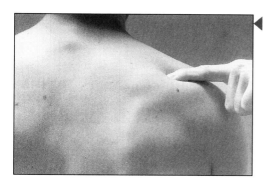

FIGURE 7-23
THE SUPRASPINOUS FOSSA

This structure, located at the posterior surface of the scapula above the scapular spine (Fig. 7-20), is the site of origin of the supraspinatus muscle (Fig. 8-11).

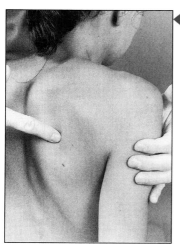

FIGURE 7-24
THE INFRASPINOUS FOSSA

This structure, located at the posterior surface of the scapula beneath the scapular spine (Fig. 7-20), is the site of origin of the infraspinatus muscle (Fig. 8-13).

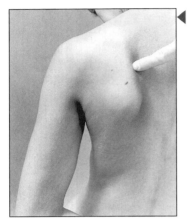

FIGURE 7-25
THE MEDIAL MARGIN OF THE SCAPULA

This is the longest of the three margins of the scapula. It is marked with an obtuse angle whose apex corresponds to the medial extremity of the scapular spine. Above this angle, the levator scapulae muscle has its insertion (see Fig. 2-21). The rhomboid minor muscle and the rhomboid major muscle have their insertions beneath this angle.

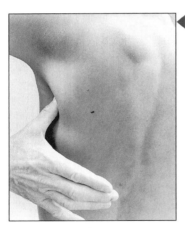

FIGURE 7-26
THE LATERAL MARGIN OF THE SCAPULA

This margin widens superiorly below the glenoid cavity to form the infraglenoid tubercle, the site of origin of the long head of the triceps brachii muscle.

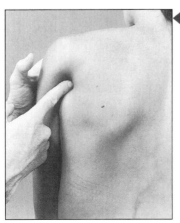

FIGURE 7-27
THE NECK OF THE SCAPULA

This structure, the glenoid cavity, which it supports, and the coracoid process (Fig. 7-28) form the lateral angle of the scapula. The posterior surface of this neck presents a groove that allows communication, lateral to the scapular spine, between the supraspinous fossa and the infraspinous fossa.

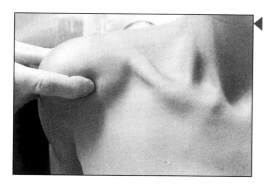

◄ FIGURE 7-28
THE CORACOID PROCESS

This structure is located just medial to the humeral head and below the clavicle, as shown in this figure. The apex and the medial border of this structure may be palpated. This bony structure is the site of attachment of the pectoralis minor muscle (Fig. 8-6), the coracobrachialis muscle (see Fig. 9-8), and the tendon of the short head of the biceps brachii muscle (see Figs 9-4 and 9-5).

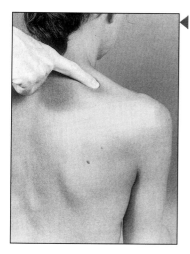

◄ FIGURE 7-29
THE SUPERIOR MARGIN OF THE SCAPULA

This short and thin structure ends laterally with the scapular notch, where the suprascapular nerve runs. The omohyoid muscle inserts medial to this notch on the superior margin.

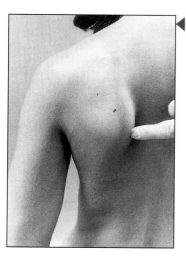

◄ FIGURE 7-30
THE INFERIOR ANGLE OF THE SCAPULA

This angle, which is thick, rough, and rounded, is located at the junction of the medial and lateral margins. It is an inconstant site of attachment of a fasciculus of the latissimus dorsi muscle.

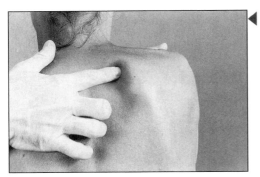

◄ **FIGURE 7-31**
THE SUPERIOR ANGLE OF THE SCAPULA — POSTERIOR (OR DORSAL) APPROACH

With the subject seated, take hold of the anterior part of the subject's shoulder with one hand and push it back and upward to make the medial margin of the scapula protrude. The index finger indicates the angle of interest.

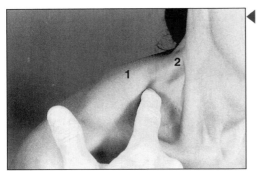

◄ **FIGURE 7-32**
THE SUPERIOR ANGLE OF THE SCAPULA — ANTERIOR APPROACH

With the subject seated, place the subject's arm in retropulsion (actively or passively) in order to slide the scapula upward and forward on the rib cage so that the angle of interest appears under your fingers through the mass of the trapezius muscle (1).

Comment: The muscle that inserts into this angle is the levator scapulae muscle (2).

THE PROXIMAL END OF THE HUMERUS

The notable structures accessible by palpation are

- The humerus—global grip of the humeral head (Fig. 7-34)
- Global approach to three structures of the humerus— the lesser tubercle, the intertubercular groove, and the greater tubercle (Fig. 7-35)
- Global approach to three structures of the humerus— the lesser tubercle, the intertubercular groove, and the greater tubercle (other method) (Fig. 7-36)

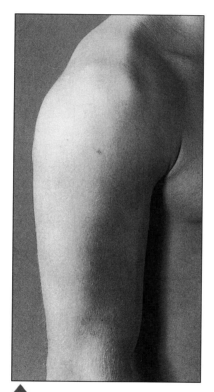

▲

FIGURE 7-33
PRESENTATION OF THE
PROXIMAL END OF THE HUMERUS

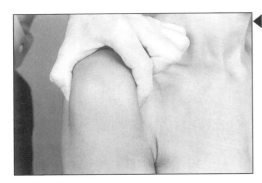

FIGURE 7-34

THE HUMERUS — GLOBAL GRIP OF THE HUMERAL HEAD

In this figure, the global grip on the lateral end of the clavicle and on the acromion surrounds the humeral head. Ask the subject to alternate medial and lateral shoulder rotations; the elbow may be flexed at 90°. The humeral head rolls under your fingers.

Comment: From an initial position of an internal rotation of the subject's shoulder, you can clearly feel the passage of the greater tubercle and the lesser tubercle (see also Figs. 7-35 and 7-36). Between those two tubercles, the intertubercular groove (see also Figs. 7-35 and 7-36) can also be clearly felt.

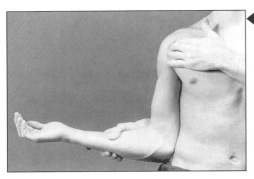

FIGURE 7-35

GLOBAL APPROACH TO THREE STRUCTURES OF THE HUMERUS — THE LESSER TUBERCLE, THE INTERTUBERCULAR GROOVE, AND THE GREATER TUBERCLE

The subject is seated, with the arm pressed against the body, the elbow flexed at 90°, the hand in supination. Place four fingers on the pectoralis major muscle and on the anterior fasciculus of the deltoid muscle. With the other hand, bring the subject's upper limb in external rotation. In this position, you will feel the coracoid process under your fingers (see Fig. 7-28) and, just lateral to this structure, the lesser tubercle. Rotate the subject's arm medially in order to feel, in a lateral position, first the intertubercular groove and then the greater tubercle.

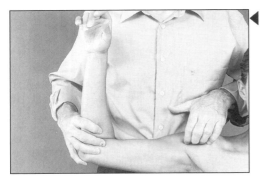

FIGURE 7-36

GLOBAL APPROACH TO THREE STRUCTURES OF THE HUMERUS — THE LESSER TUBERCLE, THE INTERTUBERCULAR GROOVE, AND THE GREATER TUBERCLE (OTHER METHOD)

With the subject seated, with the shoulder abducted at 90° and the elbow flexed at 90°, stand behind the subject and place four fingers at the level of the deltopectoral groove. With your other hand, grasp the subject's elbow and perform rapid, small-amplitude movements of external and internal rotation of the shoulder. The medial density that you feel under your fingers is the lesser tubercle; the lateral density is the greater tubercle; and the depression between those two structures is the intertubercular groove.

CHAPTER
Eight

MYOLOGY

THE ANTERIOR MUSCULAR GROUP

This group consists of the pectoralis major muscle, the pectoralis minor muscle, and the subclavius muscle. The notable structures accessible by palpation are

- The clavicular part of the pectoralis major muscle (Fig. 8-2)
- The sternocostal part of the pectoralis major muscle (Fig. 8-3)

- The abdominal part of the pectoralis major muscle (Fig. 8-4)
- The subclavius muscle (Fig. 8-5)
- The pectoralis minor muscle (Fig. 8-6)

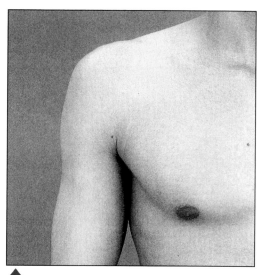

▲
FIGURE 8-1
THE SHOULDER — THE ANTERIOR
MUSCULAR GROUP

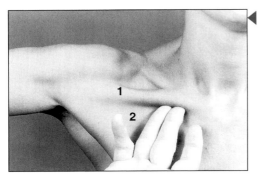

◄ FIGURE 8-2
THE CLAVICULAR PART OF THE PECTORALIS MAJOR MUSCLE

Abduct the subject's arm at 90°, with the elbow flexed at 90° and the forearm pointing upward. Apply resistance at the medial aspect of the arm and ask the subject to adduct the arm horizontally. Place two fingers under the clavicle to find a groove that separates the clavicular bundle (1) from the sternocostochondral bundle (2) (Fig. 8-3), as shown in this figure.

Comment: This bundle inserts into the medial two-thirds of the anterior border of the clavicle.

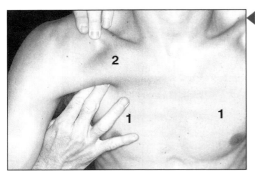

◄ FIGURE 8-3
THE STERNOCOSTAL PART OF THE PECTORALIS MAJOR MUSCLE

Abduct the subject's arm at 90°. Apply resistance against the horizontal adduction of the arm; the bundle of interest (1) appears under the groove that separates it from the clavicular part (2) (see Fig. 8-2).

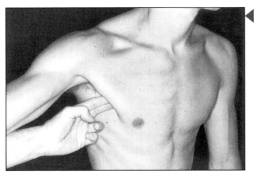

◄ FIGURE 8-4
THE ABDOMINAL PART OF THE PECTORALIS MAJOR MUSCLE

Abduct the subject's upper limb at 90°. Oppose the adduction of the shoulder by applying resistance at the medial aspect of the arm. The bundle of interest is the inferolateral border of the pectoralis major muscle.

Comment: This bundle attaches to the aponeurosis of the rectus abdominis muscle.

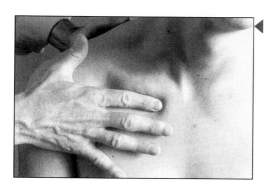

FIGURE 8-5
THE SUBCLAVIUS MUSCLE

In this figure, the index finger indicates globally the position of the subclavius muscle, a muscle that is hardly perceptible under the fingers. It extends from the lower surface of the clavicle to the first costal cartilage.

Comment: As a true active ligament of the sternocostal articulation, this muscle is a key element of the different movements of the clavicle.

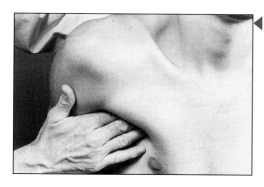

FIGURE 8-6
THE PECTORALIS MINOR MUSCLE

The subject is seated or in a supine position. Cradle the subject's forearm and support the upper limb. The subject's elbow is flexed at 90° and rests on your forearm. This supportive grip allows you to move the subject's shoulder upward and inward to maximally relax the pectoralis major muscle. Once this muscle is relaxed, slide your fingers under the pectoralis major muscle, as shown in this figure. You will find a rather imposing muscular cord that is the muscle of interest. The pectoralis minor muscle is easily felt, even in a relaxed position. Nevertheless, you can activate this muscle in order to feel it better: ask the subject to perform fast, repeated inspirations to mobilize the third, fourth, and fifth ribs, which are the medial sites of insertion of this muscle. (In this case, the fixed point is the coracoid process.) Or you can ask the subject to move the shoulder forward (as in this figure), since this is an action of the pectoralis minor muscle if the fixed point is at the ribs.

THE INTERNAL MUSCULAR GROUP

This group consists of a single muscle: the serratus anterior muscle.

The notable structure accessible by palpation is

• The serratus anterior muscle—palpation on the ribs (Fig. 8-8)

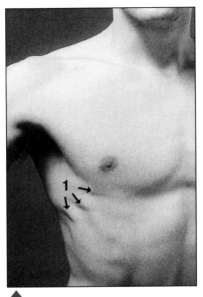

FIGURE 8-7
ANTEROLATERAL VIEW OF THE
TRUNK — THE INTERNAL MUSCULAR
GROUP OF THE SHOULDER

(1) Serratus anterior muscle

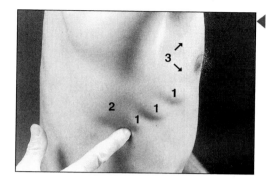

FIGURE 8-8
THE SERRATUS ANTERIOR MUSCLE —
PALPATION ON THE RIBS

While the subject is standing or sitting, ask him to perform brief, repeated inspirations so that the muscular digitations (1), which originate from the ribs, appear between the latissimus dorsi muscle (2) in back and the pectoralis major muscle (3) in front (see also Figs. 5-20 and 5-21).

THE POSTERIOR MUSCULAR GROUP

This group consists of the six muscles of the posterior side of the axillary fossa. They are in direct contact with the scapula. Of these muscles, only one is positioned at the anterior surface of that bone: the subscapularis muscle. The other five (the supraspinatus, infraspinatus, teres minor, teres major, and latissimus dorsi muscles) are located posterior to the scapula.

The notable structures accessible by palpation are

- The subscapularis muscle (Fig. 8-10)
- The supraspinatus muscle (Fig. 8-11)
- The humeral insertion of the supraspinatus muscle (Fig. 8-12)
- The infraspinatus muscle (Fig. 8-13)

- The teres minor muscle (Fig. 8-14)
- The humeral insertions of the infraspinatus muscle and the teres minor muscle (Fig. 8-15)
- The teres major muscle (Fig. 8-16)
- The latissimus dorsi muscle (Fig. 8-17)

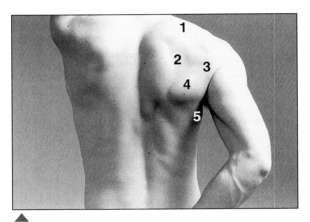

▲
FIGURE 8-9
THE POSTERIOR MUSCULAR GROUP

(1) Supraspinatus muscle
(2) Infraspinatus muscle
(3) Teres minor muscle
(4) Teres major muscle
(5) Latissimus dorsi muscle

Comment: The position of the subscapularis muscle cannot be seen in this figure (it is located on the anterior surface of the scapula).

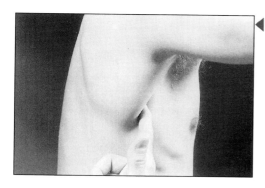

FIGURE 8-10
THE SUBSCAPULARIS MUSCLE

To access this muscle, separate the scapula from the rib cage and slide your finger on the anterior surface of the scapula (see Fig. 7-12), between the latissimus dorsi muscle laterally and the pectoralis major muscle medially and anteriorly.

Comment: The nerves and vessels of the axillary fossa are located at the anterior surface of this muscle. This muscle is part of the muscular group that is classically called the rotator cuff. The other muscles of this group are the supraspinatus muscle, the infraspinatus muscle, and the teres minor muscle.

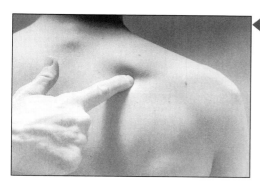

FIGURE 8-11
THE SUPRASPINATUS MUSCLE

This muscle is perceptible only through the trapezius muscle, above the scapular spine, in the supraspinous fossa. An abduction of the subject's arm allows a better perception of this muscle, since it acts as a stabilizer of the shoulder during this movement.

Comment: This muscle is part of what is classically called the rotator cuff.

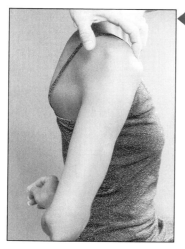

FIGURE 8-12
THE HUMERAL INSERTION OF THE SUPRASPINATUS MUSCLE

Place the subject's upper limb as shown in this picture: the shoulder in internal rotation and in retropulsion (the dorsum of the hand and the posterior aspect of the forearm are placed against the back). The superior surface of the greater tubercle of the humerus, which is the site of insertion of the structure of interest, is palpable in front of the apex of the acromion (see Fig. 7-18).

Comment: This muscle helps form the acromioclavicular arch and is part of what is classically called the rotator cuff.

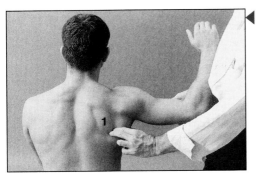

FIGURE 8-13
THE INFRASPINATUS MUSCLE

With the subject seated, support his or her arm (shoulder abducted at 90°, elbow flexed at 90°) and ask him or her to rotate the shoulder externally (the subject moves the posterior aspect of the forearm upward and backward), as shown in this figure. You will feel the contraction in the infraspinous fossa of the scapula, to which this muscle is attached (1).

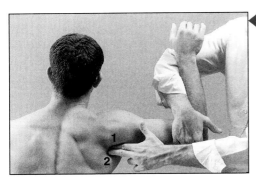

FIGURE 8-14
THE TERES MINOR MUSCLE

With the subject seated, support his or her arm (shoulder abducted at 90°, elbow flexed at 90°), with his or her forearm placed in pronation and resting on your arm (see figure). Place a bidigital grip at the lateral border of the scapula, between the posterior bundle of the deltoid muscle (1) above (see Fig. 8-19) and the teres minor muscle (2) below (see Fig. 8-16). Ask the subject to perform successive movements of external rotation of the shoulder to allow you to feel the contractions of the muscle under your fingers.

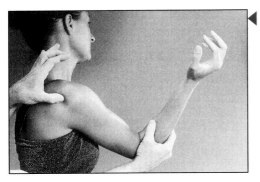

FIGURE 8-15
THE HUMERAL INSERTIONS OF THE INFRASPINATUS MUSCLE AND THE TERES MINOR MUSCLE

To palpate the tendons of these muscles at the humeral level, first place the subject's shoulder in flexion, adduction, and external rotation. Then place your thumb under the posterior inferior border of the acromion (Fig. 7-16), in contact with the middle and posterior surfaces of the greater tubercle of the humerus.

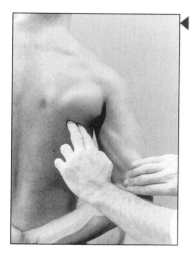

FIGURE 8-16
THE TERES MAJOR MUSCLE

With the subject seated or in a prone position, with the dorsum of the hand and the posterior aspect of the forearm resting on the sacrum, apply resistance at the medial aspect of the arm and resist the retropulsion of the arm. The muscle of interest, indicated by the index finger, usually bulges out prominently.

Comment: This muscle originates from the inferior third of the lateral quarter of the infraspinous fossa.

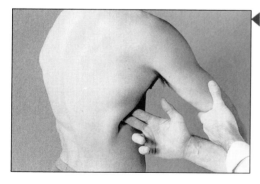

FIGURE 8-17
THE LATISSIMUS DORSI MUSCLE

Oppose an adduction of the arm by applying resistance at the medial aspect of the arm. The muscle bulges at the posterolateral aspect of the thorax (see also Figs. 5-6, 5-7, and 5-8).

THE EXTERNAL MUSCULAR GROUP

This group consists of a single muscle located at the lateral aspect of the shoulder: the deltoid muscle.
The notable structures accessible by palpation are

• The posterior (or spinous) bundle of the deltoid muscle (Fig. 8-19)

• The intermediate (or acromial) bundle of the deltoid muscle (Fig. 8-20)

• The anterior (or clavicular) bundle of the deltoid muscle (Fig. 8-21)

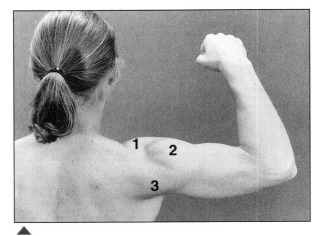

▲
FIGURE 8-18
POSTERIOR VIEW OF THE SHOULDER REGION

(1) Anterior (or clavicular) bundle of the deltoid muscle

(2) Intermediate (or acromial) bundle of the deltoid muscle

(3) Posterior (or spinous) bundle of the deltoid muscle

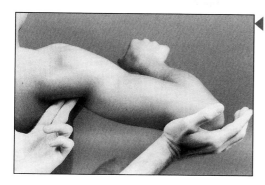

FIGURE 8-19
THE POSTERIOR (OR SPINOUS)
BUNDLE OF THE DELTOID MUSCLE

Position the subject's arm at 90° of abduction, with the elbow flexed. Apply resistance at the posterior and inferior aspect of the arm, above the elbow, as shown in the figure. Ask the subject to perform a horizontal retropulsion. The muscle belly, indicated by the bidigital grip, appears or is felt at the posterior aspect of the shoulder.

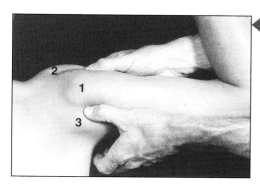

FIGURE 8-20
THE INTERMEDIATE (OR ACROMIAL)
BUNDLE OF THE DELTOID MUSCLE

The initial position of the subject is the same as that described in Figure 8-19. In this figure, the two thumbs separate the intermediate bundle (1) from the anterior (2) and posterior (3) bundles. Ask the subject to abduct the arm, against which you may apply resistance.

Comment: The deltoid muscle covers the shoulder joint and is separated from it by the subdeltoid bursa.

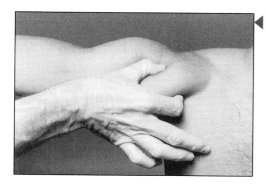

FIGURE 8-21
THE ANTERIOR (OR CLAVICULAR)
BUNDLE OF THE DELTOID MUSCLE

The subject's shoulder is still abducted at 90°, with the elbow flexed. In this figure, the anterior bundle is held between the thumb and the index finger. Ask the subject to perform a horizontal flexion of the shoulder, which you resist.

THE ARM

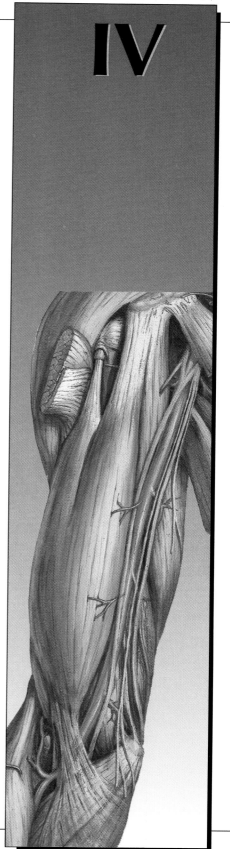

BRACHIAL ARTERY IN SITU

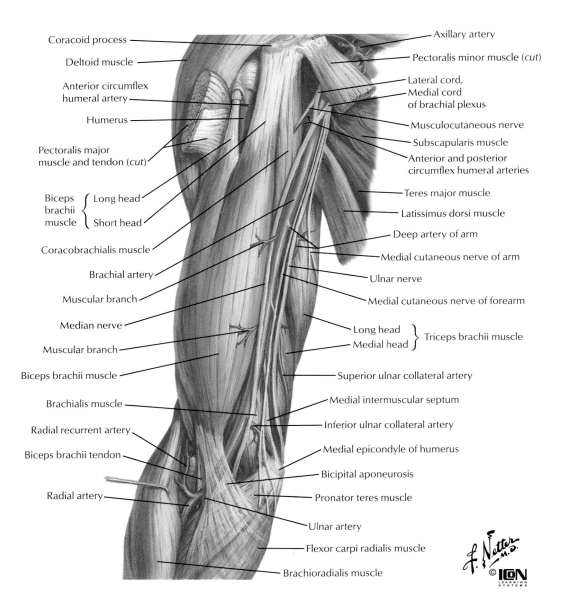

Coracoid process

Deltoid muscle

Anterior circumflex humeral artery

Humerus

Pectoralis major muscle and tendon (*cut*)

Biceps brachii muscle { Long head / Short head

Coracobrachialis muscle

Brachial artery

Muscular branch

Median nerve

Muscular branch

Biceps brachii muscle

Brachialis muscle

Radial recurrent artery

Biceps brachii tendon

Radial artery

Axillary artery

Pectoralis minor muscle (*cut*)

Lateral cord, Medial cord of brachial plexus

Musculocutaneous nerve

Subscapularis muscle

Anterior and posterior circumflex humeral arteries

Teres major muscle

Latissimus dorsi muscle

Deep artery of arm

Medial cutaneous nerve of arm

Ulnar nerve

Medial cutaneous nerve of forearm

Long head / Medial head } Triceps brachii muscle

Superior ulnar collateral artery

Medial intermuscular septum

Inferior ulnar collateral artery

Medial epicondyle of humerus

Bicipital aponeurosis

Pronator teres muscle

Ulnar artery

Flexor carpi radialis muscle

Brachioradialis muscle

MUSCLES OF ARM: POSTERIOR VIEWS

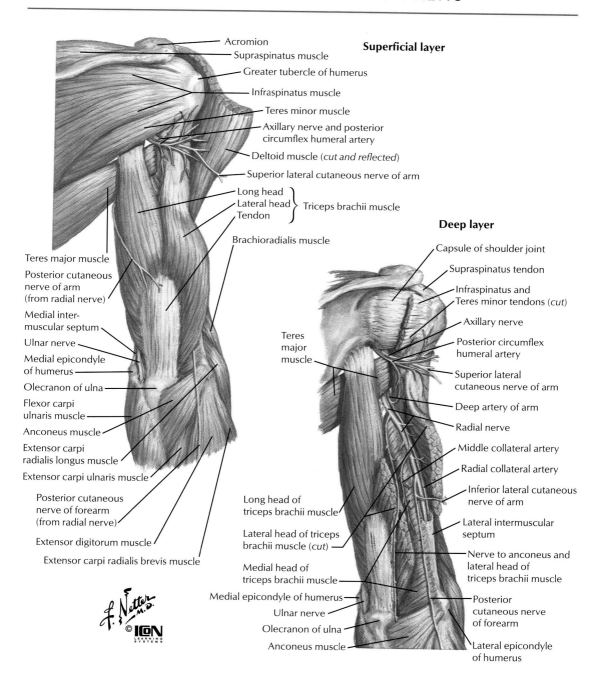

Superficial layer

Acromion
Supraspinatus muscle
Greater tubercle of humerus
Infraspinatus muscle
Teres minor muscle
Axillary nerve and posterior circumflex humeral artery
Deltoid muscle (*cut and reflected*)
Superior lateral cutaneous nerve of arm
Long head
Lateral head } Triceps brachii muscle
Tendon
Brachioradialis muscle

Teres major muscle
Posterior cutaneous nerve of arm (from radial nerve)
Medial inter-muscular septum
Ulnar nerve
Medial epicondyle of humerus
Olecranon of ulna
Flexor carpi ulnaris muscle
Anconeus muscle
Extensor carpi radialis longus muscle
Extensor carpi ulnaris muscle
Posterior cutaneous nerve of forearm (from radial nerve)
Extensor digitorum muscle
Extensor carpi radialis brevis muscle

Deep layer

Capsule of shoulder joint
Supraspinatus tendon
Infraspinatus and Teres minor tendons (*cut*)
Axillary nerve
Posterior circumflex humeral artery
Superior lateral cutaneous nerve of arm
Deep artery of arm
Radial nerve
Middle collateral artery
Radial collateral artery
Inferior lateral cutaneous nerve of arm
Lateral intermuscular septum
Nerve to anconeus and lateral head of triceps brachii muscle
Posterior cutaneous nerve of forearm
Lateral epicondyle of humerus

Teres major muscle

Long head of triceps brachii muscle
Lateral head of triceps brachii muscle (*cut*)
Medial head of triceps brachii muscle
Medial epicondyle of humerus
Ulnar nerve
Olecranon of ulna
Anconeus muscle

F. Netter M.D.
© ICON
LEARNING
SYSTEMS

TOPOGRAPHIC PRESENTATION OF THE ARM

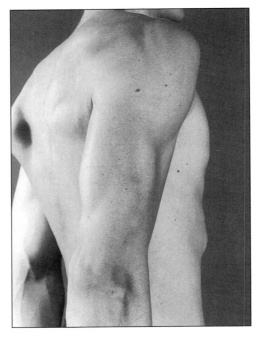

FIGURE 9-1
POSTEROLATERAL VIEW OF THE ARM REGION

C H A P T E R
N i n e

MYOLOGY

THE ANTERIOR MUSCULAR GROUP

This group includes three muscles: the biceps brachii muscle, the coracobrachialis muscle, and the brachialis muscle. These three muscles appear in two planes: a superficial plane and a deep plane.

The notable structures accessible by palpation are

• The superficial plane
- the belly of the long head of the biceps brachii muscle (Fig. 9-3)
- the belly of the short head of the biceps brachii muscle (Figs. 9-4 and 9-5)
- the tendon of the biceps brachii muscle (Fig. 9-6)
- the bicipital aponeurosis (Fig. 9-7)

• The deep plane
- the belly of the coracobrachialis muscle (Fig. 9-8)
- the belly of the brachialis muscle in the distal third of the arm (Fig. 9-9)
- the brachialis muscle in the lateral bicipital groove of the elbow (Fig. 9-10)
- the brachialis muscle in the medial bicipital groove of the elbow (Fig. 9-11)
- the brachialis muscle—global approach (Fig. 9-12)

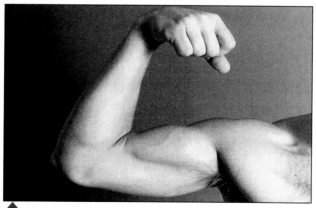

▲
FIGURE 9-2
THE ANTERIOR REGION OF THE ARM

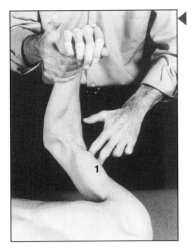

◀ FIGURE 9-3
THE BELLY OF THE LONG HEAD OF THE BICEPS BRACHII MUSCLE

You can palpate this muscle (1), as shown in the figure, without any difficulty along the entire anterior aspect of the arm, from the elbow region up
to where it disappears under the deltoid muscle. Ask the subject to con-
tract and relax this muscle while flexing the elbow against resistance, with
the forearm in supination, and you will find the belly even more easily (see
also Fig. 9-4).

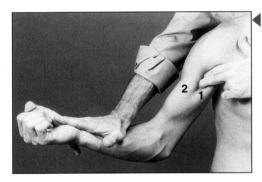

◀ FIGURE 9-4
THE BELLY OF THE SHORT HEAD
OF THE BICEPS BRACHII MUSCLE

To distinguish the short head (1) from the long head (2),
apply light resistance against the flexion of the forearm,
with the forearm in supination. With the other hand, place
a bi- or tridigital grip at the proximal third of the anterior
aspect of the arm and in contact with the pectoralis major
muscle. From this position, move your grip toward the
elbow (downward and inward) to find a groove that separates the muscle bellies of the long head and the short head
of the biceps. To find this groove more easily, ask the subject for a series of contractions and relaxations with the
elbow flexed.

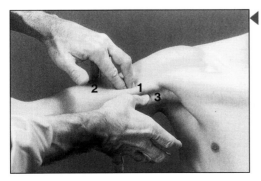

◀ FIGURE 9-5
THE SHORT HEAD OF THE BICEPS BRACHII MUSCLE

Hold the subject's forearm between your rib cage and your
arm. In this way, the subject's arm is supported, but your
hands are free for the examination. As this figure shows, the
short head (1) of the biceps brachial muscle is isolated from
the long head (2) (see also Fig. 9-4) and from the coracobrachialis muscle (3), on which the right thumb rests.

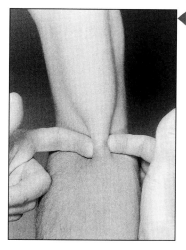

◀ **FIGURE 9-6**
THE TENDON OF THE BICEPS BRACHII MUSCLE

This very strong tendon is easily palpated at the elbow fold. Apply resistance against the flexion of the forearm (which is placed in supination) to help you to locate this tendon.

Comment: The tendon inserts into the posterior aspect of the radial tuberosity.

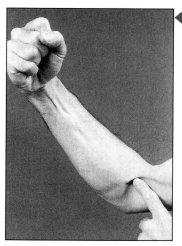

◀ **FIGURE 9-7**
THE BICIPITAL APONEUROSIS

After asking the subject to flex the forearm (which has been placed in supination) on the arm, place your index finger at the medial aspect of the elbow against the tendon of the biceps brachii muscle to feel this aponeurosis. It detaches from the medial border and from the anterior aspect of this tendon to disappear in the aponeurosis of the medial epicondylar muscles.

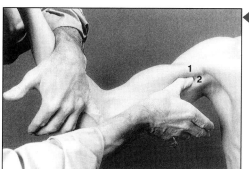

◀ **FIGURE 9-8**
THE BELLY OF THE CORACOBRACHIALIS MUSCLE

Place a bi- or tridigital grip at the medial aspect of the arm, behind the short head (1) (Fig. 9-5) of the biceps brachii muscle. Ask the subject to flex and adduct the shoulder, as shown in this figure, with the elbow previously placed in flexion to maximally relax the biceps brachii muscle. You can feel a muscular cord (2) tighten under your fingers.

Comment: This muscle extends from the coracoid process to the medial aspect of the humerus.

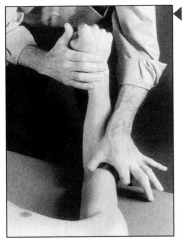

FIGURE 9-9

THE BELLY OF THE BRACHIALIS MUSCLE IN THE DISTAL THIRD OF THE ARM

As shown in this figure, place a global grip with your thumb and your other fingers on the lateral and medial aspect of the arm, behind the biceps brachii muscle. Ask the subject to flex the elbow against resistance, with the forearm previously placed in pronation.

Comment: This muscle extends from the humerus to the ulnar tuberosity (see also Figs. 9-10, 9-11, and 9-12).

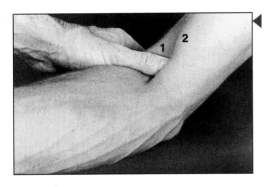

FIGURE 9-10

THE BRACHIALIS MUSCLE IN THE LATERAL BICIPITAL GROOVE OF THE ELBOW

At this level, the muscle of interest is located medial to the brachioradialis muscle (1) and behind and lateral to the biceps brachii muscle (2). To make these two muscles protrude, ask the subject to flex the elbow against resistance, with the forearm placed in a neutral position. After locating these two muscles, slide your thumb between them and push your thumb to the floor of the lateral groove, in contact with the brachialis muscle. Move your palpating finger(s) behind the tendon of the biceps brachii muscle (Fig. 9-6) to better feel this structure in its entirety.

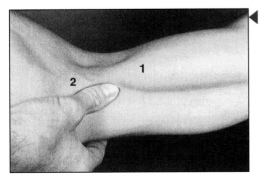

FIGURE 9-11

THE BRACHIALIS MUSCLE IN THE MEDIAL BICIPITAL GROOVE OF THE ELBOW

The position of the forearm and the muscular action are identical to those described above. The brachialis muscle is palpated in the same way between the biceps brachii muscle (1) laterally and the pronator teres muscle (2) medially.

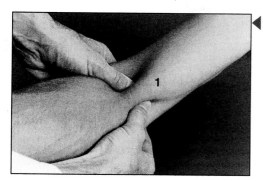

FIGURE 9-12
THE BRACHIALIS MUSCLE — GLOBAL APPROACH

For a global approach, place your thumbs on either side of the distal extremity of the biceps brachii muscle (1). Ask the subject to flex the forearm on the arm while you resist this movement (see also Figs. 9-10 and 9-11).

THE POSTERIOR MUSCULAR GROUP

This group consists of a single muscle: the triceps brachii muscle.

The notable structures accessible by palpation are

- The proximal tendon of the long head of the triceps brachii muscle (Fig. 9-14)
- The belly of the long head of the triceps brachii muscle (Fig. 9-15)
- The lateral head of the triceps brachii muscle (Fig. 9-16)
- The medial head of triceps brachii muscle—posterior view (Fig. 9-17)
- The medial head of triceps brachii muscle—medial view (Fig. 9-18)
- The distal tendon of the triceps brachii muscle (Fig. 9-19)

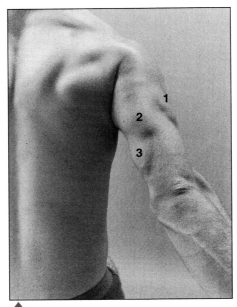

▲
FIGURE 9-13
THE POSTERIOR REGION OF THE ARM

(1) Lateral head of the triceps brachii muscle

(2) Long head of the triceps brachii muscle

(3) Medial head of the triceps brachii muscle

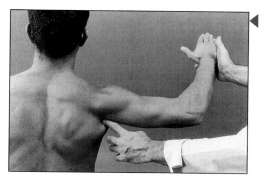

FIGURE 9-14

THE PROXIMAL TENDON OF THE LONG HEAD OF THE TRI-CEPS BRACHII MUSCLE

The subject is seated. Stand next to the subject and place a uni- or bidigital grip at the posterior aspect of the shoulder, in contact with the posterior bundle of the deltoid muscle (see Fig. 8-19) and lateral to the teres minor muscle (see Fig. 8-14). The subject's upper limb is positioned as shown in this figure: shoulder abducted at 90°, elbow flexed at 90°. Apply resistance at the distal aspect of the forearm and ask the subject to extend the elbow. You will feel the tendon under your fingers at the posterior aspect of the shoulder.

Comment: The long head of the triceps brachii muscle originates proximally from the infraglenoid tubercle and the proximal extremity of the lateral margin of the scapula.

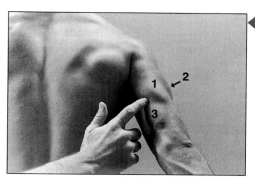

FIGURE 9-15

THE BELLY OF THE LONG HEAD OF THE TRICEPS BRACHII MUSCLE

This belly (1) should not be confused with the lateral head of the triceps brachii muscle (2), which is located lateral to and in front of it, nor with the medial head of the triceps brachii muscle (3), which is located below and medial to it. To make the belly protrude and to palpate it in contraction, ask the subject to extend the forearm against resistance.

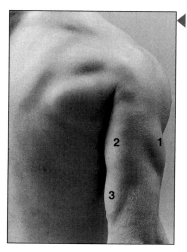

FIGURE 9-16

THE LATERAL HEAD OF THE TRICEPS BRACHII MUSCLE

This head (1) is located at the lateral aspect of the arm, lateral to and in front of the long head (2) of the triceps brachii muscle. Ask the subject to extend the forearm on the arm against resistance to help you visualize it. The medial head of the triceps brachii muscle is shown (3).

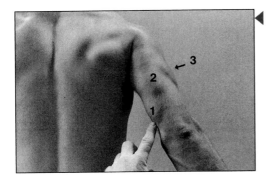

◀ FIGURE 9-17
THE MEDIAL HEAD OF THE TRICEPS BRACHII MUSCLE — POSTERIOR VIEW

Ask the subject to perform a sequence of contractions and relaxations, extending the forearm on the arm, to allow you to visualize and feel this muscle (1), which is located in the distal extension of the long head (2) and medial to it. The lateral head of triceps brachii muscle is shown (3).

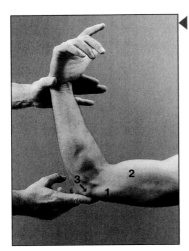

◀ FIGURE 9-18
THE MEDIAL HEAD OF THE TRICEPS BRACHII MUSCLE — MEDIAL VIEW

In this figure, the muscle belly of the medial head (1) is visible at the medial aspect of the arm, behind and medial to the biceps brachii muscle (2), above the medial epicondyle (3) (see Figs. 11-7 and 11-8). Ask the subject to extend the forearm on the arm against resistance to help you visualize and feel the medial head.

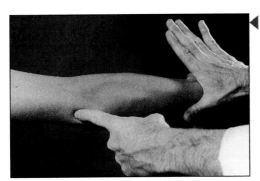

◀ FIGURE 9-19
THE DISTAL TENDON OF THE TRICEPS BRACHII MUSCLE

The distal tendon is usually flattened from front to back, but it can also exist as a full cylindrical cord, perceptible at the posterior aspect of the elbow, just before its insertion into the superior surface of the olecranon. Ask the subject to extend the forearm on the arm against resistance to help you feel this tendon.

C H A P T E R
T e n

NERVES
AND VESSELS

The notable structures accessible by palpation are

- The brachial artery (Fig. 10-2)
- The median nerve and the brachial artery in the distal aspect (Fig. 10-3)

- The ulnar nerve in the distal aspect of the arm (Fig. 10-4)

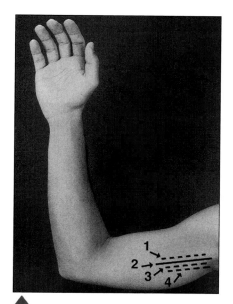

▲
FIGURE 10-1
MEDIAL VIEW OF THE ARM

(1) Median nerve
(2) Brachial artery
(3) Radial nerve
(4) Ulnar nerve

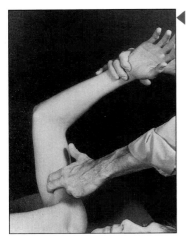

◄ FIGURE 10-2
THE BRACHIAL ARTERY

After locating the coracobrachialis muscle (Fig. 9-8) with the help of a flexion and an adduction of the shoulder, as shown in this figure, place a grip behind this muscle belly, and you will feel the pulse of the brachial artery.

Comment: Be careful while taking the pulse, as the median nerve is located over the brachial artery.

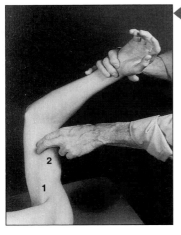

◄ FIGURE 10-3
THE MEDIAN NERVE AND THE BRACHIAL ARTERY IN THE DISTAL ASPECT

After locating the belly of the coracobrachialis muscle (1) (Fig. 9-8) with the help of a flexion and an adduction of the shoulder, place your fingertips behind that belly and bring the upper limb in horizontal abduction; the forearm may be placed in flexion and pronation. You can follow this nerve along its entire course to the anteromedial aspect of the arm, right down to the elbow, while pushing the biceps brachii muscle (2) laterally so you can roll the nerve under your fingers. In its distal course, the brachial artery can be followed with the median nerve, at the medial aspect of the arm. You can feel the pulse of this artery all the way down to the elbow fold.

Comment: Be careful while taking the pulse, as the median nerve is located over the brachial artery. Very rarely, this nerve is located behind the artery.

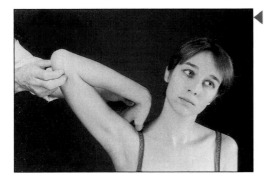

◄ FIGURE 10-4
THE ULNAR NERVE IN THE DISTAL ASPECT OF THE ARM

At the junction of the superior third and the middle third of the arm, this nerve is directed downward, backward, and inward. It perforates the medial intermuscular septum of the arm. From this level down to the epicondylar–olecranon groove, it is located in the posterior compartment of the arm and it can be rolled under the fingers on the medial head of the triceps brachii muscle (Fig. 9-18). To better feel this nerve under your fingers, position the subject's arm in maximal shoulder flexion, with or without an abduction, with the elbow maximally flexed, the forearm in pronation, and the wrist in extension. Be careful not to leave the subject in this position too long, because the intraneural compression is maximal in this "biomechanical position" (see also Figs. 12-1 and 12-2).

THE

ELBOW

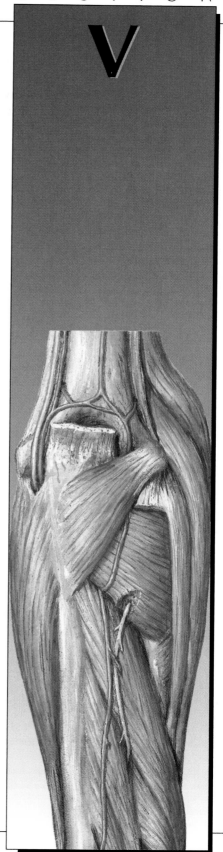

MUSCLES OF THE FOREARM (DEEP LAYER): POSTERIOR VIEW

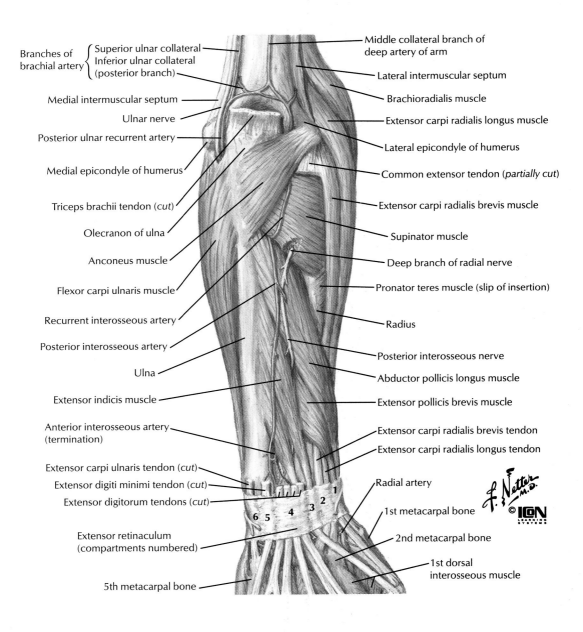

Branches of brachial artery
{ Superior ulnar collateral
Inferior ulnar collateral
(posterior branch)

Medial intermuscular septum

Ulnar nerve

Posterior ulnar recurrent artery

Medial epicondyle of humerus

Triceps brachii tendon (cut)

Olecranon of ulna

Anconeus muscle

Flexor carpi ulnaris muscle

Recurrent interosseous artery

Posterior interosseous artery

Ulna

Extensor indicis muscle

Anterior interosseous artery
(termination)

Extensor carpi ulnaris tendon (cut)

Extensor digiti minimi tendon (cut)

Extensor digitorum tendons (cut)

Extensor retinaculum
(compartments numbered)

5th metacarpal bone

Middle collateral branch of
deep artery of arm

Lateral intermuscular septum

Brachioradialis muscle

Extensor carpi radialis longus muscle

Lateral epicondyle of humerus

Common extensor tendon (partially cut)

Extensor carpi radialis brevis muscle

Supinator muscle

Deep branch of radial nerve

Pronator teres muscle (slip of insertion)

Radius

Posterior interosseous nerve

Abductor pollicis longus muscle

Extensor pollicis brevis muscle

Extensor carpi radialis brevis tendon

Extensor carpi radialis longus tendon

Radial artery

1st metacarpal bone

2nd metacarpal bone

1st dorsal
interosseous muscle

6 5 4 3 2 1

MUSCLES OF THE FOREARM (SUPERFICIAL LAYER): ANTERIOR VIEW

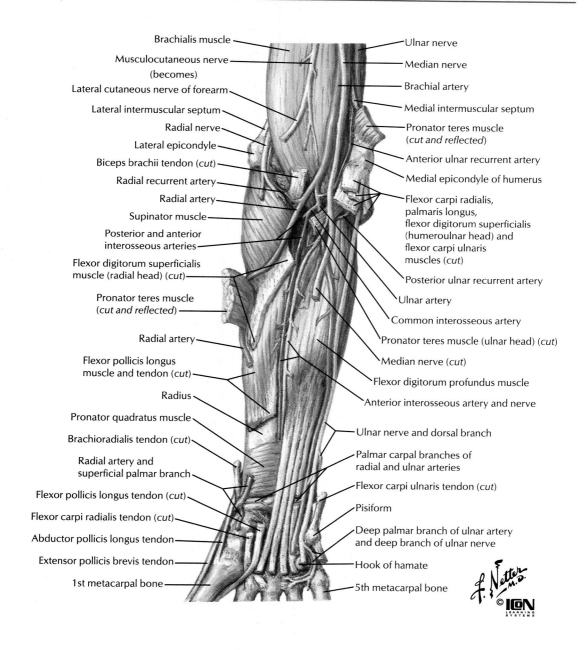

Brachialis muscle

Musculocutaneous nerve (becomes)

Lateral cutaneous nerve of forearm

Lateral intermuscular septum

Radial nerve

Lateral epicondyle

Biceps brachii tendon (cut)

Radial recurrent artery

Radial artery

Supinator muscle

Posterior and anterior interosseous arteries

Flexor digitorum superficialis muscle (radial head) (cut)

Pronator teres muscle (cut and reflected)

Radial artery

Flexor pollicis longus muscle and tendon (cut)

Radius

Pronator quadratus muscle

Brachioradialis tendon (cut)

Radial artery and superficial palmar branch

Flexor pollicis longus tendon (cut)

Flexor carpi radialis tendon (cut)

Abductor pollicis longus tendon

Extensor pollicis brevis tendon

1st metacarpal bone

Ulnar nerve

Median nerve

Brachial artery

Medial intermuscular septum

Pronator teres muscle (cut and reflected)

Anterior ulnar recurrent artery

Medial epicondyle of humerus

Flexor carpi radialis, palmaris longus, flexor digitorum superficialis (humeroulnar head) and flexor carpi ulnaris muscles (cut)

Posterior ulnar recurrent artery

Ulnar artery

Common interosseous artery

Pronator teres muscle (ulnar head) (cut)

Median nerve (cut)

Flexor digitorum profundus muscle

Anterior interosseous artery and nerve

Ulnar nerve and dorsal branch

Palmar carpal branches of radial and ulnar arteries

Flexor carpi ulnaris tendon (cut)

Pisiform

Deep palmar branch of ulnar artery and deep branch of ulnar nerve

Hook of hamate

5th metacarpal bone

F. Netter M.D.

© ICON
LEARNING
SYSTEMS

BONES OF THE ELBOW

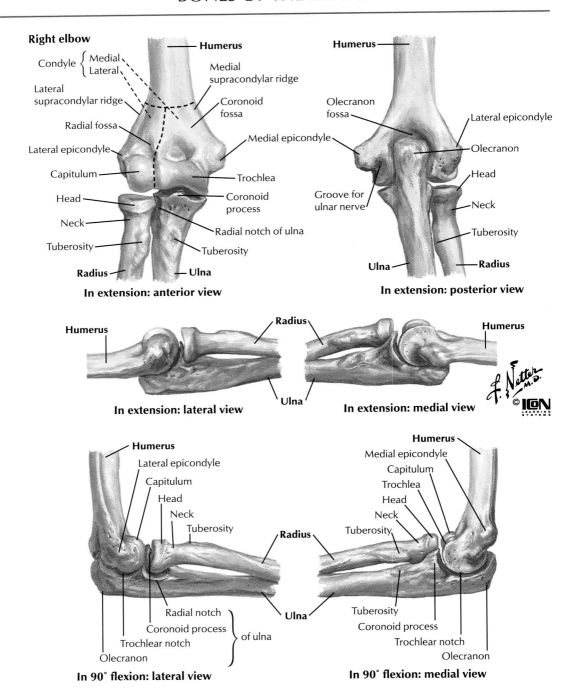

Right elbow

Condyle { Medial, Lateral }

Humerus

Medial supracondylar ridge

Lateral supracondylar ridge

Coronoid fossa

Radial fossa

Medial epicondyle

Lateral epicondyle

Capitulum

Trochlea

Head

Coronoid process

Neck

Radial notch of ulna

Tuberosity

Tuberosity

Radius

Ulna

In extension: anterior view

Humerus

Olecranon fossa

Lateral epicondyle

Olecranon

Head

Groove for ulnar nerve

Neck

Tuberosity

Ulna

Radius

In extension: posterior view

Humerus

Radius

Humerus

Ulna

In extension: lateral view

In extension: medial view

Humerus

Lateral epicondyle

Capitulum

Head

Neck

Tuberosity

Radius

Radial notch
Coronoid process } of ulna
Trochlear notch

Olecranon

In 90° flexion: lateral view

Humerus

Medial epicondyle

Capitulum

Trochlea

Head

Neck

Tuberosity

Radius

Tuberosity

Coronoid process

Trochlear notch

Olecranon

Ulna

In 90° flexion: medial view

LIGAMENTS OF THE ELBOW

Right elbow

Anterior view

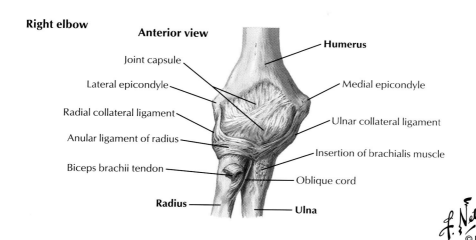

Humerus

Joint capsule

Lateral epicondyle

Medial epicondyle

Radial collateral ligament

Ulnar collateral ligament

Anular ligament of radius

Insertion of brachialis muscle

Biceps brachii tendon

Oblique cord

Radius

Ulna

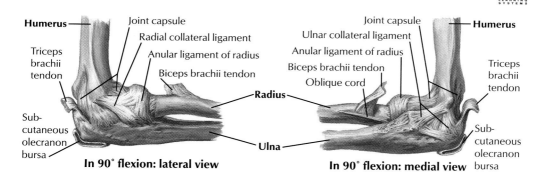

Humerus

Joint capsule

Radial collateral ligament

Anular ligament of radius

Biceps brachii tendon

Radius

Triceps brachii tendon

Sub-cutaneous olecranon bursa

Ulna

In 90° flexion: lateral view

Joint capsule

Ulnar collateral ligament

Anular ligament of radius

Biceps brachii tendon

Oblique cord

Humerus

Triceps brachii tendon

Sub-cutaneous olecranon bursa

In 90° flexion: medial view

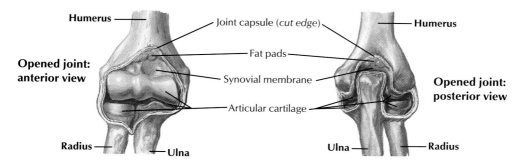

Humerus

Joint capsule (*cut edge*)

Humerus

Opened joint: anterior view

Fat pads

Synovial membrane

Articular cartilage

Opened joint: posterior view

Radius

Ulna

Ulna

Radius

TOPOGRAPHIC PRESENTATION OF THE ELBOW

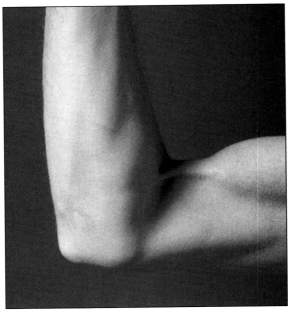

FIGURE 11-1
MEDIAL VIEW OF THE ELBOW REGION

CHAPTER
Eleven
OSTEOLOGY

The notable structures accessible by palpation are

· The humerus
 — the capitulum of the humerus (Fig. 11-3)
 — the lateral epicondyle of the humerus (Fig. 11-4)
 — the lateral supracondylar crest (Fig. 11-5)
 — the olecranon fossa (Fig. 11-6)
 — the medial epicondyle (Fig. 11-7)
 — posterior view of the medial epicondyle (Fig. 11-8)
 — the medial supracondylar crest (Fig. 11-9)
 — the groove for the ulnar nerve (Fig. 11-10)

· The radius
 — the head of the radius (Fig. 11-11)
 — the neck of the radius (Fig. 11-12)
 — the radial tuberosity (Fig. 11-13)

· The ulna
 — visualization of the olecranon at the level of the elbow (Fig. 11-14)
 — the superior surface of the olecranon (Fig. 11-15)
 — the medial surface of the olecranon (Fig. 11-16)
 — the lateral surface of the olecranon (Fig. 11-17)
 — the posterior border of the shaft of the ulna (Fig. 11-18)
 — the coronoid process of the ulna (Fig. 11-19)

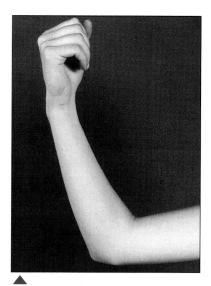

▲
FIGURE 11-2
GENERAL PRESENTATION OF THE ELBOW

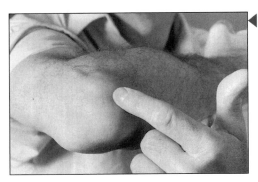

FIGURE 11-3
THE CAPITULUM OF THE HUMERUS

This structure, which is located at the distal and lateral end of the humerus, articulates with the radial fovea. Ask the subject to flex the elbow to allow you to feel the maximum expanse of the capitulum under your fingers. This action allows you to examine the posterior and inferior aspect of the structure of interest. It feels smooth under your fingers.

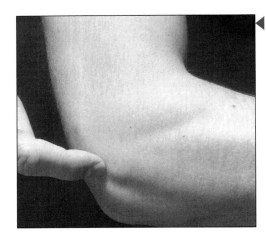

FIGURE 11-4
THE LATERAL EPICONDYLE OF THE HUMERUS

This structure is located above and lateral to the capitulum of the humerus (Fig. 11-3) and below the distal extremity of the lateral supracondylar crest (Fig. 11-5). It feels rough under the fingers. It is the site of origin of the lateral epicondylar muscles and attachment of the radial collateral ligament.

Comment: The epicondylar muscles consist of the following muscles: anconeus, extensor carpi radialis brevis, extensor digitorum, extensor digiti minimi, extensor carpi ulnaris, and supinator. The anconeus muscle has its own distinct tendon at the posterior surface of the lateral epicondyle of the humerus. The other muscles have a common tendon.

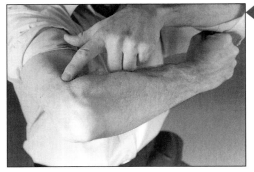

FIGURE 11-5
THE LATERAL SUPRACONDYLAR CREST

This crest is felt as a sharp edge, directly accessible under the skin above the lateral epicondyle (Fig. 11-4). This crest is much more pronounced than the medial supracondylar crest.

Comment: This crest is continued proximally by the lateral border of the humerus (which appears very pronounced under the fingers) up to the deltoid tuberosity.

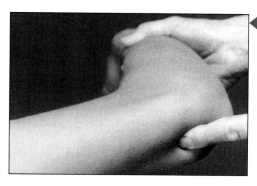

FIGURE 11-6
THE OLECRANON FOSSA

This structure, which is situated at the distal end of the posterior surface of the humerus, receives the proximal extremity of the olecranon during the extension of the forearm on the arm. It is much easier to feel if the subject's elbow is flexed at 130° to 140° to relax the tendon of the triceps brachii muscle. Place a bidigital grip on the capitulum of the humerus (Fig. 11-3) and move your grip backward, pushing the tendon of the triceps brachii muscle medially. You will feel the fossa under your fingers above the olecranon.

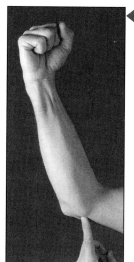

FIGURE 11-7
THE MEDIAL EPICONDYLE

This structure is located above and medial to the trochlea of the humerus, at the distal end of the medial border of the shaft of the bone (see also Fig. 11-8).

Comment: The anterior surface and the apex of the medial epicondyle are the site of origin for the following muscles: pronator teres, flexor carpi radialis, palmaris longus, flexor carpi ulnaris, and flexor digitorum superficialis. The posterior surface of the medial epicondyle is smooth. It presents a vertical groove for the passage of the ulnar nerve. The inferior border is the site of insertion of the ulnar collateral ligament.

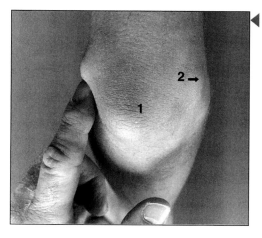

FIGURE 11-8
POSTERIOR VIEW OF THE MEDIAL EPICONDYLE

This figure shows the position of the medial epicondyle, indicated by the index finger, in relation to the olecranon (1) and the lateral epicondyle (2).

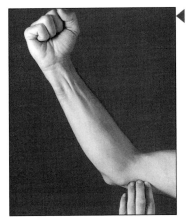

◀ **FIGURE 11-9**
THE MEDIAL SUPRACONDYLAR CREST

This structure is much less pronounced than the lateral supracondylar crest. It is felt under the fingers as a blunt edge above the medial epicondyle. It is easy to access.

Comment: This crest is continued proximally by the medial border of the humerus.

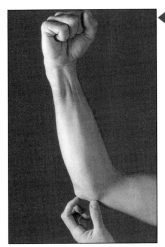

◀ **FIGURE 11-10**
THE GROOVE FOR THE ULNAR NERVE

This vertical groove is located at the posterior surface of the medial epicondyle. In this figure, the thumb–index finger grip indicates the boundary of the structure of interest: the thumb is placed medially on the medial epicondyle, and the index finger is placed on the olecranon.

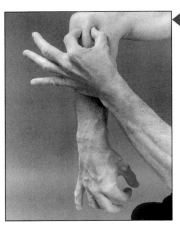

◀ **FIGURE 11-11**
THE HEAD OF THE RADIUS

After placing your thumb and your index finger at the level of the capitulum of the humerus (Fig. 11-3) (with the elbow flexed at 90°), slide your grip downward without losing contact with the skin. You will feel the humeroradial interspace under your fingers, and just below it, you can grip the head of the radius. If in doubt, ask the subject to perform movements of pronation–supination and you will feel the head rotate under your fingers.

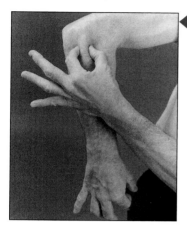

FIGURE 11-12
THE NECK OF THE RADIUS

Starting with the thumb–index finger grip of the radial head (described in Fig. 11-11), move your grip about one finger's breadth downward, and your fingertips will feel a narrow section, which is the structure of interest.

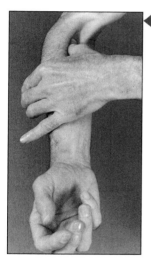

FIGURE 11-13
THE RADIAL TUBEROSITY

Place your thumb on the floor of the lateral groove of the elbow fold (see comment), lateral to the distal end of the tendon of the biceps brachii muscle (as shown in this figure), and you will be in contact with the bony structure of interest. Note that supination of the subject's forearm brings the radial tuberosity in contact with your grip; pronation moves it away.

Comment: The lateral groove of the elbow fold is directed obliquely downward and inward. It is formed by the lateral aspect of the biceps brachii muscle medially and anteriorly, the brachioradialis muscle laterally, and the brachialis muscle posteriorly. The radial tuberosity is an oval structure located at the anteromedial aspect of the bone, at the union of the neck and the body of the radius. The posterior surface is a site of insertion of the biceps brachii muscle.

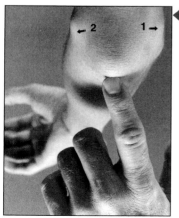

FIGURE 11-14
VISUALIZATION OF THE OLECRANON AT THE LEVEL OF THE ELBOW

This is the posterior vertical process of the proximal end of the ulna. This figure allows the visualization of the topographic situation of the olecranon (indicated by the index finger) in relation to the lateral epicondyle (1) and the medial epicondyle (2). These are three of the most important bony structures of the elbow.

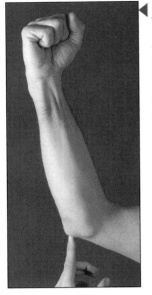

FIGURE 11-15

THE SUPERIOR SURFACE OF THE OLECRANON

This structure, which is directly under the skin, is very easy to access. Anteriorly, it is continued by a process that fits in the olecranon fossa of the humerus while the subject extends the forearm on the arm.

Comment: The tendon of the triceps brachii muscle is inserted into the posterior aspect of this surface.

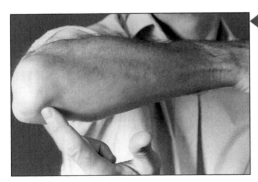

FIGURE 11-16

THE MEDIAL SURFACE OF THE OLECRANON

This surface, indicated by the index finger, is noteworthy because it is the site of insertion of the posterior fasciculus of the ulnar collateral ligament and an origin of the flexor carpi ulnaris muscle.

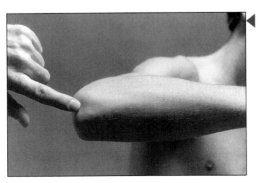

FIGURE 11-17

THE LATERAL SURFACE OF THE OLECRANON

This is the site of insertion of the radial collateral ligament of the elbow, as well as of the anconeus muscle.

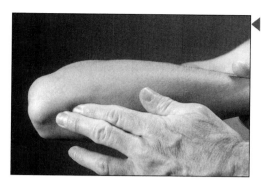

FIGURE 11-18
THE POSTERIOR BORDER OF THE SHAFT OF THE ULNA

This bony structure extends distally from the posterior surface of the olecranon. It is easy to examine.

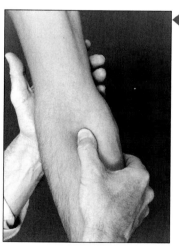

FIGURE 11-19
THE CORONOID PROCESS OF THE ULNA

Place one hand on the posterior surface of the olecranon (Fig. 11-14); with the subject's elbow slightly flexed, place your other hand on the medial border of the proximal end of the ulna, with your thumb placed medial to the distal tendon of the biceps brachii muscle (see Fig. 9-6). With your other fingers, cover the posterior border of the ulna. Your thumb is facing the coronoid process, a bony structure that can be approached only indirectly through the considerable muscular mass of the anterior muscular group of the forearm.

Comment: The coronoid process is one of the two processes of the proximal end of the ulna; the other process is the olecranon (Fig. 11-14). These two bony structures are joined together to form a hook-shaped cavity: the trochlear notch.

CHAPTER
Twelve

NERVES AND VESSELS

The notable structures accessible by palpation are

· The ulnar nerve in the groove for the ulnar nerve (Fig. 12-2)
· The ulnar nerve in the proximal aspect of the forearm (Fig. 12-3)

· The median nerve at the level of the medial bicipital groove (Fig. 12-4)
· The brachial artery at the level of the medial bicipital groove (Fig. 12-5)

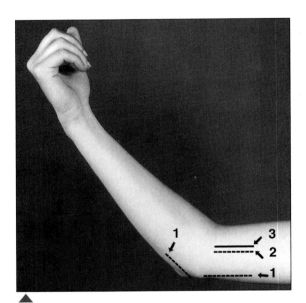

▲
FIGURE 12-1
VISUALIZATION OF THE ROUTES OF THE PRINCIPAL
NERVES AND VESSELS AT THE MEDIAL ASPECT
OF THE ELBOW

(1) Ulnar nerve
(2) Median nerve
(3) Brachial artery

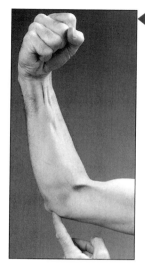

◀ FIGURE 12-2
THE ULNAR NERVE IN THE GROOVE FOR THE ULNAR NERVE

This nerve is easy to access. Place your index finger in the groove for the ulnar nerve (Fig. 11-10) to be in direct contact with the structure of interest. You will feel it under your fingers as a full cylindrical cord; approach it very carefully. This nerve (see Fig. 12-1) is positioned in the groove for the ulnar nerve, and then it passes through the arch that unites the medial epicondylar portion of the flexor carpi ulnaris muscle with the ulnar portion.

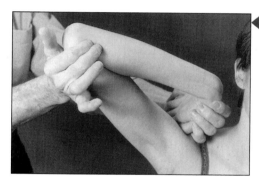

◀ FIGURE 12-3
THE ULNAR NERVE IN THE PROXIMAL ASPECT
OF THE FOREARM

Beyond the groove for the ulnar nerve (Fig. 12-2), this nerve is also palpable at the proximal aspect of the forearm (see also Fig. 12-1). To palpate this nerve, flex the subject's arm, with the forearm in pronation and the hand in extension. The nerve is palpable in the extension of the groove for the ulnar nerve, in the proximal third of the forearm. You will feel it under your fingers as a full cylindrical cord.

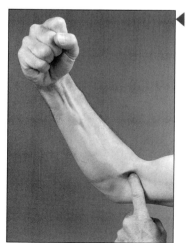

◀ FIGURE 12-4
THE MEDIAN NERVE AT THE LEVEL OF THE MEDIAL BICIPITAL GROOVE

As shown in this figure, place a bidigital grip medial to the tendon of the biceps brachii muscle to feel the structure as a full cylindrical cord that you can roll under your fingers.

Comment: The brachial artery is located lateral to this nerve.

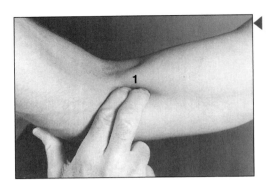

FIGURE 12-5
THE BRACHIAL ARTERY AT THE LEVEL
OF THE MEDIAL BICIPITAL GROOVE

Place a bidigital grip in the fold of the elbow, medial to and behind the tendon of the biceps brachii muscle (1) to feel the pulse of the brachial artery (the median nerve is located medial to this artery).

THE
FOREARM

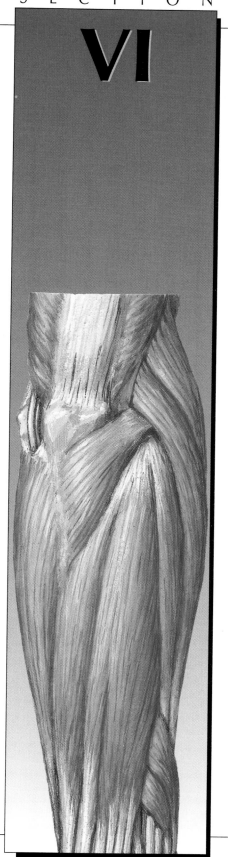

MUSCLES OF FOREARM (SUPERFICIAL LAYER): POSTERIOR VIEW

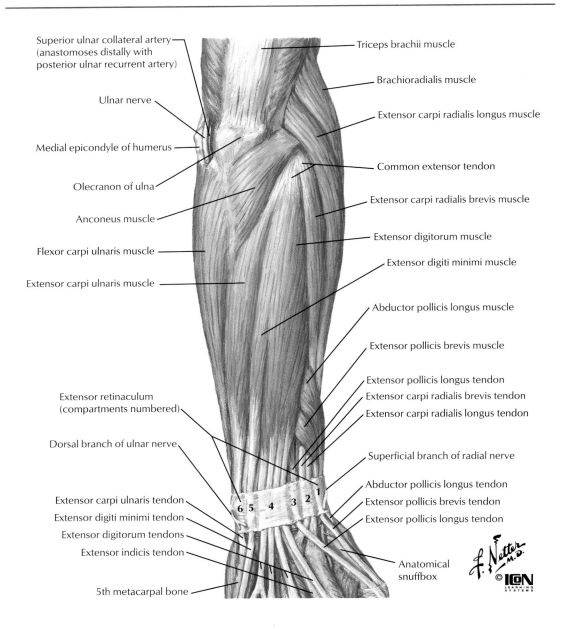

Superior ulnar collateral artery (anastomoses distally with posterior ulnar recurrent artery)

Ulnar nerve

Medial epicondyle of humerus

Olecranon of ulna

Anconeus muscle

Flexor carpi ulnaris muscle

Extensor carpi ulnaris muscle

Extensor retinaculum (compartments numbered)

Dorsal branch of ulnar nerve

Extensor carpi ulnaris tendon
Extensor digiti minimi tendon
Extensor digitorum tendons
Extensor indicis tendon

5th metacarpal bone

Triceps brachii muscle

Brachioradialis muscle

Extensor carpi radialis longus muscle

Common extensor tendon

Extensor carpi radialis brevis muscle

Extensor digitorum muscle

Extensor digiti minimi muscle

Abductor pollicis longus muscle

Extensor pollicis brevis muscle

Extensor pollicis longus tendon
Extensor carpi radialis brevis tendon
Extensor carpi radialis longus tendon

Superficial branch of radial nerve

Abductor pollicis longus tendon
Extensor pollicis brevis tendon
Extensor pollicis longus tendon

Anatomical snuffbox

6 5 4 3 2 1

MUSCLES OF FOREARM (SUPERFICIAL LAYER): ANTERIOR VIEW

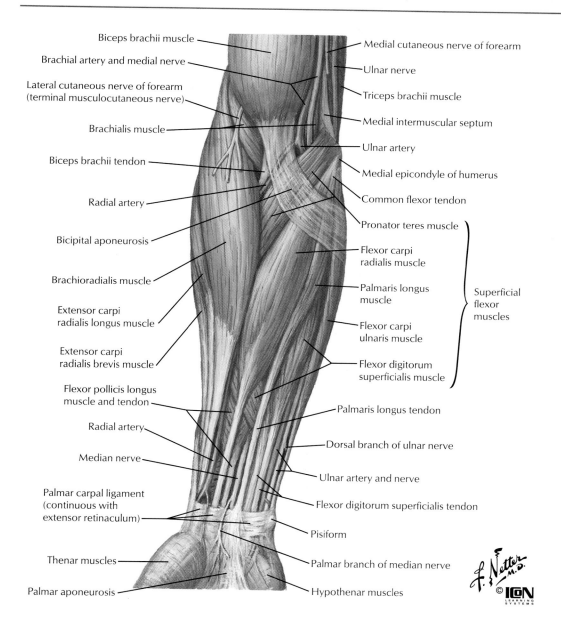

Biceps brachii muscle

Brachial artery and medial nerve

Lateral cutaneous nerve of forearm
(terminal musculocutaneous nerve)

Brachialis muscle

Biceps brachii tendon

Radial artery

Bicipital aponeurosis

Brachioradialis muscle

Extensor carpi
radialis longus muscle

Extensor carpi
radialis brevis muscle

Flexor pollicis longus
muscle and tendon

Radial artery

Median nerve

Palmar carpal ligament
(continuous with
extensor retinaculum)

Thenar muscles

Palmar aponeurosis

Medial cutaneous nerve of forearm

Ulnar nerve

Triceps brachii muscle

Medial intermuscular septum

Ulnar artery

Medial epicondyle of humerus

Common flexor tendon

Pronator teres muscle

Flexor carpi
radialis muscle

Palmaris longus
muscle

Flexor carpi
ulnaris muscle

Flexor digitorum
superficialis muscle

Superficial
flexor
muscles

Palmaris longus tendon

Dorsal branch of ulnar nerve

Ulnar artery and nerve

Flexor digitorum superficialis tendon

Pisiform

Palmar branch of median nerve

Hypothenar muscles

131

FLEXOR TENDONS, ARTERIES AND NERVES AT WRIST

Palmar view

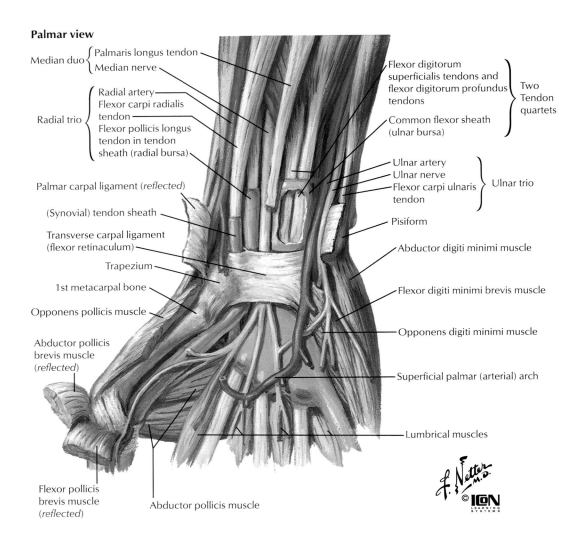

Median duo { Palmaris longus tendon
             Median nerve

Radial trio { Radial artery
              Flexor carpi radialis tendon
              Flexor pollicis longus tendon in tendon sheath (radial bursa)

Palmar carpal ligament (*reflected*)

(Synovial) tendon sheath

Transverse carpal ligament (flexor retinaculum)

Trapezium

1st metacarpal bone

Opponens pollicis muscle

Abductor pollicis brevis muscle (*reflected*)

Flexor pollicis brevis muscle (*reflected*)

Abductor pollicis muscle

Flexor digitorum superficialis tendons and flexor digitorum profundus tendons
} Two Tendon quartets

Common flexor sheath (ulnar bursa)

Ulnar artery
Ulnar nerve
Flexor carpi ulnaris tendon
} Ulnar trio

Pisiform

Abductor digiti minimi muscle

Flexor digiti minimi brevis muscle

Opponens digiti minimi muscle

Superficial palmar (arterial) arch

Lumbrical muscles

TOPOGRAPHIC PRESENTATION OF THE FOREARM

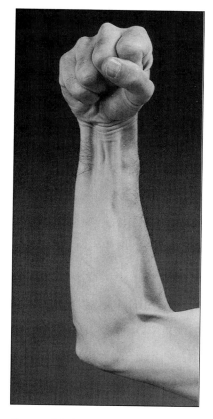

FIGURE 13-1
THE ANTERIOR (VENTRAL) SURFACE
OF THE FOREARM

CHAPTER
Thirteen

MYOLOGY

THE LATERAL MUSCULAR GROUP

The notable structures accessible by palpation are

- The proximal aspect of the brachioradialis muscle (Fig. 13-3)
- The belly of the brachioradialis muscle (Fig. 13-4)
- The insertion of the brachioradialis muscle (Fig. 13-5)
- The origin of the extensor carpi radialis longus muscle (Fig. 13-6)
- The belly of the extensor carpi radialis longus muscle at the elbow (Fig. 13-7)
- The tendon of the extensor carpi radialis longus muscle (Fig. 13-8)
- Visualization of the tendon of the extensor carpi radialis longus muscle at the wrist (Fig. 13-9)

- Distal palpation of the tendon of the extensor carpi radialis longus muscle—step 1 (Fig. 13-10)
- Distal palpation of the tendon of the extensor carpi radialis longus muscle—step 2 (Fig. 13-11)
- The origin of the extensor carpi radialis brevis muscle (Fig. 13-12)
- Topographic relationships of the extensor carpi radialis brevis muscle (Fig. 13-13)
- The extensor carpi radialis brevis muscle at the distal third of the forearm (Fig. 13-14)
- The insertion of the extensor carpi radialis brevis muscle (Fig. 13-15)
- The supinator muscle (Fig. 13-16)

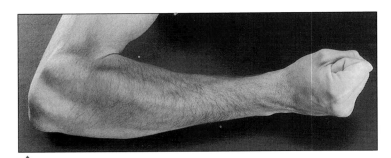

▲
FIGURE 13-2
VIEW OF THE LATERAL MUSCULAR GROUP

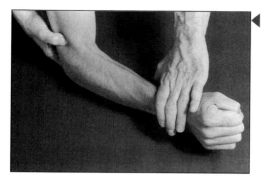

◀ **FIGURE 13-3**

THE PROXIMAL ASPECT OF THE BRACHIORADIALIS MUSCLE

Place the subject's forearm in a neutral position with regard to pronation–supination. Ask the subject to flex the forearm on the arm and apply resistance at the distal third of the radius. You will feel the contraction at the distal aspect of the lateral border of the humerus.

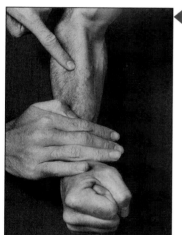

◀ **FIGURE 13-4**

THE BELLY OF THE BRACHIORADIALIS MUSCLE

The action requested and your resistance are identical to those described in Figure 13-3. The muscle belly appears as a pronounced projection, as shown in this figure.

Comment: In its downward course, this muscle belly covers the extensor carpi radialis longus and brevis muscles, as well as the distal end of the pronator teres muscle.

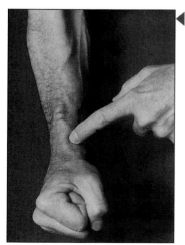

◀ **FIGURE 13-5**

THE INSERTION OF THE BRACHIORADIALIS MUSCLE

This muscle inserts into the base of the styloid process of the radius through a flattened tendon. The insertion is indicated by the index finger.

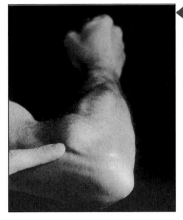

◀ FIGURE 13-6
THE ORIGIN OF THE EXTENSOR CARPI RADIALIS LONGUS MUSCLE

Ask the subject to perform an extension and a radial deviation of the wrist (with the elbow flexed). You will feel the muscular contraction at the lateral border of the humerus, at three fingers' breadth below the origin of the brachioradialis muscle.

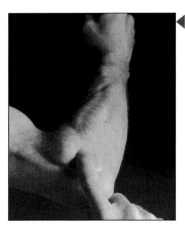

◀ FIGURE 13-7
THE BELLY OF THE EXTENSOR CARPI RADIALIS LONGUS MUSCLE
AT THE ELBOW

In many subjects, this muscle belly appears clearly at the external aspect of the elbow when they perform an extension and a radial deviation of the wrist. In other subjects, you can feel the contraction at the lateral aspect of the elbow, lateral to the proximal aspect of the brachioradialis muscle (Fig. 13-3) (at the level of the elbow fold).

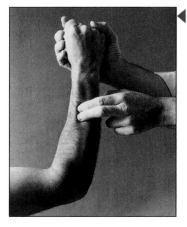

◀ FIGURE 13-8
THE TENDON OF THE EXTENSOR CARPI RADIALIS LONGUS MUSCLE

At the level of the middle third of the forearm, the muscle belly is continued by a tendon. It is located at the anterolateral aspect of the body of the extensor carpi radialis brevis muscle. More distally, using a bidigital grip, you can distinguish the two tendons by making them roll them on the body of the radius.

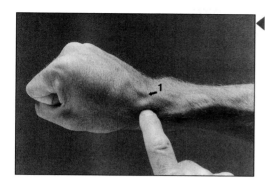

◀ FIGURE 13-9

VISUALIZATION OF THE TENDON OF THE EXTENSOR CARPI RADIALIS LONGUS MUSCLE AT THE WRIST

In some subjects, this tendon, which inserts into the lateral aspect of the dorsal surface of the base of the second metacarpal, is clearly visible (as is the case in this figure) lateral to the tendon of the extensor carpi radialis brevis muscle (1) (Fig. 13-15) if the subject clenches the fist.

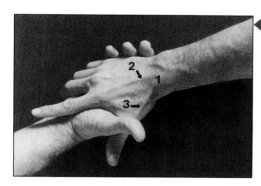

◀ FIGURE 13-10

DISTAL PALPATION OF THE TENDON OF THE EXTENSOR CARPI RADIALIS LONGUS MUSCLE — STEP 1

This figure shows a triangle with a distal base and a proximal apex (1) where the tendons of the long and short extensor carpi radialis muscles are palpated. This triangle is formed by a distal base (the first commissure), an ulnar side (the tendon of the extensor digitorum muscle for the index finger) (2), and a radial side (the tendon of the extensor pollicis longus muscle) (3).

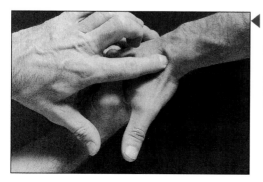

◀ FIGURE 13-11

DISTAL PALPATION OF THE TENDON OF THE EXTENSOR CARPI RADIALIS LONGUS MUSCLE — STEP 2

Place a fingertip at the ulnar border of the tendon of the extensor pollicis longus muscle and push it toward the radius to find the structure of interest (see also Fig. 15-16).

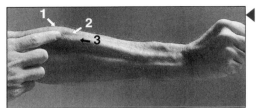

◀ **FIGURE 13-12**
THE ORIGIN OF THE EXTENSOR CARPI RADIALIS
BREVIS MUSCLE

At the proximal aspect of the forearm, the muscle of interest is covered by the belly of the extensor carpi radialis longus muscle (1). The index finger indicates the "point" where the belly of the extensor carpi radialis brevis muscle (2), located lateral to the extensor digitorum muscle (3), emerges at the posterolateral aspect of the forearm.

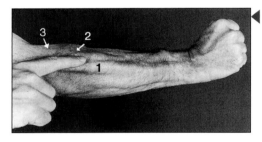

◀ **FIGURE 13-13**
TOPOGRAPHIC RELATIONSHIPS OF THE EXTENSOR CARPI
RADIALIS BREVIS MUSCLE

The muscle belly indicated by the index finger is located lateral to the extensor digitorum muscle (1). At this level, it adjoins the tendon of the extensor carpi radialis longus muscle (2) (not visible in this figure), which is located lateral to it. The brachioradialis muscle (3) (Fig. 13-4) is also located lateral to it.

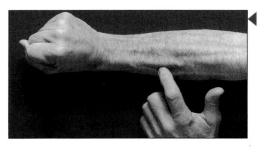

◀ **FIGURE 13-14**
THE EXTENSOR CARPI RADIALIS BREVIS MUSCLE AT THE
INFERIOR THIRD OF THE FOREARM

At this level, the tendon, which is accompanied by the tendon of the extensor carpi radialis longus muscle, passes in front of the abductor pollicis longus muscle (Fig. 13-36) and more distally in front of the extensor pollicis brevis muscle (Fig. 13-38).

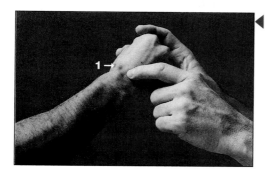

FIGURE 13-15

THE INSERTION OF THE EXTENSOR CARPI RADIALIS BREVIS MUSCLE

In this figure, the tendon of interest, indicated by the index finger, is located medial to the tendon of the extensor carpi radialis longus muscle (1) (see also Fig. 13-9).

Comment: The tendon of the muscle of interest is attached to the styloid process of the third metacarpal (see also Fig. 15-16).

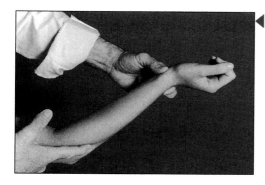

FIGURE 13-16

THE SUPINATOR MUSCLE

After locating the neck of radius (see also Fig. 11-12), place a uni- or bidigital grip on that structure (this grip overlaps the adjacent muscular mass). The subject's elbow is flexed at 45° (so you can better visualize the muscle of interest), and the forearm is placed in supination. Starting from this position, ask the subject to perform repeated brief, quick movements of supination. You will feel the contraction of this deep muscle under your fingers.

THE POSTERIOR MUSCULAR GROUP

The notable structures accessible by palpation are

- The extensor digitorum muscle in its proximal aspect (Fig. 13-18)
- The extensor digitorum muscle at the level of the forearm (Fig. 13-19)
- The extensor digitorum muscle in its distal aspect (Fig. 13-20)
- The extensor digitorum muscle at the level of the wrist (Fig. 13-21)
- The tendons of the extensor digitorum muscle in the dorsum of the hand (Fig. 13-22)
- The terminations of the extensor digitorum muscle at the level of the phalanges (Fig. 13-23)
- The extensor indicis muscle in the dorsum of the hand (Fig. 13-24)
- Topographic relationships of the extensor indicis muscle and the extensor digitorum muscle (Fig. 13-25)
- The tendon of the extensor digitorum muscle for the index finger and the aponeurotic expansions (Fig. 13-26)
- The origin of the extensor digiti minimi muscle (Fig. 13-27)
- The belly of the extensor digiti minimi muscle (Fig. 13-28)
- The tendon of the extensor digiti minimi muscle (Fig. 13-29)
- The tendon of the extensor digiti minimi muscle in the dorsum of the hand (Fig. 13-30)

- The aponeurotic extension of the extensor digitorum muscle on the tendon of the extensor digiti minimi muscle (Fig. 13-31)
- The origin of the extensor carpi ulnaris muscle (Fig. 13-32)
- The belly of the extensor carpi ulnaris muscle (Fig. 13-33)
- The extensor carpi ulnaris muscle in its distal aspect (Fig. 13-34)
- The anconeus muscle (Fig. 13-35)
- The belly of the abductor pollicis longus muscle (Fig. 13-36)
- The tendon of the abductor pollicis longus muscle (Fig. 13-37)
- The belly of the extensor pollicis brevis muscle (Fig. 13-38)
- The tendon of the extensor pollicis brevis muscle at the wrist (Fig. 13-39)
- The insertion of the extensor pollicis brevis muscle (Fig. 13-40)
- The extensor pollicis longus muscle at the posterior surface of the radius (Fig. 13-41)
- The tendon of the extensor pollicis longus muscle at the wrist (Fig. 13-42)
- The insertion of the extensor pollicis longus muscle (Fig. 13-43)

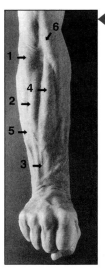

◀ FIGURE 13-17
POSTERIOR VIEW OF THE FOREARM

(1) Anconeus muscle

(2) Extensor carpi ulnaris muscle

(3) Extensor digiti minimi muscle

(4) Extensor digitorum muscle

(5) Flexor carpi ulnaris muscle

(6) Extensor carpi radialis longus muscle

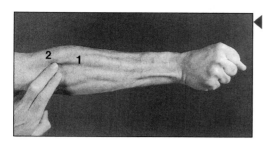

◀ FIGURE 13-18
THE EXTENSOR DIGITORUM MUSCLE
IN ITS PROXIMAL ASPECT

This muscle (1) is located behind and medial to the extensor carpi radialis longus muscle (2) (Fig. 13-7). Ask the subject to perform repeated extensions of the wrist and the fingers to demonstrate the structure of interest.

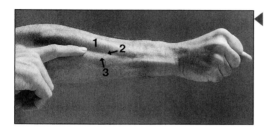

◀ FIGURE 13-19
THE EXTENSOR DIGITORUM MUSCLE
AT THE LEVEL OF THE FOREARM

This muscle (1) has a central position on the posterior aspect of the forearm. It descends superficial to the supinator muscle and the four muscles of the deep plane of the posterior region of the forearm. The extensor digiti minimi muscle (2) (not visible in this figure) (see also Fig. 13-28) and the extensor carpi ulnaris muscle (3) (see Fig. 13-33) run along this muscle medially. Ask the subject for the same muscular action as described in Fig. 13-18.

Comment: At this level, four muscular bundles make up the muscular body.

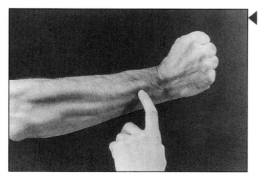

◀ FIGURE 13-20
THE EXTENSOR DIGITORUM MUSCLE IN ITS DISTAL ASPECT

In the distal posterior aspect of the forearm, this muscle is made up of four tendons that extend the four muscular bundles described above.

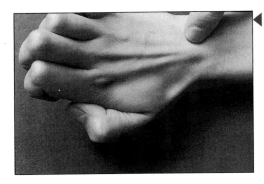

FIGURE 13-21
THE EXTENSOR DIGITORUM MUSCLE
AT THE LEVEL OF THE WRIST

At this level, the four tendons and the tendon of the extensor indicis muscle join together in a conduction canal (which is part of the extensor retinaculum), where the tendons are held down at the posterior surface of the radius before they enter the dorsal aspect of the hand.

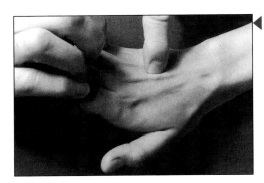

FIGURE 13-22
THE TENDONS OF THE EXTENSOR DIGITORUM MUSCLE
IN THE DORSUM OF THE HAND

Place the subject's hand in extension and apply resistance at the posterior aspect of the proximal phalanges (as shown in this figure) to make the tendons protrude in the dorsum of the hand.

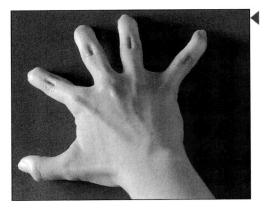

FIGURE 13-23
THE TERMINATIONS OF THE EXTENSOR DIGITORUM MUSCLE
AT THE LEVEL OF THE PHALANGES

Each tendon ends on the base of the phalanges of its corresponding finger.

Comment: This figure shows a tendon of the extensor digitorum muscle that is divided into two at the level of the phalanges, which is an exception.

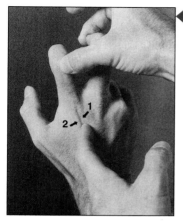

◀ **FIGURE 13-24**
THE EXTENSOR INDICIS MUSCLE IN THE DORSUM OF THE HAND

This muscle extends from the ulna to the index finger. At the dorsal aspect of the wrist and the hand, the tendon of this muscle (1) is located medial to the tendon of the extensor digitorum muscle for the index finger (2). In most cases, these two tendons are joined together at the level of the metacarpophalangeal joint.

Comment: In this figure, the index finger is intercalated between the two tendons mentioned above.

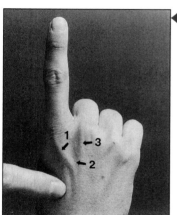

◀ **FIGURE 13-25**
TOPOGRAPHIC RELATIONSHIPS OF THE EXTENSOR INDICIS MUSCLE AND THE EXTENSOR DIGITORUM MUSCLE

If the metacarpophalangeal joints are flexed and the subject is asked to extend the index finger, the tendon of the extensor digitorum muscle for the index finger (1) "skips" over the tendon of the extensor indicis muscle of the index finger (indicated by the examiner), since it is pulled by an aponeurotic expansion (2) that binds this tendon to the tendon of the extensor digitorum muscle for the middle finger (3). This traction moves the tendon of the extensor digitorum muscle for the index finger to the ulnar border of the tendon of the extensor indicis muscle.

Comment: The tendon that forms an italic S (1) on the dorsum of the hand during the gesture described above is therefore the tendon of the extensor digitorum muscle for the index finger.

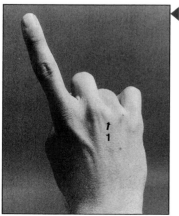

◀ **FIGURE 13-26**
THE TENDON OF THE EXTENSOR DIGITORUM MUSCLE FOR THE INDEX FINGER AND THE APONEUROTIC EXPANSIONS (1)

In the dorsum of the hand, the tendons of the extensor digitorum muscle are joined together by fibrous bands (1) that may be transverse or oblique (see also Fig. 13-25).

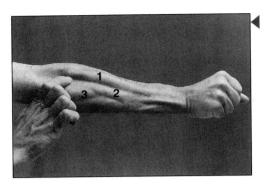

◄ **FIGURE 13-27**
THE ORIGIN OF THE EXTENSOR DIGITI MINIMI MUSCLE

This origin is located at the level of the lateral epicondyle of the humerus, medial to the extensor digitorum muscle (1).

(1) Extensor digitorum muscle
(2) Extensor carpi ulnaris muscle
(3) Anconeus muscle

In this figure, the index finger shows the position of the extensor digiti minimi muscle in the groove between the extensor digitorum muscle (1) and the extensor carpi ulnaris muscle (2).

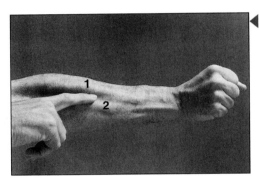

◄ **FIGURE 13-28**
THE BELLY OF THE EXTENSOR DIGITI MINIMI MUSCLE

This very long and very thin belly is located in the depression between the bellies of the extensor digitorum muscle (1) and the extensor carpi ulnaris (2) muscle. To feel the contraction, place a bi- or tridigital grip in this depression and ask the subject to perform repeated extensions of the little finger.

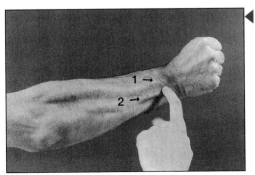

◄ **FIGURE 13-29**
THE TENDON OF THE EXTENSOR DIGITI MINIMI MUSCLE

Place your index finger or a bi- or tridigital grip medial to the tendon of the extensor digitorum muscle (1) and lateral to the tendon of the extensor carpi ulnaris muscle (2) in order to feel the tendon of interest under your fingers. The subject's repeated extensions of the proximal phalanx of the fifth finger (with the other two phalanges flexed) may help you to feel this structure.

Comment: The tendon passes in its own sheath over the head of the ulna and posterior to the wrist joint.

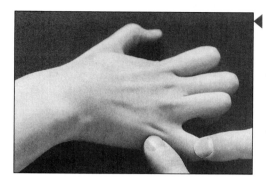

FIGURE 13-30

**THE TENDON OF THE EXTENSOR DIGITI MINIMI MUSCLE
IN THE DORSUM OF THE HAND**

The tendon of the extensor digiti minimi muscle is usually divided in two. This characteristic appears clearly in the figure. To demonstrate it, ask the subject to hyperextend the metacarpophalangeal joint of the little finger while you apply resistance.

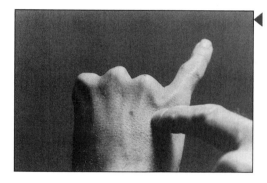

FIGURE 13-31

**THE APONEUROTIC EXTENSION OF THE EXTENSOR
DIGITORUM MUSCLE ON THE TENDON OF THE
EXTENSOR DIGITI MINIMI MUSCLE**

As the index finger indicates, a connection normally exists between the tendon of the extensor digitorum muscle for the ring finger and the tendon of the extensor digiti minimi muscle.

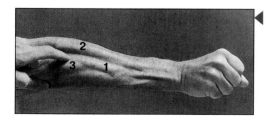

FIGURE 13-32

THE ORIGIN OF THE EXTENSOR CARPI ULNARIS MUSCLE

The index finger indicates the proximal aspect of the muscle of interest (1). After locating the extensor digitorum muscle (2), place your grip medial to it and ask the subject to perform repeated extensions of the wrist together with an ulnar deviation to allow you to feel the muscle under your fingers. It may be helpful to locate the anconeus muscle (3) to ensure the correct positioning of your fingers.

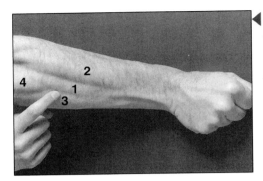

◄ FIGURE 13-33
THE BELLY OF THE EXTENSOR CARPI ULNARIS MUSCLE

The index finger shows this muscle belly (1), which is located medial to the body of the extensor digitorum muscle (2) and lateral to the body of the flexor carpi ulnaris muscle (3). The anconeus muscle (4) is located proximal and medial to it.

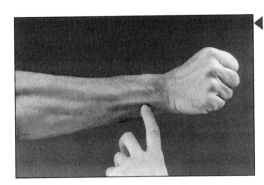

◄ FIGURE 13-34
THE EXTENSOR CARPI ULNARIS MUSCLE IN ITS DISTAL ASPECT

The tendon of the extensor carpi ulnaris muscle, indicated by the index finger, passes through an osteofibrous sheath posterior to the distal end of the ulna before it inserts into the medial tubercle of the fifth metacarpal.

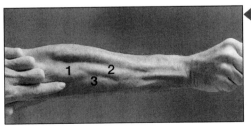

◄ FIGURE 13-35
THE ANCONEUS MUSCLE

To better palpate this muscle, place a tridigital grip at the lateral border of the olecranon and slide it downward and outward without losing contact with the skin. You can feel a muscular relief under your fingers. Ask the subject to perform repeated extensions of the elbow so that you can better feel the muscle belly.

In this figure, the index finger is placed over the anconeus muscle (1), which is located medial to the body of the extensor carpi ulnaris muscle (2) and lateral to the flexor carpi ulnaris muscle (3).

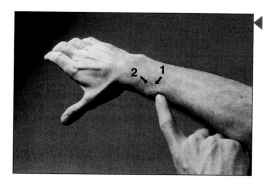

FIGURE 13-36
THE BELLY OF THE ABDUCTOR POLLICIS LONGUS MUSCLE

The belly of this muscle is palpated at the posterior surface of the radius. It is visible in this figure, as indicated by the index finger, at its passage on the lateral surface of the radius. Ask the subject to perform repeated abductions of the thumb so that you can better feel the contraction.

Comment: An oblique groove (1) separates the abductor pollicis longus muscle from the extensor pollicis brevis muscle (2).

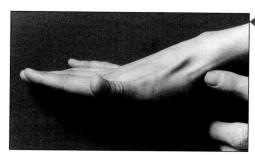

FIGURE 13-37
THE TENDON OF THE ABDUCTOR POLLICIS LONGUS MUSCLE

To find this tendon, indicated by the index finger, ask the subject to abduct the thumb. This tendon inserts into the lateral aspect of the base of the first metacarpal.

Comment: It is not always easy to distinguish the tendon of the abductor pollicis longus muscle from the tendon of the extensor pollicis brevis muscle (Fig. 13-39). Often, these two tendons are coupled and present as a single tendon. Keep in mind that the abductor pollicis longus muscle is in a more anterior position.

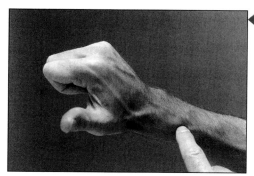

FIGURE 13-38
THE BELLY OF THE EXTENSOR POLLICIS BREVIS MUSCLE

This muscle is located below the abductor pollicis longus muscle at the posterior aspect of the forearm. Like the abductor pollicis longus muscle, the extensor pollicis brevis muscle passes around the external surface of the radius. In most cases, it is difficult to distinguish these two muscle bellies. Remember that the belly of the extensor pollicis brevis muscle is located more distally. It is also possible to palpate an oblique groove (Fig. 13-36) that separates these two muscle bellies at the posterolateral aspect of the radius. To find the structure of interest below this groove, ask the subject to abduct the thumb repeatedly to allow you to feel the muscular contraction.

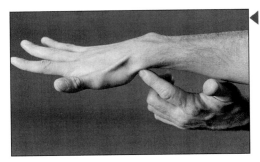

◀ FIGURE 13-39
THE TENDON OF THE EXTENSOR POLLICIS BREVIS MUSCLE AT THE WRIST

At this level, it is often difficult to distinguish this tendon from the tendon of the abductor pollicis longus muscle (Fig. 13-37) because the two are coupled. To make this tendon protrude at the lateral aspect of the wrist, ask the subject to abduct the thumb while it is extended. Keep in mind that the tendon of interest is located behind the tendon of the abductor pollicis longus muscle.

Comment: This tendon constitutes the anterolateral border of the anatomical snuffbox (see comment Fig. 13-42).

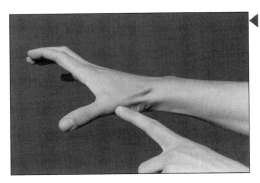

◀ FIGURE 13-40
THE INSERTION OF THE EXTENSOR POLLICIS BREVIS MUSCLE

As seen in this figure, after following the dorsal surface of the first metacarpal, this tendon inserts into the dorsal aspect of the base of the proximal phalanx.

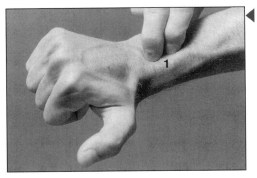

◀ FIGURE 13-41
THE EXTENSOR POLLICIS LONGUS MUSCLE AT THE POSTERIOR SURFACE OF THE RADIUS

Place a bidigital grip at the posterior surface of the distal radius, medial to the body of the extensor pollicis brevis muscle (1) (Fig. 13-38). Ask the subject to move the thumb behind the plane of the hand so that you can feel this tendon tighten under your fingers.

Comment: The body of the extensor pollicis longus muscle has an oblique route downward and outward at the posterior aspect of the forearm. It is located under the extensor pollicis brevis muscle to which it is joined.

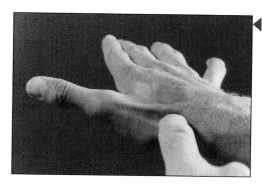

FIGURE 13-42
THE TENDON OF THE EXTENSOR POLLICIS
LONGUS MUSCLE AT THE WRIST

The requested muscular action to make this tendon protrude is the same as that described in Fig. 13-41. This tendon constitutes the posterolateral border of the anatomical snuffbox. The anterolateral border is formed by the tendon of the extensor pollicis brevis muscle.

Comment: The anatomical snuffbox is a triangular depression that appears at the posterolateral aspect of the wrist during the contraction of the extensor muscles of the thumb. The floor of this depression is the scaphoid bone.

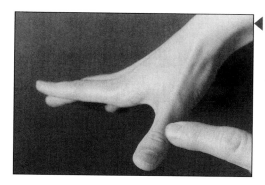

FIGURE 13-43
THE INSERTION OF THE EXTENSOR POLLICIS
LONGUS MUSCLE

As shown in this figure, after following the dorsal surface of the first metacarpal and the proximal phalanx, this tendon inserts into the dorsal aspect of the base of the distal phalanx.

THE ANTERIOR MUSCULAR GROUP

The notable structures accessible by palpation are

- Location of the medial epicondylar muscles (Fig. 13-45)
- The common tendon of origin of the medial epicondylar muscles (Fig. 13-46)
- The belly of the pronator teres muscle (Fig. 13-47)
- The distal aspect of the pronator teres muscle (Fig. 13-48)
- The belly of the flexor carpi radialis muscle (Fig. 13-49)
- The tendon of the flexor carpi radialis muscle (Fig. 13-50)
- The distal tendon of the distal flexor carpi radialis muscle (Fig. 13-51)
- The belly of the palmaris longus muscle (Fig. 13-52)
- The palmaris longus tendon (Fig. 13-53)
- The proximal aspect of the flexor carpi ulnaris muscle (Fig. 13-54)
- The flexor carpi ulnaris muscle at the medial aspect of the forearm (Fig. 13-55)

- The tendon of the flexor carpi ulnaris muscle (Fig. 13-56)
- The flexor digitorum superficialis muscle, superficial plane—the tendon for the fourth finger (Fig. 13-57)
- The flexor digitorum superficialis muscle, superficial plane—the tendon for the third finger (Fig. 13-58)
- The flexor digitorum superficialis muscle, deep plane— the tendons for the fifth finger and the index fingers (Fig. 13-59)
- The distal belly of the flexor digitorum superficialis muscle (Fig. 13-60)
- The tendons of the flexor digitorum superficialis muscle at the palm of the hand (Fig. 13-61)
- The belly of the flexor pollicis longus muscle (Fig. 13-62)
- The tendon of the flexor pollicis longus muscle (Fig. 13-63)

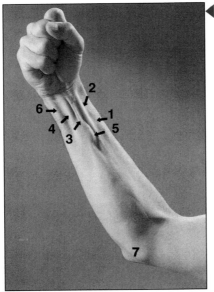

◀ **FIGURE 13-44**
ANTERIOR VIEW OF THE FOREARM

(1) Flexor pollicis longus muscle

(2) Flexor carpi radialis tendon

(3) Palmaris longus tendon

(4) Flexor digitorum superficialis tendon

(5) Palmaris longus muscle belly

(6) Flexor carpi ulnaris muscle

(7) Common tendon of origin of the medial epicondylar muscles

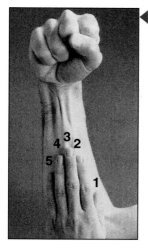

FIGURE 13-45
LOCATION OF THE MEDIAL EPICONDYLAR MUSCLES

With the subject's elbow flexed, wrist in a neutral position or slightly flexed, and fist clenched and in a neutral position with regard to pronation–supination, place your hand with the fingers together at the medial aspect of the elbow, with the thenar eminence resting on the medial epicondyle.

(1) The thumb shows the direction of the pronator teres muscle
(2) The index finger shows the direction of the flexor carpi radialis muscle
(3) The middle finger shows the direction of the palmaris longus muscle
(4) The ring finger shows the direction of the flexor digitorum superficialis muscle
(5) The little finger shows the direction of the flexor carpi ulnaris muscle

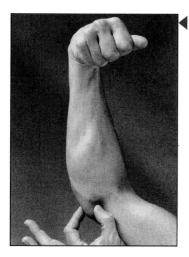

FIGURE 13-46
THE COMMON TENDON OF ORIGIN OF THE MEDIAL EPICONDYLAR MUSCLES

Place your thumb and your index finger at the level of the medial epicondyle and ask the subject to flex the wrist together with an ulnar deviation. You will feel the contraction of the common tendon under your fingers.

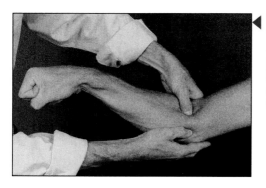

FIGURE 13-47
THE BELLY OF THE PRONATOR TERES MUSCLE

Place your grip just medial to the tendon of the biceps brachii muscle (see Fig. 9-6) and ask the subject to perform a pronation of the forearm with the fist clenched. You will feel the muscle belly tighten under your fingers.

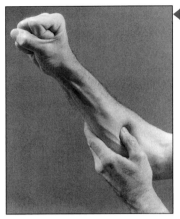

► **FIGURE 13-48**
THE DISTAL ASPECT OF THE PRONATOR TERES MUSCLE

After locating the muscle belly (Fig. 13-47), follow it obliquely downward and outward to the distal insertion at the middle third of the lateral surface of the radius. To help you locate this structure, ask the subject to perform a pronation of the forearm with the fist clenched.

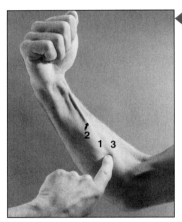

► **FIGURE 13-49**
THE BELLY OF THE FLEXOR CARPI RADIALIS MUSCLE

Ask the subject to flex the wrist together with a radial deviation and you will feel the muscle belly (1) that is continuous with the tendon (2), medial to the pronator teres muscle (3) (Fig. 13-48).

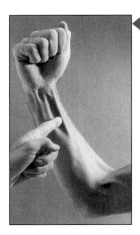

► **FIGURE 13-50**
THE TENDON OF THE FLEXOR CARPI RADIALIS MUSCLE

The action requested is identical to that described in Figure 13-49. The tendon of interest is the most lateral of the visible tendons on the distal third of the anterior aspect of the forearm.

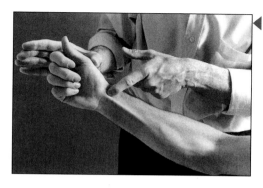

◀ FIGURE 13-51
THE DISTAL TENDON OF THE FLEXOR
CARPI RADIALIS MUSCLE

The action requested is a slight flexion of the wrist together with a radial deviation. In this figure, resistance is applied against the radial deviation.

Comment: This muscle inserts distally at the anterior aspect of the base of the second and third metacarpals.

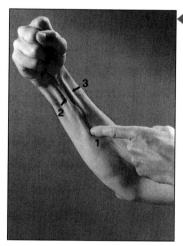

◀ FIGURE 13-52
THE BELLY OF THE PALMARIS LONGUS MUSCLE

Ask the subject to flex the wrist. The muscle belly (1) is perceived to be continuous with the tendon (2), as indicated by the index finger, medial to the flexor carpi radialis muscle (3). This muscle is not always present.

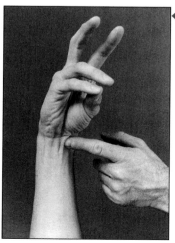

◀ FIGURE 13-53
THE PALMARIS LONGUS TENDON

Ask the subject to oppose the thumb and the little finger and to slightly flex the wrist to make the tendon of interest protrude more. This is a very long tendon that occupies the distal two thirds of the anterior aspect of the forearm.

Comment: This tendon ends on the flexor retinaculum and on the palmar aponeurosis.

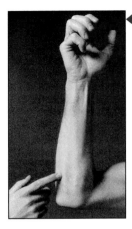

FIGURE 13-54
THE PROXIMAL ASPECT OF THE FLEXOR CARPI ULNARIS MUSCLE

Ask the subject to perform a flexion and an ulnar deviation of the wrist. You will feel the muscle belly, indicated by the index finger, medial to the palmaris longus muscle, close to the ulna.

Comment: At the proximal aspect of the forearm, it is difficult to distinguish this muscle from the epicondylar muscles.

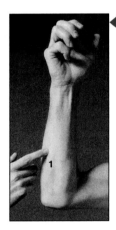

FIGURE 13-55
THE FLEXOR CARPI ULNARIS MUSCLE AT THE
MEDIAL ASPECT OF THE FOREARM

The two portions of this muscle (the humeral portion originates from the medial epicondyle and the ulnar portion originates from the medial border of the olecranon and the superior two thirds of the posterior border of the ulna) join to form one muscle belly (1) that descends in the medial aspect of the forearm and ends with a single tendon (see Fig. 13-56).

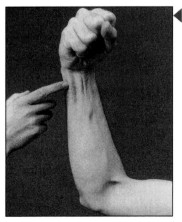

FIGURE 13-56
THE TENDON OF THE FLEXOR CARPI ULNARIS MUSCLE

This tendon is the most medial of all tendons visible at the anterior aspect of the forearm. To make it protrude, ask the subject to flex the wrist together with an ulnar deviation.

Comment: This tendon inserts into the pisiform with expansions for the hook of the hamate, the fifth metacarpal, and the palmar radiocarpal ligament.

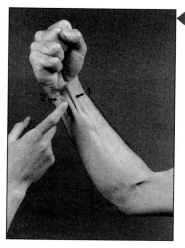

◀ FIGURE 13-57
THE FLEXOR DIGITORUM SUPERFICIALIS MUSCLE:
SUPERFICIAL PLANE — THE TENDON FOR THE FOURTH FINGER

In this figure, the index finger points to the tendon for the ring finger, medial to the tendon of the palmaris longus muscle (1). Place your index finger at the radial border of the tendon of the flexor carpi ulnaris muscle (2) and ask the subject to clench the fist and to perform brief, repeated flexions of the wrist (see also Fig. 15-5).

Comment: The tendons for the ring finger and the middle finger constitute the superficial plane of the flexor digitorum superficialis muscle.

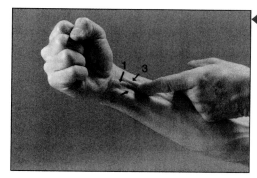

◀ FIGURE 13-58
THE FLEXOR DIGITORUM SUPERFICIALIS MUSCLE,
SUPERFICIAL PLANE — THE TENDON FOR THE THIRD FINGER

In this figure, the index finger pushes the tendon of the palmaris longus muscle (1) outward (toward the radius) in order to make contact with the tendon for the middle finger (2), which is located at the radial border of the tendon for the ring finger of the flexor digitorum superficialis muscle. Ask the subject to oppose the thumb and the middle finger (not shown in this figure) and to flex the wrist briefly and repeatedly to allow you to better feel this tendon under your fingers. Another method for perceiving this structure is to ask the subject to clench the fist and perform brief flexions of the wrist with a slight ulnar deviation (see also Fig. 15-6).

(1) Palmaris longus muscle

(2) Tendon for the middle finger

(3) Tendon of the flexor carpi radialis muscle

Comment: The tendons for the ring finger and the middle finger constitute the superficial plane of the flexor digitorum superficialis muscle.

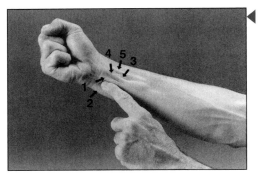

◀ **FIGURE 13-59**

THE FLEXOR DIGITORUM SUPERFICIALIS MUSCLE: DEEP PLANE — THE TENDONS FOR THE FIFTH AND THE INDEX FINGERS

The tendon for the little finger: In this figure, the index finger is placed at the ulnar border of the tendon for the ring finger (1) in order to make contact with the tendon for the little finger, which is located lateral to the tendon of the flexor carpi ulnaris muscle (2) and medial to the tendon for the ring finger (1) (already mentioned above). Ask the subject to clench the fist and to perform brief, repeated flexions of the wrist to let you feel this tendon tighten (see also Fig. 15-7).

The tendon for the index finger: In this figure, the tendon for the index finger (3) is visible lateral to the tendon of the palmaris longus muscle (4) and medial to the tendon of the flexor carpi radialis muscle (5). For a better perception of this tendon, ask the subject for the same muscular action as that described above (fist clenched and brief, repeated flexions of the wrist) (see also Fig. 15-8).

Comment: The two tendons described above form the deep plane of the flexor digitorum superficialis muscle.

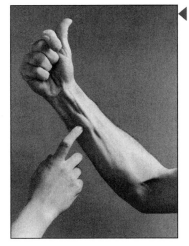

◀ **FIGURE 13-60**

THE DISTAL BELLY OF THE FLEXOR DIGITORUM SUPERFICIALIS MUSCLE

In this figure, the index finger indicates a belly of the deep plane of the flexor digitorum superficialis muscle. This plane contains the tendons for the index finger and the little finger. The superficial plane contains tendons for the middle finger and the ring finger. To make this muscle belly protrude, ask the subject to clench the third, fourth, and fifth fingers and, with the wrist in slight flexion, to perform brief, repeated flexions of the index finger.

Comment: This muscular plane is not accessible in all subjects.

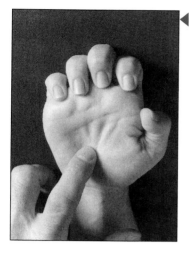

FIGURE 13-61
THE TENDONS OF THE FLEXOR DIGITORUM SUPERFICIALIS MUSCLE IN THE PALM OF THE HAND

The tendons in the palm of the hand are usually very visible when the subject hyperextends the metacarpophalangeal joints and flexes the middle and distal phalanges. If the tendons are not visible, they are easily palpated.

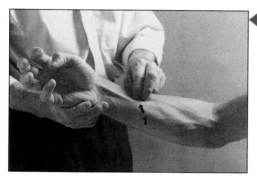

FIGURE 13-62
THE BELLY OF THE FLEXOR POLLICIS LONGUS MUSCLE

Place a uni- or bidigital grip lateral to the flexor carpi radialis muscle (1) (Fig. 13-50). Ask the subject to perform repeated flexions of the distal phalanx of the thumb on the proximal phalanx to allow you to feel the contraction under your fingers.

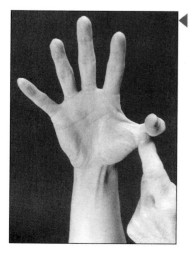

FIGURE 13-63
THE TENDON OF THE FLEXOR POLLICIS LONGUS MUSCLE

This tendon can be plainly perceived at the palmar surface of the proximal phalanx of the thumb when the subject performs rapid, repeated flexions of the distal phalanx on the proximal phalanx.

THE WRIST AND THE HAND

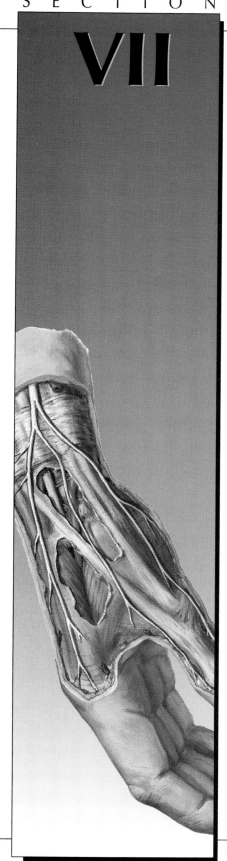

WRIST AND HAND: DEEPER PALMAR DISSECTIONS

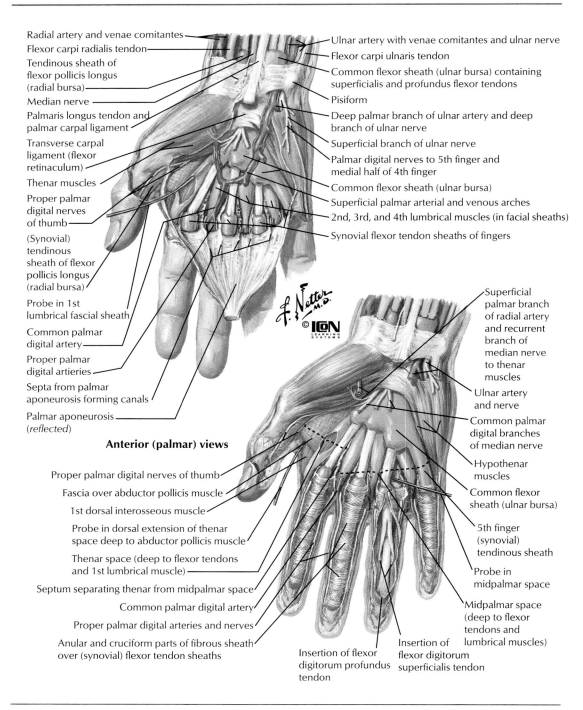

Radial artery and venae comitantes

Flexor carpi radialis tendon

Tendinous sheath of flexor pollicis longus (radial bursa)

Median nerve

Palmaris longus tendon and palmar carpal ligament

Transverse carpal ligament (flexor retinaculum)

Thenar muscles

Proper palmar digital nerves of thumb

(Synovial) tendinous sheath of flexor pollicis longus (radial bursa)

Probe in 1st lumbrical fascial sheath

Common palmar digital artery

Proper palmar digital arteries

Septa from palmar aponeurosis forming canals

Palmar aponeurosis (reflected)

Ulnar artery with venae comitantes and ulnar nerve

Flexor carpi ulnaris tendon

Common flexor sheath (ulnar bursa) containing superficialis and profundus flexor tendons

Pisiform

Deep palmar branch of ulnar artery and deep branch of ulnar nerve

Superficial branch of ulnar nerve

Palmar digital nerves to 5th finger and medial half of 4th finger

Common flexor sheath (ulnar bursa)

Superficial palmar arterial and venous arches

2nd, 3rd, and 4th lumbrical muscles (in facial sheaths)

Synovial flexor tendon sheaths of fingers

Anterior (palmar) views

Proper palmar digital nerves of thumb

Fascia over abductor pollicis muscle

1st dorsal interosseous muscle

Probe in dorsal extension of thenar space deep to abductor pollicis muscle

Thenar space (deep to flexor tendons and 1st lumbrical muscle)

Septum separating thenar from midpalmar space

Common palmar digital artery

Proper palmar digital arteries and nerves

Anular and cruciform parts of fibrous sheath over (synovial) flexor tendon sheaths

Insertion of flexor digitorum profundus tendon

Insertion of flexor digitorum superficialis tendon

Superficial palmar branch of radial artery and recurrent branch of median nerve to thenar muscles

Ulnar artery and nerve

Common palmar digital branches of median nerve

Hypothenar muscles

Common flexor sheath (ulnar bursa)

5th finger (synovial) tendinous sheath

Probe in midpalmar space

Midpalmar space (deep to flexor tendons and lumbrical muscles)

WRIST AND HAND: SUPERFICIAL RADIAL DISSECTION

Lateral (radial view)

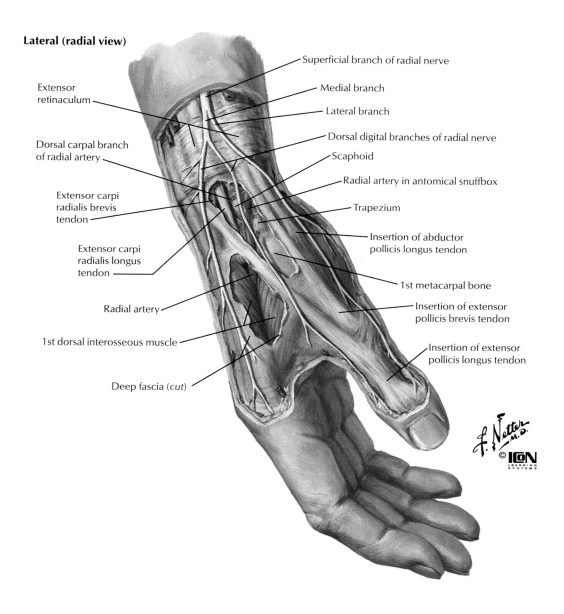

Superficial branch of radial nerve

Medial branch

Lateral branch

Dorsal digital branches of radial nerve

Scaphoid

Radial artery in antomical snuffbox

Trapezium

Insertion of abductor pollicis longus tendon

1st metacarpal bone

Insertion of extensor pollicis brevis tendon

Insertion of extensor pollicis longus tendon

Extensor retinaculum

Dorsal carpal branch of radial artery

Extensor carpi radialis brevis tendon

Extensor carpi radialis longus tendon

Radial artery

1st dorsal interosseous muscle

Deep fascia (*cut*)

EXTENSOR TENDONS AT WRIST

Posterior (dorsal) view

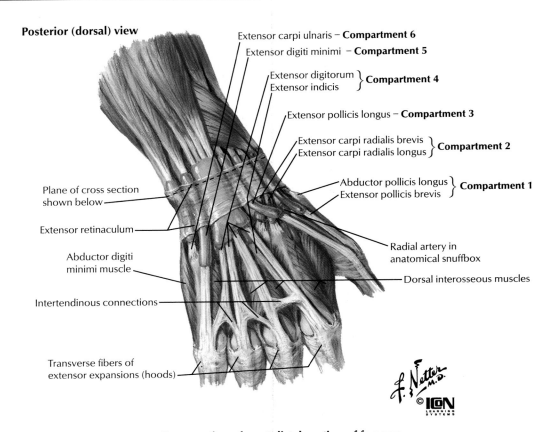

Extensor carpi ulnaris – **Compartment 6**

Extensor digiti minimi – **Compartment 5**

Extensor digitorum }
Extensor indicis } **Compartment 4**

Extensor pollicis longus – **Compartment 3**

Extensor carpi radialis brevis }
Extensor carpi radialis longus } **Compartment 2**

Abductor pollicis longus }
Extensor pollicis brevis } **Compartment 1**

Plane of cross section shown below

Extensor retinaculum

Abductor digiti minimi muscle

Intertendinous connections

Transverse fibers of extensor expansions (hoods)

Radial artery in anatomical snuffbox

Dorsal interosseous muscles

Cross section of most distal portion of forearm

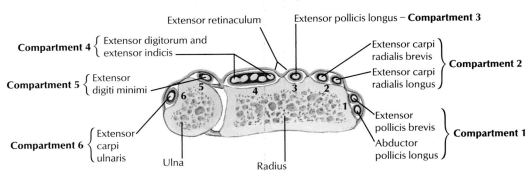

Extensor retinaculum

Extensor pollicis longus – **Compartment 3**

Compartment 4 { Extensor digitorum and extensor indicis

Compartment 5 { Extensor digiti minimi

Compartment 6 { Extensor carpi ulnaris

Ulna

Radius

Extensor carpi radialis brevis }
Extensor carpi radialis longus } **Compartment 2**

Extensor pollicis brevis }
Abductor pollicis longus } **Compartment 1**

FLEXOR AND EXTENSOR TENDONS IN FINGERS

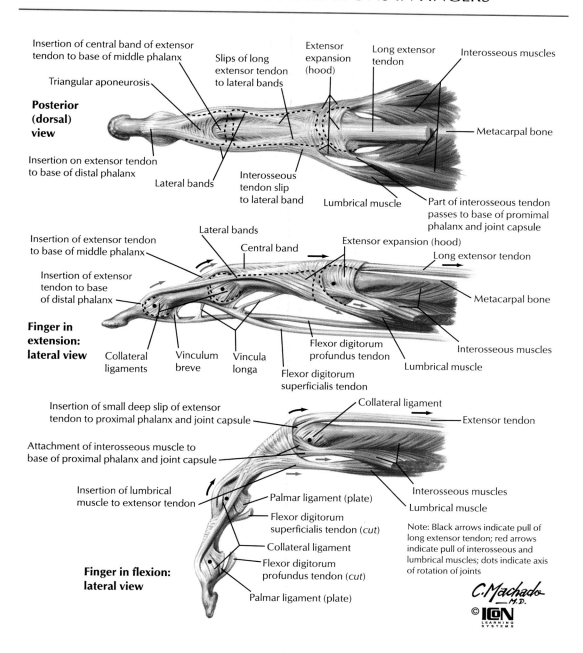

Insertion of central band of extensor tendon to base of middle phalanx

Triangular aponeurosis

Posterior (dorsal) view

Insertion on extensor tendon to base of distal phalanx

Lateral bands

Slips of long extensor tendon to lateral bands

Interosseous tendon slip to lateral band

Extensor expansion (hood)

Long extensor tendon

Interosseous muscles

Metacarpal bone

Lumbrical muscle

Part of interosseous tendon passes to base of promimal phalanx and joint capsule

Insertion of extensor tendon to base of middle phalanx

Insertion of extensor tendon to base of distal phalanx

Finger in extension: lateral view

Lateral bands

Central band

Collateral ligaments

Vinculum breve

Vincula longa

Flexor digitorum superficialis tendon

Extensor expansion (hood)

Long extensor tendon

Metacarpal bone

Flexor digitorum profundus tendon

Lumbrical muscle

Interosseous muscles

Insertion of small deep slip of extensor tendon to proximal phalanx and joint capsule

Attachment of interosseous muscle to base of proximal phalanx and joint capsule

Insertion of lumbrical muscle to extensor tendon

Finger in flexion: lateral view

Collateral ligament

Extensor tendon

Palmar ligament (plate)

Flexor digitorum superficialis tendon (cut)

Collateral ligament

Flexor digitorum profundus tendon (cut)

Palmar ligament (plate)

Interosseous muscles

Lumbrical muscle

Note: Black arrows indicate pull of long extensor tendon; red arrows indicate pull of interosseous and lumbrical muscles; dots indicate axis of rotation of joints

C. Machado
M.D.

© ICON
LEARNING SYSTEMS

TOPOGRAPHIC PRESENTATION OF THE HAND

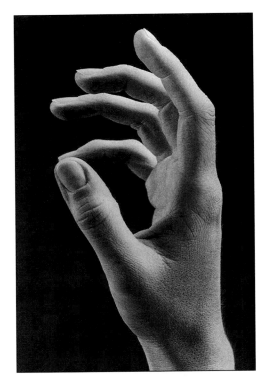

FIGURE 14-1
GENERAL PRESENTATION OF THE HAND

CHAPTER Fourteen

OSTEOLOGY

THE DISTAL END OF THE TWO BONES OF THE FOREARM

The notable structures accessible by palpation are

- The distal end or head of the ulna (Fig. 14-2)
- The distal end or head of the ulna and the styloid process (Fig. 14-3)
- The distal end of the radius (Fig. 14-4)

- The distal end of the radius—the ulnar or medial border (Fig. 14-5)
- The distal end of the radius—the lateral surface and the styloid process of the radius (Fig. 14-6)
- The dorsal tubercle of the radius—posterior view (Fig. 14-7)

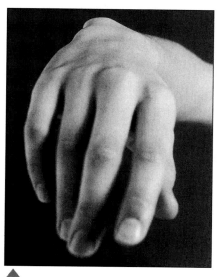

▲

FIGURE 14-2

THE DISTAL END OR HEAD OF THE ULNA

This figure demonstrates the distal end of the ulna, which feels like a bulge under the fingers and overlooks the medial portion of the proximal row of the carpal bones. Cylindrical in shape, it consists of two projections separated by a groove: the styloid process (Fig. 14-3) and the lateral projection, which articulates with the ulnar notch of the radius.

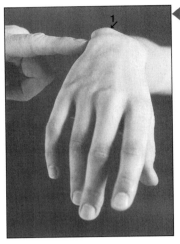

◀ **FIGURE 14-3**
THE DISTAL END OR HEAD OF THE ULNA AND THE STYLOID PROCESS

The distal end (1) bears the styloid process, also called the posteromedial eminence, indicated by the index finger. It forms a sort of beak at the distal end of the ulna, easily accessible at this level with a thumb–index finger grip. This bony structure is separated from the lateral surface (which articulates with the ulnar notch of the radius) by a sagittal groove, where the tendon of the extensor carpi ulnaris muscle passes.

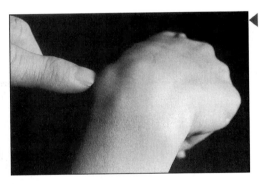

▶ **FIGURE 14-4**
THE DISTAL END OF THE RADIUS

This figure demonstrates the distal end of the radius, which overlooks and articulates with the lateral portion of the first row of carpal bones. The inferior surface of the distal end articulates laterally with the scaphoid and medially with the lunate.

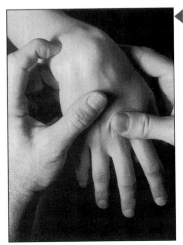

◀ **FIGURE 14-5**
THE DISTAL END OF THE RADIUS — THE ULNAR OR MEDIAL BORDER

The ulnar notch, a concave articular surface intended to receive the head of the ulna, is located at the level of this border. With the subject's wrist in a neutral position, place your index finger on the posterior surface of the head of the ulna, pointing toward the distal end of the radius. Ask the subject to flex the wrist to allow the structure of interest to "appear" under your finger.

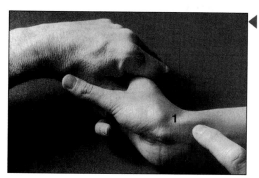

FIGURE 14-6
THE DISTAL END OF THE RADIUS — THE LATERAL SURFACE AND THE STYLOID PROCESS OF THE RADIUS

The lateral surface indicated by the index finger presents two vertical grooves: an anterior groove, where the tendons of the abductor pollicis longus and the extensor pollicis brevis muscles pass, and a posterior groove, where the tendons of the extensor carpi radialis longus and the extensor carpi radialis brevis muscles pass. The lateral surface ends distally with the styloid process of the radius (1).

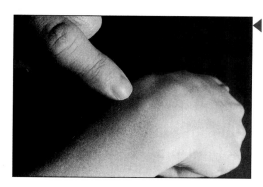

FIGURE 14-7
THE DORSAL TUBERCLE OF THE RADIUS — POSTERIOR VIEW

This tubercle is an important landmark at the posterior aspect of the wrist. It separates two grooves: a lateral groove, where the tendon of the extensor pollicis longus muscle passes, and a medial groove, where the tendons of the extensor digitorum muscle and the extensor indicis muscle pass. The bony structure of interest (1) is located in the middle of the posterior surface of the distal end of the radius, medially limited by its ulnar border (see Fig. 14-5).

THE CARPAL BONES
The Bones of the Proximinal Row

The notable structures accessible by palpation are

- Presentation of the anatomical snuffbox (Fig. 14-9)
- The scaphoid: lateral approach—step 1(Fig. 14-10)
- The scaphoid: lateral approach—step 2 (Fig. 14-11)
- The scaphoid—anterior approach (Fig. 14-12)
- The scaphoid—other anterior approach (Fig. 14-13)
- The scaphoid tubercle (Fig. 14-14)
- The scaphoid: posterior approach—step 1. Topographic visualization (Fig. 14-15)
- The scaphoid: posterior approach—step 2 (Fig. 14-16)

- The scaphoid—global approach (Fig. 14-17)
- The lunate—topographic visualization (Fig. 14-18)
- The lunate—proximal approach (Fig. 14-19)
- The lunate—distal approach (Fig. 14-20)
- The triquetrum—step 1 (Fig. 14-21)
- The triquetrum—step 2 (Fig. 14-22)
- The triquetrum—global approach (Fig. 14-23)
- The pisiform (Fig. 14-24)
- The pisiform (Fig. 14-25)

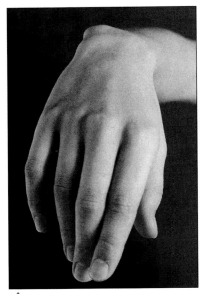

▲
FIGURE 14-8
DISTAL (OR INFERIOR) VIEW
OF THE CARPAL BONES—FIRST ROW

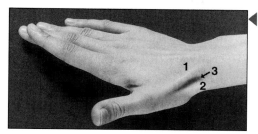

FIGURE 14-9
PRESENTATION OF THE ANATOMICAL SNUFFBOX

The tendons of the extensor pollicis longus muscle (1) and the extensor pollicis brevis muscle (2) move away from one another in the wrist region and mark the boundaries of a triangular area with a proximal base and a distal apex. This area is called the anatomical snuffbox. The floor (3) of this area is occupied by the scaphoid proximally and the trapezium distally. The tendon of the abductor pollicis longus muscle, attached anteriorly to the tendon of the extensor pollicis brevis muscle, is also part of the snuffbox (see also Figs. 15-11, 15-12, and 15-13).

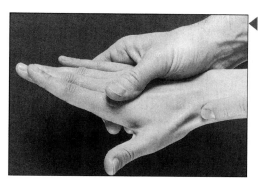

FIGURE 14-10
THE SCAPHOID: LATERAL APPROACH — STEP 1

The subject's hand is in a neutral position. After locating the anatomical snuffbox (Fig. 14-9), slide your index finger down the back of this depression limited by the extensor tendons of the thumb (Fig. 14-9). In this figure, the index finger is placed between the styloid process of the radius (Fig. 14-6) and the scaphoid.

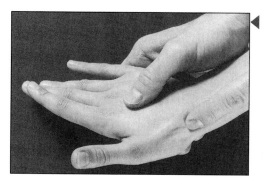

FIGURE 14-11
THE SCAPHOID: LATERAL APPROACH — STEP 2

Starting with the same technique of approach as in Figure 14-10, move your index finger further distally in the anatomical snuffbox (Fig. 14-9). With your other hand, bend the subject's hand toward the ulna. The lateral surface of the scaphoid is now under your index finger.

Comment: This surface presents a groove where the radial artery runs.

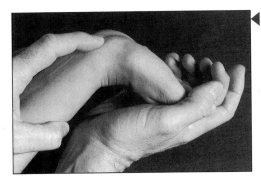

FIGURE 14-12
THE SCAPHOID — ANTERIOR APPROACH

In this figure, the wrist is in extension in order to expose the anterior (or palmar) surface of the scaphoid. You will feel this structure as a convexity (a bulge) under your index finger.

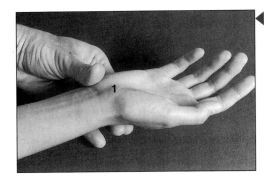

FIGURE 14-13
THE SCAPHOID — OTHER ANTERIOR APPROACH

Place the interphalangeal joint of your thumb on the radial aspect of the pisiform (Fig. 14-25), in the extension of the first cutaneous palmar fold. The flexion of the interphalangeal joint brings your thumb in contact with the palmar surface of the scaphoid (1).

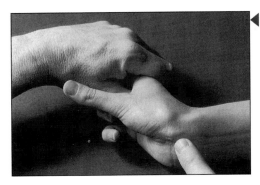

FIGURE 14-14
THE SCAPHOID TUBERCLE

In this figure, the left thumb is in contact with the scaphoid tubercle. This bony structure extends laterally the anterior (or palmar) surface of the scaphoid. Place your grip at the anterior aspect of the tendon of the abductor pollicis longus muscle (1) to feel this tubercle. Repeated ulnar deviations will help you feel this structure.

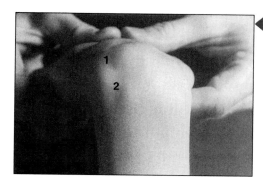

FIGURE 14-15

THE SCAPHOID: POSTERIOR APPROACH — STEP 1.
TOPOGRAPHIC VISUALIZATION

The dorsal surface of the scaphoid (1) is found in the extension of the distal end of the radius (2) (at the lateral aspect).

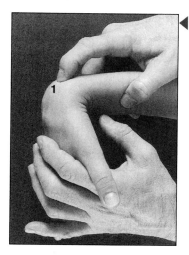

FIGURE 14-16
THE SCAPHOID: POSTERIOR APPROACH — STEP 2

Place your index finger on the radiocarpal interspace. With your other hand, bring the subject's hand in palmar flexion. You will feel the dorsal surface of the scaphoid as a convexity (1) below the radiocarpal interspace.

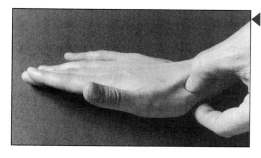

FIGURE 14-17
THE SCAPHOID — GLOBAL APPROACH

This figure shows a global approach to the scaphoid; it is held with a thumb–index finger grip at its palmar and lateral surfaces. To locate the palmar surface, see Figures. 14-12, 14-13, and 14-14. The lateral surface of the scaphoid, where the thumb is, corresponds to the floor of the anatomical snuffbox (see Figs. 14-9, 14-10, and 14-11).

Comment: The scaphoid can also be globally approached with a thumb–index finger grip on the palmar and dorsal surfaces.

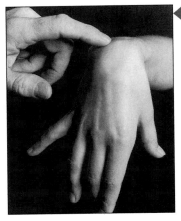

FIGURE 14-18
THE LUNATE — TOPOGRAPHIC VISUALIZATION

This bony structure is indicated by the index finger. To make the lunate protrude, ask the subject to flex the wrist to free it from the articular carpal surface located at the distal end of the radius.

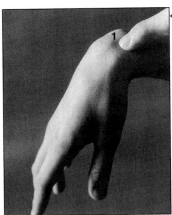

FIGURE 14-19
THE LUNATE — PROXIMAL APPROACH

First locate the dorsal tubercle of the radius (see Fig. 14-7). Then place your index finger medial (ulnar side) to this structure in the radiocarpal interspace, pointing toward the third metacarpal. Ask the subject to flex the wrist to make the lunate (1) appear under your index finger.

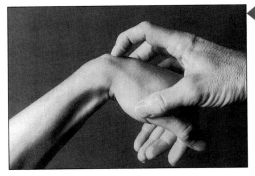

FIGURE 14-20
THE LUNATE — DISTAL APPROACH

After locating the capitate (Figs. 14-36 through 14-43), position your index finger in the capitate depression (located just above the base of the third metacarpal). Now slide your index finger onto the head of the capitate, which you will feel as a convexity under your finger, toward the distal end of the radius, between the tendon of the extensor digitorum muscle medially (ulnar side) and an imaginary line that extends distally from the dorsal tubercle of the radius, laterally (radial side) (Fig. 14-7). With the subject's wrist flexed, you will feel the lunate between the head of the capitate and the posterior border of the radius.

Comments: If you slide your grip too far laterally (radially), you will end up on the dorsal surface of the scaphoid (see Figs. 14-15 and 14-16). If you do not slide your grip far enough toward the radius, you will end up on the head of the capitate (see Fig. 14-41).

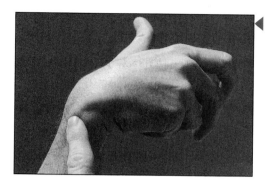

FIGURE 14-21
THE TRIQUETRUM — STEP 1

Place the subject's hand in palmar flexion, with the forearm in supination. The index finger indicates the styloid process of the ulna (Fig. 14-3), the most distal bony projection of the medial border of the forearm or ulna.

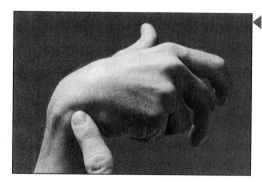

FIGURE 14-22
THE TRIQUETRUM — STEP 2

Place the subject's forearm and hand as described in Figure 14-21. The index finger indicates the triquetrum, which immediately follows the styloid process of the ulna at the medial border of the wrist.

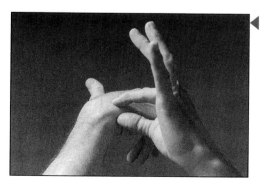

FIGURE 14-23
THE TRIQUETRUM — GLOBAL APPROACH

After locating the bony structures described in Figures 14-21 and 14-22, you can grasp the triquetrum globally. Place your thumb on the medial surface of this bone and your index finger on the dorsal surface.

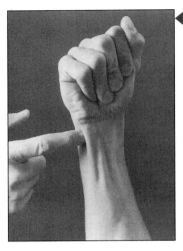

FIGURE 14-24
THE PISIFORM

The index finger indicates the tendon of the flexor carpi ulnaris muscle (Fig. 15-9). This tendon is an important structure in the examination of the pisiform, as it inserts into the anterior surface of that bone. Keep in mind that the pisiform is located at the base of the hypothenar eminence (Fig. 15-22).

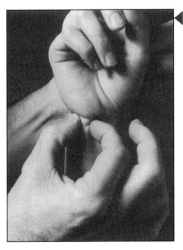

FIGURE 14-25
THE PISIFORM

The posterior surface of the pisiform articulates with the triquetrum (Figs. 14-21, 14-22, and 14-23); the anterior surface projects beneath the skin. In this figure, the thumb–index finger grip holds the bone of interest.

Comment: To better feel this structure, ask the subject to let the wrist bend naturally in palmar flexion in order to relax the tendon of the flexor carpi ulnaris muscle.

The Bones of the Distal Row

The notable structures accessible by palpation are

- The trapezium: step 1—location of the anatomical snuffbox (Fig. 14-27)
- The trapezium—step 2 (Fig. 14-28)
- The trapezium—global approach (Fig. 14-29)
- The tubercle of the trapezium—step 1 (Fig. 14-30)
- The tubercle of the trapezium—step 2 (Fig. 14-31)
- The tubercle of the trapezium—step 3 (Fig. 14-32)
- The trapezoid—topographic situation (Fig. 14-33)
- The trapezoid—step 1 (Fig. 14-34)
- The trapezoid—step 2 (Fig. 14-35)
- The capitate: constitution and topographic situation—dorsal view (Fig. 14-36)
- The capitate: step 1—dorsal view (Fig. 14-37)

- The capitate: step 2—dorsal view (Fig. 14-38)
- Visualization of the notable bony landmarks for the palpation of the capitate—lateral view (Fig. 14-39)
- The depression of the capitate—lateral view (Fig. 14-40)
- The head of the capitate—lateral view (Fig. 14-41)
- The capitate and the lunate (Fig. 14-42)
- The capitate—global approach (Fig. 14-43)
- The hamate—medial approach (Fig. 14-44)
- The hamate—dorsal approach (Fig. 14-45)
- The hamulus (hook) of the hamate—step 1 (Fig. 14-46)
- The hamulus (hook) of the hamate—step 2 (Fig. 14-47)
- The hamulus (hook) of the hamate—step 3 (Fig. 14-48)

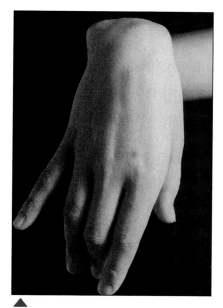

▲
FIGURE 14-26
TOPOGRAPHIC LOCATION OF THE
CARPAL BONES — DISTAL ROW

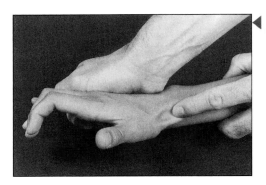

FIGURE 14-27
THE TRAPEZIUM: STEP 1— LOCATION OF THE ANATOMICAL SNUFFBOX

After locating the anatomical snuffbox (see Fig. 14-9), place your thumb on the scaphoid, located in the floor of that structure.

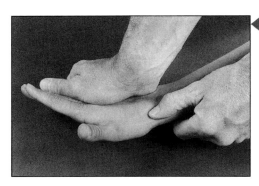

FIGURE 14-28
THE TRAPEZIUM — STEP 2

After completing the first step (fig. 14-27), move your thumb distally until you make contact with the base of the first metacarpal. You will feel the trapezium under your thumb.

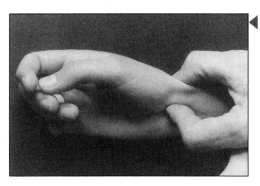

FIGURE 14-29
THE TRAPEZIUM— GLOBAL APPROACH

In this figure, the trapezium is held globally between the thumb and the index finger. Place your grip just above the base of the first metacarpal. To be certain the position is correct, ask the subject to mobilize the first metacarpal: this helps locate the trapezium, which does not move under your fingers during that action.

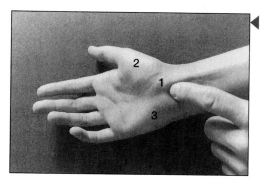

◀ FIGURE 14-30
THE TUBERCLE OF THE TRAPEZIUM — STEP 1

First locate the scaphoid (1) (see also Figs. 14-12 and 14-13) and the space between the thenar (2) and the hypothenar (3) eminences, just at the level of the wrist fold. In this figure, the index finger indicates the convexity formed by the scaphoid on the anterior aspect of the wrist.

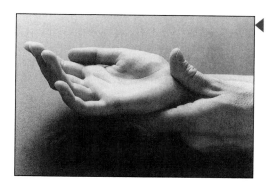

◀ FIGURE 14-31
THE TUBERCLE OF THE TRAPEZIUM — STEP 2

In this step, place the interphalangeal joint of your thumb between the thenar and the hypothenar eminences on the anterior aspect of the subject's wrist (Fig. 14-30), in contact with the scaphoid. Your thumb points toward the subject's thumb.

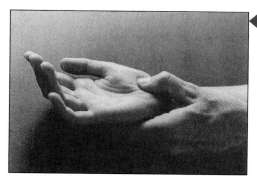

◀ FIGURE 14-32
THE TUBERCLE OF THE TRAPEZIUM — STEP 3

After completing steps 1 and 2 (Figs. 14-30 and 14-31), flex your thumb and press it down toward the subject's thumb. You will feel the tubercle of the trapezium directly under your finger, just above the base of the first metacarpal.

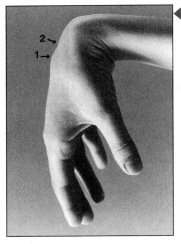

FIGURE 14-33
THE TRAPEZOID — TOPOGRAPHIC SITUATION

This figure shows both the base of the second metacarpal (1) and the position of the trapezoid (2) on the dorsal aspect of the hand.

Comment: On the dorsal aspect of the hand, do not mistake the bony projection that is the base of the second metacarpal for the dorsal surface of the trapezoid, which is located in a depression.

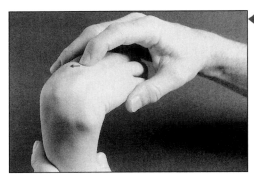

FIGURE 14-34
THE TRAPEZOID — STEP 1

In this figure, the index finger pushes (arrow) against the base of the second metacarpal, which is the bony projection indicated in Figure 14-33.

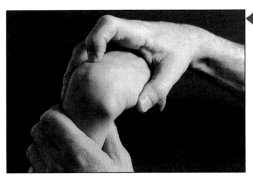

FIGURE 14-35
THE TRAPEZOID — STEP 2

After completing step 1, slide your index finger in the depression located above (proximally). Slide your grip between the two tendons of the extensor carpi radialis longus and brevis muscles (see Figs. 15-15 and 15-16).

Comment: Contact with the dorsal surface of this bone is not always possible, since it is set quite far back from the base of the second metacarpal.

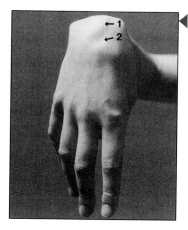

FIGURE 14-36
THE CAPITATE: CONSTITUTION AND TOPOGRAPHIC SITUATION —
DORSAL VIEW

This is the largest of all the carpals, and its major axis corresponds to the axis of the hand. It consists of a proximal portion, the head (1); a distal portion, the body (2); and a zone between these two structures, the neck.

Comment: Proximally, the capitate is embedded under the scaphoid and the lunate. Distally, it articulates with the second, third, and fourth metacarpals. The lateral surface articulates proximally with the scaphoid and distally with the trapezoid. The medial surface articulates with the hamate.

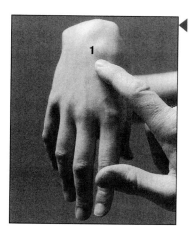

FIGURE 14-37
THE CAPITATE: STEP 1 — DORSAL VIEW

In this first step, it is necessary to find the base of the third metacarpal (1) since the capitate is located in the proximal extension of that structure.

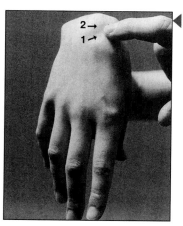

FIGURE 14-38
THE CAPITATE: STEP 2 — DORSAL VIEW

With the first step completed, slide your index finger from the base of the third metacarpal upward into a depression (1) that belongs to the body of the capitate (see also Fig. 14-36). The convexity (2) above that depression is the head of the capitate (see also Figs. 14-39, 14-40, and 14-41).

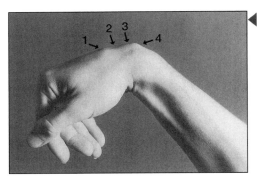

◄ **FIGURE 14-39**

VISUALIZATION OF THE NOTABLE BONY LANDMARKS FOR THE PALPATION OF THE CAPITATE — LATERAL VIEW

In this lateral view, you may clearly distinguish the base of the third metacarpal (1), the capitate depression (2), the capitate head (3), and the lunate (4), which is accessible when the wrist is flexed.

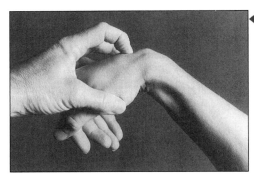

◄ **FIGURE 14-40**

THE DEPRESSION OF THE CAPITATE — LATERAL VIEW

Place your index finger in the depression in the extension of the base of the third metacarpal, lateral to the tendon of the extensor digitorum muscle.

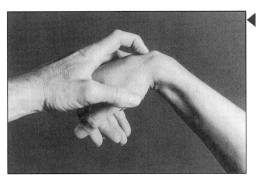

◄ **FIGURE 14-41**

THE HEAD OF THE CAPITATE — LATERAL VIEW

From the depression described in Figure 14-40, move your index finger proximally (without sliding on the skin) until you feel a convexity that is the head of the capitate.

Comment: Do not mistake this structure for the lunate (see Figs. 14-18, 14-19, 14-20, 14-39, and 14-42).

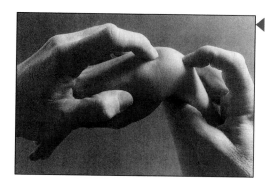

FIGURE 14-42
THE CAPITATE AND THE LUNATE

In this figure, the head of the capitate and the lunate (located more proximally) are held between the two index fingers. Do not confuse these two bony structures (see Figs. 14-18, 14-19, and 14-20 and 14-36 through 14-41).

Comment: One of the most frequent fusions involving the carpals is the fusion of the triquetrum to the lunate.

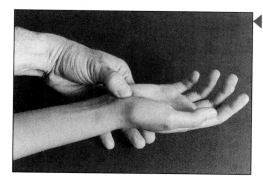

FIGURE 14-43
THE CAPITATE — GLOBAL APPROACH

The first step is to place the interphalangeal joint of your thumb on the pisiform (Figs. 14-24 and 14-25), with your thumb pointing outward. Place your index finger on the dorsum of the hand in the depression of the capitate (Figs. 14-38, 14-39, and 14-40), which is located in the extension of the base of the third metacarpal (Fig. 14-37). The second step is to flex the interphalangeal joint of your thumb to allow a global approach to the capitate.

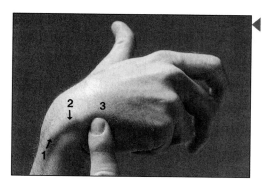

FIGURE 14-44
THE HAMATE — MEDIAL APPROACH

After locating the styloid process of the ulna (1) (see also Fig. 14-3) and the triquetrum (2) (see also Figs. 14-21, 14-22, and 14-23), place your index finger on the medial surface of the hamate between the base of the fifth metacarpal (3) and the triquetrum (2).

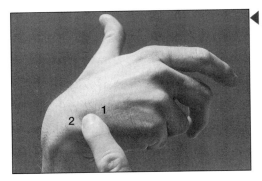

◀ FIGURE **14-45**
THE HAMATE — DORSAL APPROACH

Begin with the grip described in Figure 14-44 and slide your index finger on the dorsal surface of this bone, between the base of the fourth and fifth metacarpals (1) and the dorsal surface of the triquetrum (2).

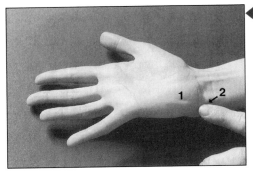

◀ FIGURE **14-46**
THE HAMULUS (HOOK) OF THE HAMATE — STEP **1**

First, locate the pisiform (indicated by the index finger), situated at the base of the hypothenar eminence (1) at the ulnar extremity of the first anterior palmar fold (2) (see also Figs. 14-24 and 14-25).

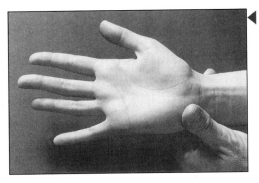

◀ FIGURE **14-47**
THE HAMULUS (HOOK) OF THE HAMATE — STEP **2**

Now, place the interphalangeal joint of your thumb on the pisiform (see Fig. 14-46).

Comment: Your thumb is pointing toward the subject's index finger.

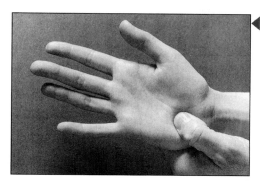

FIGURE 14-48
THE HAMULUS (HOOK) OF THE HAMATE — STEP 3

With your thumb in the position described in Figure 14-47, flex the distal phalanx on the proximal phalanx in the direction of the subject's index finger to make contact with the structure of interest, which you will feel as a protuberance under your thumb.

THE METACARPUS AND THE PHALANGES

The notable structures accessible by palpation are

- The heads of the metacarpals II to V—dorsal view (Fig. 14-50)
- The heads of the metacarpals II to V—palmar view (Fig. 14-51)
- The first metacarpal—the base (Fig. 14-52)
- The first metacarpal—the shaft or body (Fig. 14-53)
- The first metacarpal—the head (Fig. 14-54)
- The sesamoid bones of the metacarpophalangeal joint (Fig. 14-55)

- The second metacarpal (Fig. 14-56)
- The third metacarpal (Fig. 14-57)
- The fourth metacarpal (Fig. 14-58)
- The fifth metacarpal (Fig. 14-59)
- The proximal phalanx of the thumb (Fig. 14-60)
- The distal phalanx of the thumb (Fig. 14-61)

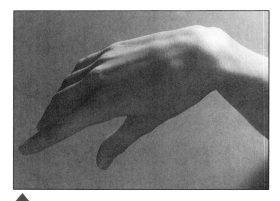

▲
FIGURE 14-49
**LATERAL VIEW OF THE METACARPALS
AND THE PHALANGES**

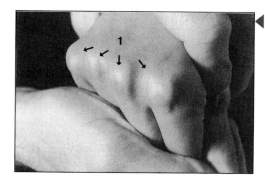

FIGURE 14-50
THE HEADS OF THE METACARPALS II TO V — DORSAL VIEW

The metacarpus consists of five bones that articulate proximally with the carpals and distally with the proximal phalanges of the fingers. In this figure, the flexion of the fingers at the level of the metacarpophalangeal joints allows the visualization of the distal aspect of the heads of the metacarpals (1).

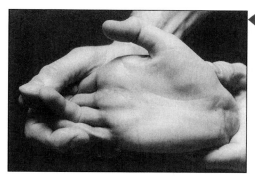

FIGURE 14-51
THE HEADS OF THE METACARPALS II TO V — PALMAR VIEW

In this figure, the extension of the fingers at the level of the metacarpophalangeal joints allows the visualization of the palmar aspect of the heads of the metacarpals.

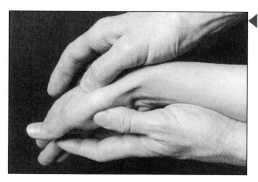

FIGURE 14-52
THE FIRST METACARPAL — THE BASE

The saddle-shaped base of the first metacarpal articulates only with the trapezium (it does not articulate with the second metacarpal). Locating this structure is thus important both in itself and for locating the trapezium (see Figs. 14-27, 14-28, and 14-29).

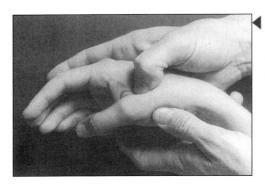

FIGURE 14-53
THE FIRST METACARPAL — THE SHAFT OR BODY

The first metacarpal is the shortest and thickest of the metacarpal bones. The shaft (diaphysis) is located between the base (Fig. 14-52) of the metacarpal and the head (Fig. 14-54).

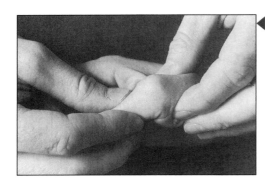

FIGURE 14-54
THE FIRST METACARPAL — THE HEAD

The head articulates with the base of the proximal phalanx. It can be demonstrated by flexing the metacarpophalangeal joint.

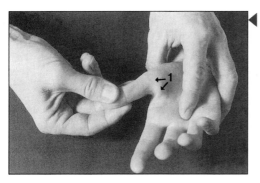

FIGURE 14-55
THE SESAMOID BONES OF THE
METACARPOPHALANGEAL JOINT

On the anterior aspect, the head of the first metacarpal presents two bumps separated by a groove. The sesamoid bones are located superficial to the two bumps. These two (lateral and medial) bony nodules (1) are always present at the level of this articulation.

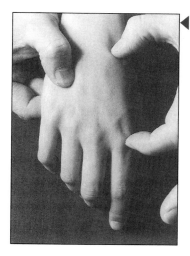

FIGURE 14-56
THE SECOND METACARPAL

The second metacarpal is the longest of the metacarpal bones. The location of its base is important for the palpation of the trapezoid (see Figs. 14-33, 14-34, and 14-35). In this figure, the grip takes hold of the second metacarpal, with the thumb at the level of the base and the index finger at the level of the head.

Comment: The base of this bone articulates with the trapezoid in the center, the trapezium laterally, and the capitate medially.

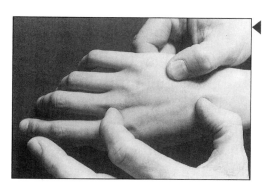

FIGURE 14-57
THE THIRD METACARPAL

The technique of approach is identical to that described in Figure 14-56. The base, which is in contact with the thumb in the thumb–index finger grip, articulates with the capitate (see Figs. 14-36 through 14-43).

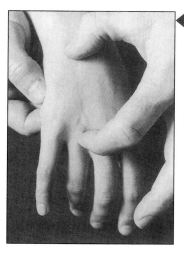

FIGURE 14-58
THE FOURTH METACARPAL

The technique of approach is identical to that described in Figure 14-56. The base articulates with the capitate (see Figs. 14-36 through 14-43) and the hamate (see Figs. 14-44 through 14-48).

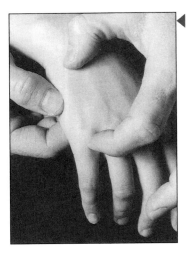

FIGURE 14-59
THE FIFTH METACARPAL

The fifth metacarpal is the shortest of all the metacarpal bones. The thumb–index finger grip is identical to that described in Figure 14-56. The thumb is in contact with the base, which articulates with the hamate (see Figs. 14-44 through 14-48), and the index finger is placed on the head of the fifth metacarpal.

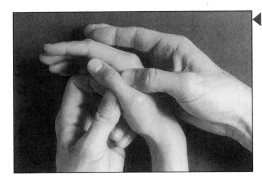

FIGURE 14-60
THE PROXIMAL PHALANX OF THE THUMB

The base has a glenoid cavity that articulates with the head of the first metacarpal. The head has a trochlea that occupies the palmar and inferior surfaces and that articulates with the base of the distal phalanx.

Comment: At the level of the other fingers, the head of the proximal phalanx articulates with the base of the middle phalanx.

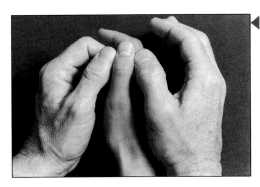

FIGURE 14-61
THE DISTAL PHALANX OF THE THUMB

The thumb has only two phalanges, whereas the other fingers have three.

Comment: At the level of the other fingers, the middle phalanx, shorter and smaller than the first, has an identical conformation. The third phalanx, also called the distal phalanx, is the smallest of the three phalanges.

CHAPTER Fifteen

MYOLOGY

THE TENDONS OF THE ANTERIOR ASPECT OF THE WRIST

The notable structures accessible by palpation are

- The tendon of the flexor pollicis longus muscle (Fig. 15-2)
- The tendon of the flexor carpi radialis muscle (Fig. 15-3)
- The tendon of the palmaris longus muscle (Fig. 15-4)
- The flexor digitorum superficialis muscle—the tendon for the fourth finger (Fig. 15-5)

- The flexor digitorum superficialis muscle—the tendon for the third finger (Fig. 15-6)
- The flexor digitorum superficialis muscle—the tendon for the fifth finger (Fig. 15-7)
- The flexor digitorum superficialis muscle—the tendon for the index finger (Fig. 15-8)
- The tendon of the flexor carpi ulnaris muscle (Fig. 15-9)

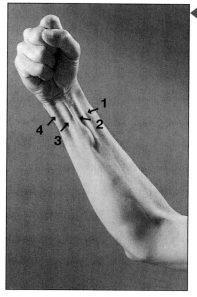

◄ **FIGURE 15-1**

GENERAL PRESENTATION OF THE TENDONS OF THE ANTERIOR ASPECT OF THE WRIST

(1) Tendon of the flexor carpi radialis muscle

(2) Tendon of the palmaris longus muscle

(3) Flexor digitorum superficialis muscle.

(4) Tendon for the ring finger

(5) Tendon of the flexor carpi ulnaris muscle

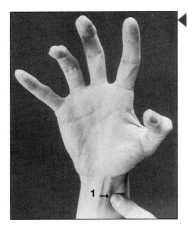

◄ FIGURE 15-2
THE TENDON OF THE FLEXOR POLLICIS LONGUS MUSCLE

Place a uni- or bidigital grip just lateral to the tendon of the flexor carpi radialis muscle (1) (Fig. 15-3). Ask the subject to perform brief, repeated flexions of the distal phalanx of the thumb and you will feel the muscular structure under your grip.

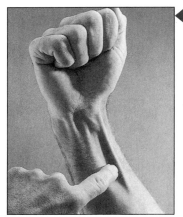

◄ FIGURE 15-3
THE TENDON OF THE FLEXOR CARPI RADIALIS MUSCLE

This tendon appears at the lateral aspect of the anterior surface of the wrist while the subject clenches the fist (the tendon is indicated by the index finger). It is located just lateral to the palmaris longus muscle (see Fig. 15-4). If this structure is not sufficiently visible, ask the subject to flex and abduct (radial deviation) the wrist together with a slight pronation of the forearm.

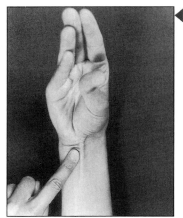

◄ FIGURE 15-4
THE TENDON OF THE PALMARIS LONGUS MUSCLE

This muscle may be absent. Ask the subject to oppose the thumb and the little finger to make this tendon protrude in the middle of the anterior aspect of the wrist. It is located medial to the flexor carpi radialis muscle (Fig. 15-3) and lateral to the flexor digitorum superficialis tendon for the ring finger (Figs. 15-5 through 15-8).

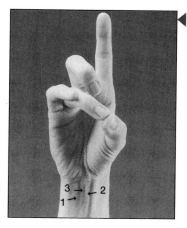

◀ FIGURE 15-5
THE FLEXOR DIGITORUM SUPERFICIALIS MUSCLE — THE TENDON
FOR THE FOURTH FINGER

This tendon (1) appears medial to the tendon of the palmaris longus muscle (2) (Fig. 15-4) while the subject clenches the fist. If the structure of interest is not visible, ask the subject to oppose the thumb and the ring finger, possibly along with a palmar flexion of the wrist, to help you locate this tendon.

Comment: In this figure, the tendon for the middle finger (3) of the flexor digitorum superficialis muscle is directly visible, which is an exception.

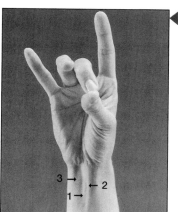

◀ FIGURE 15-6
THE FLEXOR DIGITORUM SUPERFICIALIS MUSCLE — THE TENDON
FOR THE THIRD FINGER

This tendon (1) is palpable behind the tendon of the palmaris longus muscle (2) (see Fig. 15-4) and lateral to the tendon of the flexor digitorum superficialis muscle for the ring finger (3) (Fig. 15-5). To help you find this tendon, ask the subject to oppose the thumb and the middle finger along with a palmar flexion of the wrist.

Comment: Be careful not to damage the median nerve (see also Fig. 16-3), which is very close.

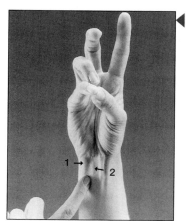

◀ FIGURE 15-7
THE FLEXOR DIGITORUM SUPERFICIALIS MUSCLE — THE TENDON
FOR THE FIFTH FINGER

This muscle is located in the groove indicated by the index finger, between the tendon of the flexor carpi ulnaris muscle (1) (see also Fig. 15-9) medially and the tendon of the flexor digitorum superficialis muscle for the ring finger (2) laterally and in front (see also Fig. 15-5). Ask the subject to oppose the thumb and the little finger so that you can better feel this structure.

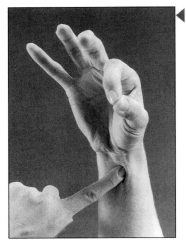

FIGURE 15-8
THE FLEXOR DIGITORUM SUPERFICIALIS MUSCLE — THE TENDON FOR THE INDEX FINGER

The tendon for the index finger is the most difficult to find. It is accessible either by pushing the palmaris longus muscle laterally, as shown in this figure, or by searching between the palmaris longus muscle (see also Fig. 15-4) and the tendon of the flexor carpi radialis muscle (Fig. 15-3). Ask the subject to oppose the thumb and the index finger so that you can better feel this structure.

Comment: Be careful not to damage the median nerve (see also Fig. 16-3), which is very close.

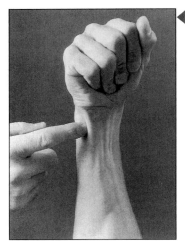

FIGURE 15-9
THE TENDON OF THE FLEXOR CARPI ULNARIS MUSCLE

Ask the subject to perform a slight flexion of the wrist and an ulnar deviation. The tendon of interest appears at the most medial aspect of the anterior surface of the wrist.

THE TENDONS OF THE LATERAL ASPECT OF THE WRIST

The notable structures accessible by palpation are

• The tendon of the abductor pollicis longus muscle (Fig. 15-11)

• The tendon of the extensor pollicis brevis muscle (Fig. 15-12)

• The tendon of the extensor pollicis longus muscle (Fig. 15-13)

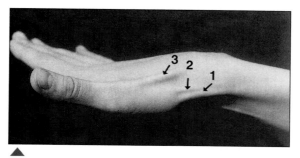

▲

FIGURE 15-10
LATERAL VIEW OF THE WRIST

(1) Tendon of the abductor pollicis longus muscle

(2) Tendon of the extensor pollicis brevis muscle

(3) Tendon of the extensor pollicis longus muscle

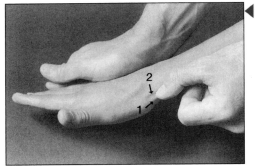

FIGURE 15-11
THE TENDON OF THE ABDUCTOR POLLICIS LONGUS MUSCLE

Place the subject's wrist in a neutral position. In some subjects, this tendon (1) appears at the anterior (or palmar) aspect of the tendon of the extensor pollicis brevis muscle (2) (Fig. 15-12) if they move the thumb away from the hand. To better visualize this muscle, ask the subject to perform a radial deviation of the hand against resistance.

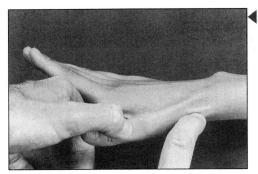

FIGURE 15-12
THE TENDON OF THE EXTENSOR POLLICIS BREVIS MUSCLE

Place the subject's wrist in a neutral position. This tendon usually appears at the lateral surface of the hand, just behind the tendon of the abductor pollicis longus muscle (see Fig. 15-11) if the subject moves the thumb away from the hand.

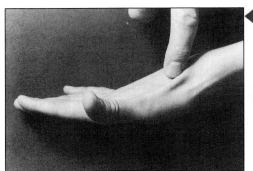

FIGURE 15-13
THE TENDON OF THE EXTENSOR POLLICIS LONGUS MUSCLE

Place the subject's wrist in a neutral position. Ask the subject to move the thumb behind the plane of the hand to make this tendon appear on the posterolateral aspect of the wrist.

THE TENDONS OF THE POSTERIOR ASPECT OF THE WRIST

The notable structures accessible by palpation are

- The tendon of the extensor carpi radialis longus muscle (Fig. 15-15)
- The tendon of the extensor carpi radialis brevis muscle (Fig. 15-16)
- The tendon of the extensor digitorum muscle (Fig. 15-17)
- The tendon of the extensor digiti minimi muscle (Fig. 15-18)
- The tendon of the extensor carpi ulnaris muscle (Fig. 15-19)

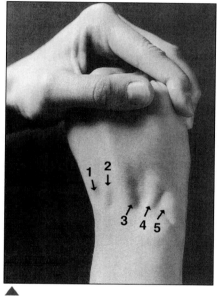

▲
FIGURE 15-14
POSTERIOR VIEW OF THE WRIST

(1) Tendon of the extensor carpi radialis longus muscle

(2) Tendon of the extensor carpi radialis brevis muscle

(3) Tendon of the extensor digitorum muscle

(4) Tendon of the extensor digiti minimi muscle

(5) Tendon of the extensor carpi ulnaris muscle

Comment: For the tendon of the extensor indicis muscle, see Figures 13-24 and 13-25.

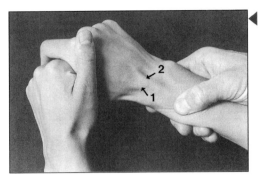

FIGURE 15-15

THE TENDON OF THE EXTENSOR CARPI RADIALIS LONGUS MUSCLE

Sometimes it is sufficient for the subject to clench the fist tightly to allow you to visualize this tendon (1). It is covered by the tendon of the extensor pollicis longus muscle (see Fig. 15-13). Place the subject's thumb on the palm to free the tendon of interest, and resist an extension and a radial deviation of the wrist (as shown in this figure).

Comment: The tendon of the extensor carpi radialis brevis muscle (2) is located medial to the muscle.

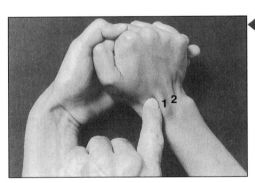

FIGURE 15-16

THE TENDON OF THE EXTENSOR CARPI RADIALIS BREVIS MUSCLE

It is usually sufficient for the subject to clench the fist tightly to let you visualize this tendon (1), which is located lateral to the tendons of the extensor digitorum muscle (2) (Fig. 15-17) and medial to the tendon of the extensor carpi radialis longus muscle (Fig. 15-15).

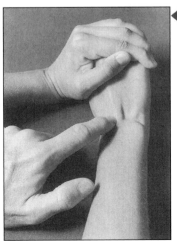

FIGURE 15-17

THE TENDON OF THE EXTENSOR DIGITORUM MUSCLE

Ask the subject to extend the wrist and the metacarpophalangeal joints against resistance. In most cases, this action is sufficient to make the tendon protrude in the middle of the posterior aspect of the wrist. The interphalangeal joints must be kept in flexion.

Comment: This structure consists of the four tendons of the extensor digitorum muscle and the tendon of the extensor indicis muscle, which is located medial to the tendon of the extensor digitorum muscle for the index finger.

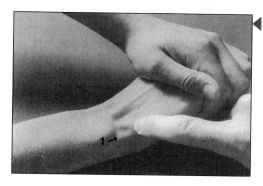

◄ **FIGURE 15-18**
THE TENDON OF THE EXTENSOR DIGITI MINIMI MUSCLE

Ask the subject to extend the wrist and the little finger while you apply resistance. The tendon (indicated by the index finger) appears at the posteromedial aspect of the wrist, lateral to the tendon of the extensor carpi ulnaris muscle (1) (Fig. 15-19).

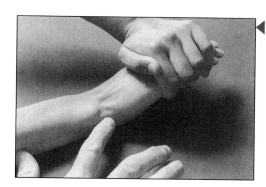

◄ **FIGURE 15-19**
THE TENDON OF THE EXTENSOR CARPI ULNARIS MUSCLE

Ask the subject to perform an ulnar deviation and an extension of the wrist while you apply resistance. The tendon (indicated by the index finger) appears at the posteromedial aspect of the wrist.

THE INTRINSIC MUSCLES OF THE HAND

The notable structures accessible by palpation are

- The thenar eminence (Fig. 15-21)
- The hypothenar eminence (Fig. 15-22)
- The flexor tendons in the palm of the hand (Fig. 15-23)
- The topographic situation of the lumbrical muscles (Fig. 15-24)

- The action of the lumbrical muscles and of the palmar and dorsal interossei muscles (Fig. 15-25)
- The action of the palmar and dorsal interossei muscles (Fig. 15-26)

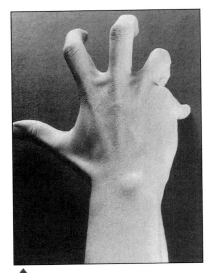

▲
FIGURE 15-20
GENERAL PRESENTATION OF THE
INTRINSIC MUSCLES OF THE HAND

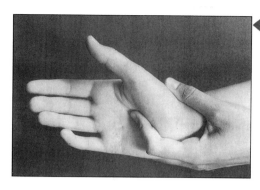

FIGURE 15-21
THE THENAR EMINENCE

This eminence, held between the thumb and the index finger, is centered over the bony "frame" formed by the first two metacarpals. It consists of three muscles arranged in two planes: the superficial plane is formed by the abductor pollicis brevis muscle, and the deep plane is formed by the opponens pollicis muscle and the flexor pollicis brevis muscle.

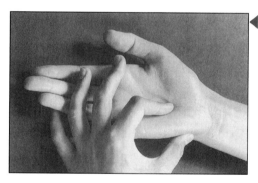

FIGURE 15-22
THE HYPOTHENAR EMINENCE

This region, held between the thumb and the index finger, lies on the fifth metacarpal. It contains four muscles, which are (from superficial to profound) the palmaris brevis muscle, the abductor digiti minimi muscle, the flexor digiti minimi brevis muscle, and the opponens digiti minimi muscle.

Comment: You can palpate the abductor digiti minimi muscle at the ulnar border of the fifth metacarpal if the subject abducts the little finger.

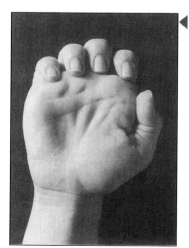

FIGURE 15-23
THE FLEXOR TENDONS IN THE PALM OF THE HAND

This figure demonstrates the tendons of the flexor muscles of the last four fingers in the palm of the hand.

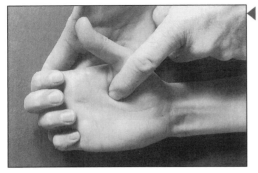

◀ FIGURE 15-24

THE TOPOGRAPHIC SITUATION OF THE LUMBRICAL MUSCLES

In this figure, the index finger pushes away the tendons of the flexor digitorum superficialis and profundus muscles for the index finger and now faces the first lumbrical muscle, which originates from the radial border of the tendon of the flexor digitorum profundus muscle for the index finger.

Comment: The second lumbrical muscle originates from the radial border of the tendon of the flexor digitorum profundus muscle for the middle finger. The third and fourth lumbrical muscles originate from the two tendons of the flexor digitorum profundus muscle of the fingers between which they are located.

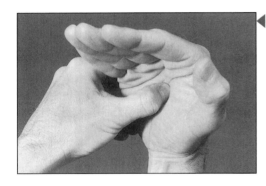

◀ FIGURE 15-25

THE ACTION OF THE LUMBRICAL MUSCLES AND OF THE PALMAR AND DORSAL INTEROSSEI MUSCLES

This group of eleven muscles (see comment for Fig. 15-24) is responsible for the flexion of the metacarpophalangeal joints of the last four fingers and for the extension of the middle and distal phalanges of these fingers (see also Fig. 15-26).

Comment: This group of intrinsic muscles of the hand consists of four lumbrical, three palmar interossei, and four dorsal interossei muscles.

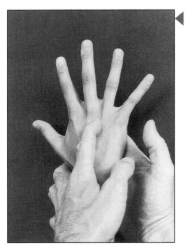

◀ FIGURE 15-26

THE ACTION OF THE PALMAR AND DORSAL INTEROSSEI MUSCLES

In addition to the action described in Figure 15-25, the dorsal interossei muscles are responsible for abducting the fingers and the palmar interossei muscles are responsible for adducting the fingers. The contraction of the interosseous muscles is felt at the dorsal aspect of the intermetacarpal spaces.

CHAPTER
Sixteen

NERVES
AND VESSELS

The notable structures accessible by palpation are

- The radial artery (pulse) at the wrist (Fig. 16-2)
- The median nerve at the anterior aspect of the wrist (Fig. 16-3)

- The ulnar artery (pulse) at the wrist (Fig. 16-4)
- The ulnar nerve at the medial aspect of the anterior surface of the wrist (Fig. 16-5)

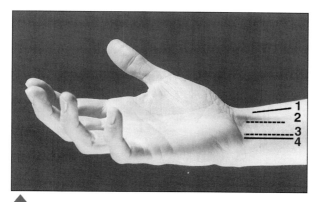

▲

FIGURE 16-1
THE NERVES AND VESSELS AT THE ANTERIOR ASPECT OF THE WRIST

(1) Radial artery
(2) Median nerve
(3) Ulnar nerve
(4) Ulnar artery

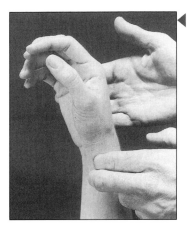

◀ FIGURE 16-2
TAKING THE RADIAL PULSE AT THE WRIST

Place your fingertips at the distal extremity of the anterior surface of the radius, lateral to the tendon of the flexor carpi radialis muscle, to feel the radial artery pulse under your fingers.

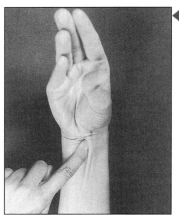

◀ FIGURE 16-3
THE MEDIAN NERVE AT THE ANTERIOR ASPECT OF THE WRIST

In the distal third of the forearm, this nerve is very close to the surface, located just deep to the antebrachial fascia, medial to the tendon of the flexor carpi radialis muscle (Fig. 15-3), lateral to the tendon of the flexor digitorum superficialis muscle for the middle finger (Fig. 15-6), and in front of the tendon of the flexor digitorum superficialis muscle for the index finger (Fig. 15-8). To palpate this nerve, push the tendon of the palmaris longus muscle laterally, as shown in this figure.

Comment: As always when palpating a nerve, be very careful during this examination.

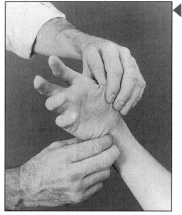

◀ FIGURE 16-4
TAKING THE ULNAR PULSE AT THE WRIST

Place a bidigital grip at the medial aspect of the anterior surface of the wrist, at the level of the palmar cutaneous folds, in contact with the lateral portion of the pisiform (see Figs. 14-24 and 14-25). Place the subject's wrist in slight extension so you can better feel the ulnar artery pulse.

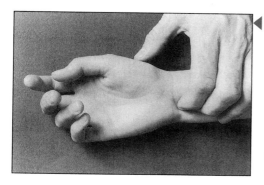

FIGURE 16-5

THE ULNAR NERVE AT THE MEDIAL ASPECT OF THE ANTERIOR SURFACE OF THE WRIST

This nerve is accessible at the lateral border of the tendon of the flexor carpi ulnaris muscle (see Fig. 15-9). It is possible to make this nerve roll on the tendon of the flexor digitorum superficialis muscle for the little finger (see Fig. 15-7).

Comment: As always when palpating a nerve, be very careful during this examination.

LOWER

EXTREMITIES

THE HIP

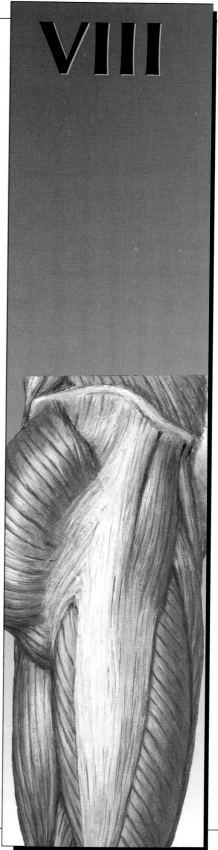

MUSCLES OF THE HIP: LATERAL VIEW

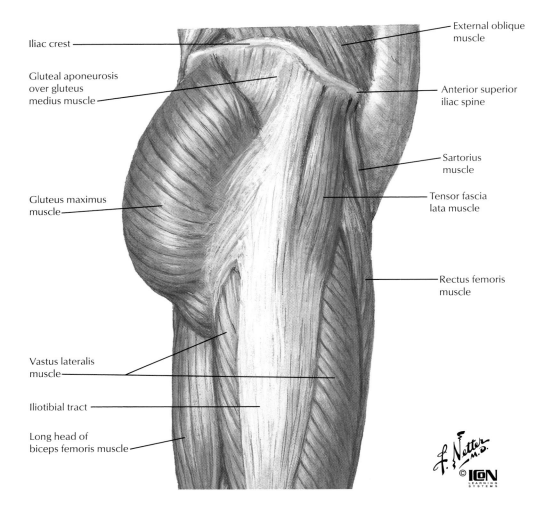

Iliac crest

Gluteal aponeurosis over gluteus medius muscle

Gluteus maximus muscle

Vastus lateralis muscle

Iliotibial tract

Long head of biceps femoris muscle

External oblique muscle

Anterior superior iliac spine

Sartorius muscle

Tensor fascia lata muscle

Rectus femoris muscle

MUSCLES OF THE HIP: POSTERIOR VIEW

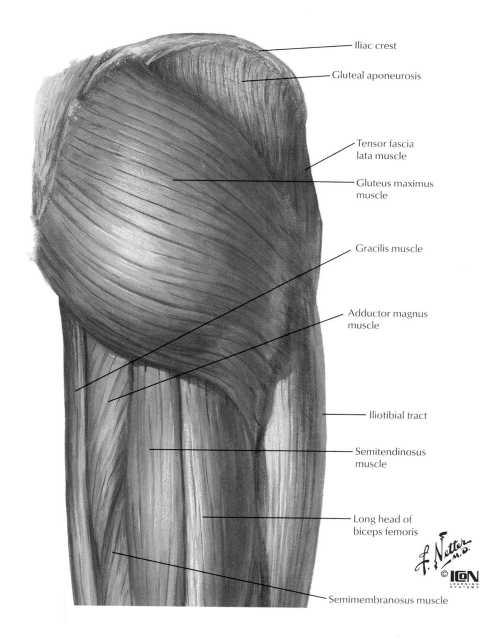

Iliac crest

Gluteal aponeurosis

Tensor fascia lata muscle

Gluteus maximus muscle

Gracilis muscle

Adductor magnus muscle

Iliotibial tract

Semitendinosus muscle

Long head of biceps femoris

Semimembranosus muscle

TOPOGRAPHIC PRESENTATION OF THE HIP

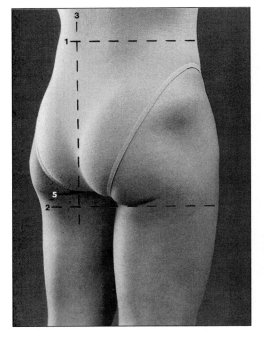

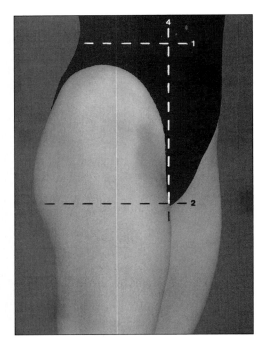

FIGURE 17-1
POSTEROLATERAL VIEW

(1) Superior border
(2) Inferior border
(3) Posteromedial border
(5) Gluteal fold

FIGURE 17-2
ANTEROLATERAL VIEW

(1) Superior border
(2) Inferior border
(4) Anteromedial border

CHAPTER
Seventeen OSTEOLOGY

THE ILIOFEMORAL REGION

The bony structures accessible by palpation are

• The iliac bone
— the iliac crest (Fig. 17-4)
— the anterosuperior iliac spine (Fig. 17-5)
— the tubercle of the iliac crest (Fig. 17-6)
— the pubic tubercle (Fig. 17-7)
— the posterosuperior iliac spine (Fig. 17-8)
— the small "coxal notch" (Fig. 17-9) and the posteroinferior iliac spine
— the ischial spine and the lesser sciatic notch (Fig. 17-10)

— the greater sciatic notch (Fig. 17-11)
— the ischial tuberosity (Fig. 17-12)
— the inferior border of the iliac bone (Fig. 17-13)

• The femur
— the femoral head (Figs. 17-14, 17-15, and 17-16)
— the greater trochanter (Figs. 17-17 and 17-18)
— the lesser trochanter (Figs. 17-19 and 17-20)

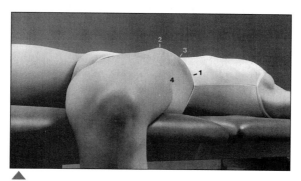

▲
FIGURE 17-3
LOW-ANGLE VIEW OF THE HIP REGION
(The patient is supine; the knee is in the foreground)

Iliac Bone
(1) Iliac crest
(2) Anterosuperior iliac spine
(3) Tubercle of the iliac crest

Femur
(4) Greater trochanter

THE ILIAC BONE

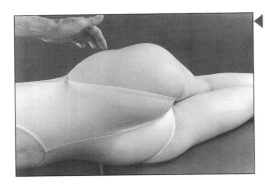

◀ **FIGURE 17-4**
THE ILIAC CREST

It is possible to perceive changes in the curvature of this structure as well as its variations in thickness. To do so, follow it from front to back and from back to front using bidigital palpation or grabbing it between your thumb and index finger.

The crest itself, as well as its lateral and medial "borders," should be followed.

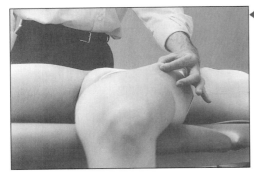

◀ **FIGURE 17-5**
THE ANTEROSUPERIOR ILIAC SPINE

This is easy to access. Begin by finding the precise location of the most anterior part of the iliac crest. Grab this structure between your thumb and index finger to delineate it clearly.

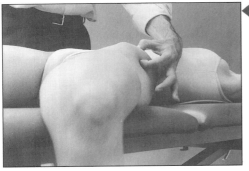

◀ **FIGURE 17-6**
THE TUBERCLE OF THE ILIAC CREST

Located on top of the anterior curvature, this structure projects toward the external iliac fossa. Follow the iliac crest from front to back between your thumb and index finger in order to perceive the thickening of the superior border of the bone.

Comment: In this photograph, the digital grip is positioned facing the investigated structure, which is palpated by the index finger.

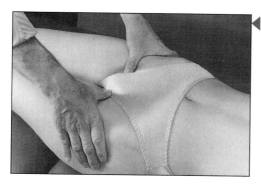

FIGURE 17-7
THE PUBIC TUBERCLE

With your hands laid flat at the level of the greater trochanter bilaterally, your thumbs move horizontally and medially, searching across the pubic region (the mons veneris) for a spine-shaped bony prominence (the pubic tubercle). This is located over the most medial part of the horizontal ramus of the pubis, next to the symphysis pubis and more precisely at the junction of the "pectineal crest" and the anterior lip of the "subpubic groove."

Comment: In male subjects, be careful with the spermatic cord during this examination.

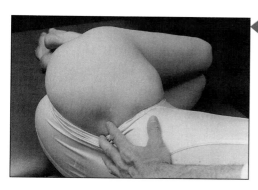

FIGURE 17-8
THE POSTEROSUPERIOR ILIAC SPINE

This structure, which faces the sacroiliac joint, corresponds to a more or less visible dimple.

It can also be demonstrated by finding the most posterior segment of the iliac crest and following it to its junction with the posterior border of the iliac bone. The latter is characterized by a slight depression representing the small "coxal notch."

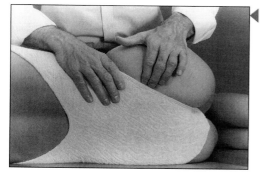

FIGURE 17-9
THE SMALL COXAL NOTCH AND
THE POSTEROINFERIOR ILIAC SPINE

The Small Coxal Notch

The small coxal notch is located between the posterosuperior iliac spine and the posteroinferior iliac spine at approximately two fingers' breadth from the latter. By moving the pelvis forward and back, this structure is more easily found.

The Posteroinferior Iliac Spine

A bidigital grip, positioned approximately two fingers' breadth from the posterosuperior iliac spine, determines its localization. It is better felt when the pelvis is alternately moved forward and back.

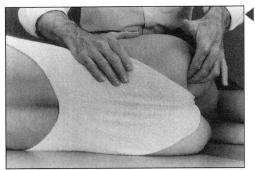

◀ **FIGURE 17-10**
THE ISCHIAL SPINE AND THE LESSER SCIATIC NOTCH

The Ischial Spine

With the subject lying on his or her side and the hip in flexion, locate the ischial tuberosity and move upward to the lesser sciatic notch, using a digital grip.

Then, apply your grip against the ischial tuberosity and slide it into the lesser sciatic notch without losing the pressure point on the skin (by this maneuver, the skin will slide on top of the underlying tissues). The ischial spine is located at the proximal end of this notch.

Comment: The gluteus maximus muscle must be relaxed.

The Lesser Sciatic Notch

The ischial tuberosity must first be located using a bidigital grip (see Fig. 17-12).

The depression palpated above the tuberosity, toward the sacrum, is the lesser sciatic notch.

Comment: This structure is located between the ischial spine and the ischial tuberosity. The gluteus maximus muscle must be relaxed. It is sometimes preferable to leave the hip in a much less flexed position than shown in this picture. This allows better penetration of the grip through the mass of the gluteal muscle, which becomes less tense.

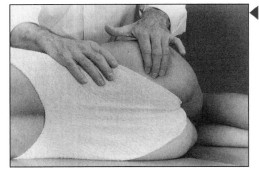

◀ **FIGURE 17-11**
THE GREATER SCIATIC NOTCH

First, locate the posteroinferior iliac spine using bidigital palpation. Lean on the external structure of the ilium. Then move your grip backward toward the greater ischial notch and the lateral border of the sacrum.

Comment: This structure, wide and deep, is located between the posteroinferior iliac spine and the ischial spine. It is examined through the muscular mass of the gluteus maximus muscle and is therefore difficult to access.

Keep in mind that its concavity is posterior and that the piriformis muscle, as well as the great ischial nerve, passes through it. The examination must be carried out accordingly.

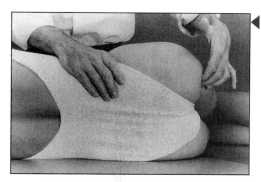

◀ **FIGURE 17-12**
THE ISCHIAL TUBEROSITY

This structure is oval with a large posterosuperior end; its narrow inferior end extends from the inferior border of the iliac bone. Flexion of the hip clears it from the gluteus maximus muscle.

It is also possible to palpate this structure with the subject prone. It is then found in the middle of the cutaneous landmark formed by the gluteal fold.

Comment: Most of the time, in sitting, one sits on the ischial tuberosities.

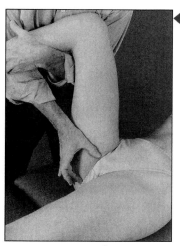

◀ **FIGURE 17-13**
THE INFERIOR BORDER OF THE ILIAC BONE

Locate the ischial tuberosity (Fig. 17-12) and the most anterior and medial part of the descending ramus of the pubis.

The inferior border of the iliac bone is easily accessible between these two bony structures.

THE FEMUR

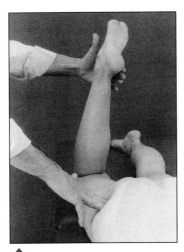

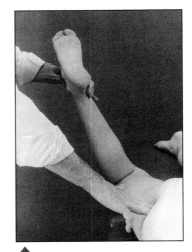

▲
FIGURE 17-14
POSTERIOR APPROACH TO THE FEMORAL HEAD

▲
FIGURE 17-15

The hip is mobilized by rotating it medially in order to push the femoral head posteriorly. The head is accessible through the muscular mass of the gluteus maximus between the greater trochanter and the lateral surface of the iliac bone.

For improved palpation of the head beneath your fingers, rotate the hip several times.

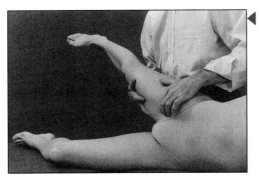

◄ **FIGURE 17-16**
ANTERIOR APPROACH TO THE FEMORAL HEAD

With the subject lying on his or her side, stand behind the subject and stabilize the pelvis with your hip (in the anteroposterior plane).

Place your proximal hand on the anterolateral aspect of the hip and grip its anterior aspect, using your finger and thumb.

Your distal hand supports the anteromedial aspect of the thigh as you slowly bring the limb into extension (stabilizing the pelvis with your hip).

The fingers of your proximal hand will gradually feel the femoral head, which is a density projecting forward.

Comment: During this mobilization, you can feel the pulse of the femoral artery, which is pushed forward by the femoral head.

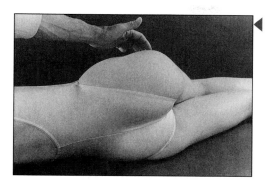

FIGURE 17-17
APPROACH TO THE GREATER TROCHANTER
WITH THE SUBJECT LYING ON HIS OR HER SIDE

In this position, the greater trochanter projects on the lateral aspect of the hip.

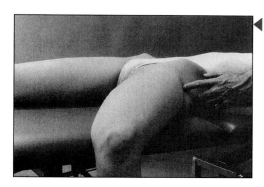

FIGURE 17-18
APPROACH TO THE GREATER TROCHANTER
WITH THE SUBJECT SUPINE

In the supine position, with the lower extremity in slight abduction, the greater trochanter is accessible in the skin depression created by the hip abduction. This position also allows optimal relaxation of the surrounding muscles, facilitating access to the different parts of the greater trochanter, including the superior border, inferior border, anterior border, posterior border, and lateral surface.

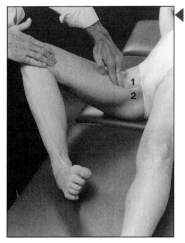

◀ **FIGURE 17-19**
**THE LESSER TROCHANTER: STEP 1 — DEMONSTRATE
THE DEPRESSION BETWEEN THE ADDUCTOR LONGUS
MUSCLE (1) AND THE GRACILIS MUSCLE (2)**

In this figure, you can see the gracilis muscle (2) in a posteromedial position.

With the subject supine, the hip and knee are flexed. As you proceed, you must resist a movement of adduction. The goal of this technique is to demonstrate these two muscular structures, between which you can make direct contact with the lesser trochanter.

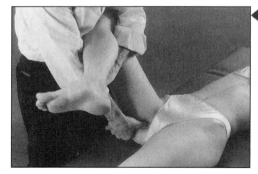

◀ **FIGURE 17-20**
THE LESSER TROCHANTER: STEP 2 — MAKE DIRECT CONTACT

The dorsal aspect of your one hand supports the lateral aspect of the leg and allows a forward movement of the lesser trochanter through an external rotation of the hip. The thumb of your other hand then slides through the soft tissues between the adductor longus and gracilis muscles, looking for a somewhat sensitive density.

CHAPTER
Eighteen

MYOLOGY

THE LATERAL INGUINOFEMORAL REGION

Triangular, with its apex proximal, this region is defined by

- The apex (proximal), formed by the anterosuperior iliac spine
- The lateral border, formed by the tensor fascia lata muscle (Fig. 18-2)
- The medial border, formed by the sartorius muscle (Fig. 18-4)

- The floor of this triangular space, formed by the rectus femoris muscle (Fig. 18-3), the proximal end of which infiltrates between the two muscles mentioned above

Comment: The muscles delineating this region belong to the topographic region of the thigh.

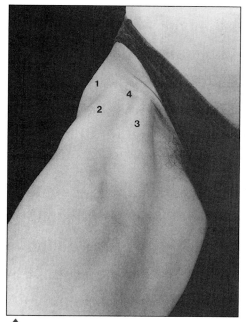

▲
FIGURE 18-1
ANTEROMEDIAL VIEW

(1) Gluteus medius muscle

(2) Tensor muscle of the fascia lata

(3) Sartorius muscle

(4) Rectus femoris muscle

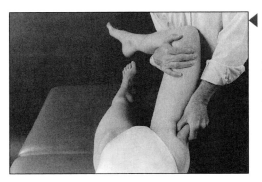

FIGURE 18-2
TENSOR MUSCLE OF THE FASCIA LATA

A resistance placed against the anteromedial aspect of the thigh in flexion demonstrates two muscles in the proximal part of the thigh. The most lateral one is the tensor fascia lata.

This muscle is located between the anterosuperior iliac spine and the greater trochanter.

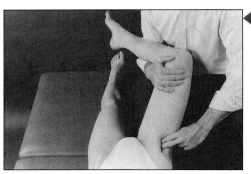

FIGURE 18-3
THE RECTUS FEMORIS MUSCLE

The most proximal portion of this muscle is found in the depression between the tensor muscle of the fascia lata laterally and the sartorius muscle medially.

Even in its relaxed state, the proximal aspect of this muscle can be palpated easily. If you request an extension of the knee, the muscular fibers will be more readily palpable.

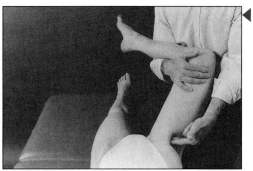

FIGURE 18-4
THE SARTORIUS MUSCLE

The technique here is similar to that used to palpate the tensor muscle of the fascia lata. The sartorius muscle corresponds to the most medial muscle mass demonstrated in the proximal portion of the thigh. The anterosuperior iliac spine is the bony landmark, since this muscle originates from it.

Comment: The sartorius muscle forms the medial border of the lateral inguinofemoral region. It is also the lateral border of the medial inguinofemoral region or femoral triangle.

THE MEDIAL INGUINOFEMORAL REGION OR FEMORAL TRIANGLE

Triangular, with an inferior apex, this region, called Scarpa's triangle, is delimited by

- The base (proximal), formed by the inguinal ligament; it joins the anterosuperior iliac spine and the pubic tubercle
- The lateral border, formed by the sartorius muscle (Fig. 18-4)
- The medial border, formed by the adductor longus muscle (Fig. 18-6)

- The apex (distal) (Fig. 18-5), formed by the junction between the sartorius and the adductor longus muscles (Fig. 18-6)
- The floor, formed medially by the pectineus muscles (Fig. 18-7) and laterally by the iliopsoas muscle (Fig. 18-8). This muscular mass forms a concave groove in which the neurovascular bundle of the lower limb lies

Comment: The sartorius, adductor longus, and pectineus muscles belong to the thigh region.

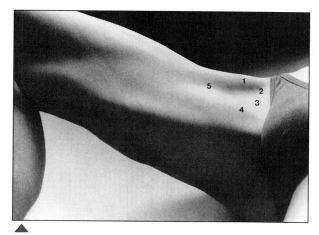

▲
FIGURE 18-5
MEDIAL VIEW

(1) Tartorius muscle

(2) Iliopsoas muscle

(3) Pectineus muscle

(4) Adductor longus muscle

(5) Apex of Scarpa's triangle, the junction point between the sartorius and adductor longus muscles

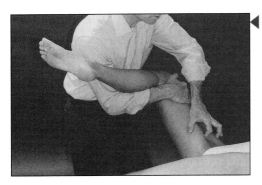

FIGURE 18-6
THE ADDUCTOR LONGUS MUSCLE

With the hip and knee in flexion, the lower extremity is abducted and your hand supports the lower thigh. Resistance against a movement of adduction demonstrates the adductor longus muscle, which appears at the superomedial aspect of the thigh.

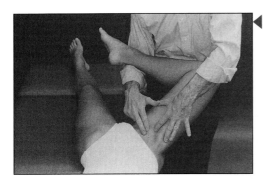

FIGURE 18-7
THE PECTINEUS MUSCLE

This muscle is found in the depression just lateral to the adductor longus muscle. It forms the medial aspect of the floor of Scarpa's triangle.

In this figure, the sartorius muscle is shown between the index and the middle fingers of the left hand (resisting the flexion and the adduction of the hip). The other hand shows the pectineus muscle.

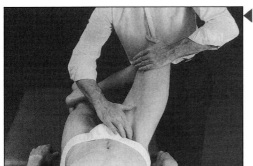

FIGURE 18-8
THE ILIOPSOAS MUSCLE IN ITS DISTAL ASPECT

Your grip must be placed medial to the proximal course of the sartorius muscle, close to its insertion on the anterosuperior iliac spine. The iliopsoas muscle is accessible at this level since it reflects on the iliopectineal surface, covering, beyond this reflection, the anterior aspect of the femoral joint. It is lined medially by the pectineus muscle. When it is placed under tension (as you resist hip flexion with your distal hand), you can palpate this muscle's contracting fibers at the level of the "iliopectineal process."

Comment: This region is sensitive and should be approached with care.

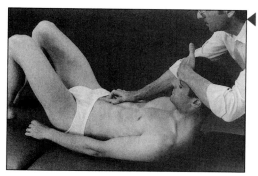

◄ **FIGURE 18-9**

THE ILIOPSOAS MUSCLE IN ITS PROXIMAL PORTION:
STEP 1 — FIND THE LANDMARKS

Resistance placed against the subject's forehead allows the abdominal muscles and therefore the lateral border of the rectus abdominis muscle to protrude. Your thumb is placed on the umbilicus and the middle finger on the anterosuperior iliac spine. Your index finger is placed in the mid portion of this line, at the lateral border of the rectus abdominis muscle.

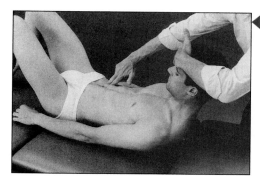

◄ **FIGURE 18-10**

THE ILIOPSOAS MUSCLE IN ITS PROXIMAL PORTION — STEP 2

The lateral border of the rectus abdominis muscle, as shown, is the optimal point at which to approach the iliopsoas muscle.

The subject's head is allowed to lie on a pillow in order to relax the abdominal muscles. You may change position and stand at the level of the subject's hip in order to perform the examination. It is essential to examine the abdominal muscles with caution and in a stepwise fashion in order to prevent guarding of the abdominal wall.

By actively flexing the subject's hip, you will create muscular tension and obtain a better idea of the structures examined.

Comment:This figure demonstrates the starting point for the examination and not the technique of palpation.

THE GLUTEAL REGION

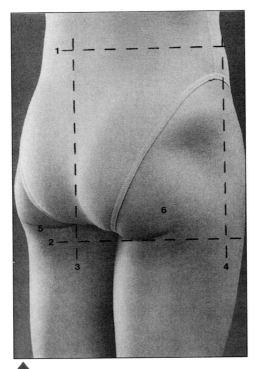

▲
FIGURE 18-11
POSTEROLATERAL VIEW

(1) Superior border: iliac crest

(2) Inferior border: gluteal fold

(3) Medial border: iliac crest and, following, the coccyx

(4) Lateral border: this is an imaginary vertical line starting at the anterosuperior iliac spine and extending downward to the level of the greater trochanter, where it joins the lateralmost aspect of the gluteal fold or its continuation

Comment: This imaginary line is noteworthy as it lines up more or less with the posterior border of the tensor muscle of the fascia lata.

(5) Gluteal fold

(6) Gluteus maximus muscle

SUPERFICIAL PLANE

The superficial plane of the gluteal region is represented by a single muscle: the gluteus maximus (Fig. 18-13).

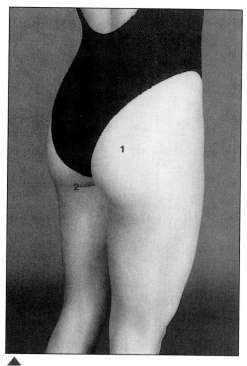

▲
FIGURE 18-12
THE GLUTEUS MAXIMUS MUSCLE

Posterolateral view
(1) Gluteus maximus muscle
(2) Gluteal fold

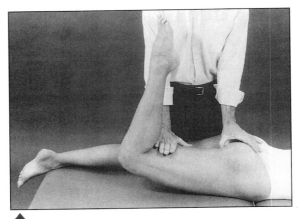

▲
FIGURE 18-13
THE GLUTEUS MAXIMUS MUSCLE

The technique demonstrated above allows visualization of the gluteus maximus muscle.

The iliac crest, the greater trochanter, and the ischial tuberosity are the essential bony landmarks surrounding the gluteal region.

The gluteal fold, which has an essentially horizontal course, corresponds approximately with the inferior border of this muscle, which follows an oblique course downward and laterally.

The subject is asked to lift the anterior aspect of the thigh off the table, keeping the knee flexed and without any compensation at the level of the lumbar region. Place resistance against the inferoposterior aspect of the thigh to prevent prompting of the knee, allowing the muscular mass to project and demonstrate the quality of the contraction as compared with that of the contralateral muscle.

Comment: The flexion of the knee, by shortening the hamstring muscles, favors the activity of the gluteus maximus muscle (i.e., extension of the hip).

MIDDLE PLANE

The middle plane of the gluteal region is represented by a single muscle: the gluteus medius (Figs. 18-15 and 18-16).

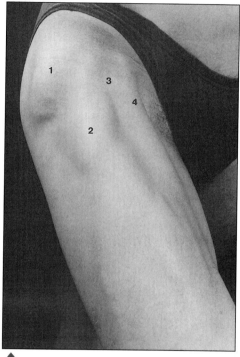

▲
FIGURE 18-14
ANTEROLATERAL VIEW OF THE HIP

(1) Gluteus medius muscle
(2) Tensor muscle of the fascia lata
(3) Rectus femoris muscle
(4) Sartorius muscle

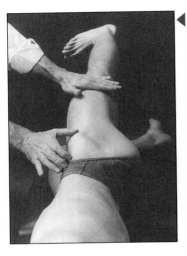

◀ **FIGURE 18-15**
THE GLUTEUS MEDIUS MUSCLE

The essential bony landmarks are the anterior part of the iliac crest and the superior border of the greater trochanter.

Place your hands as illustrated and ask the subject to abduct against resistance; the muscular body will tighten between your fingers.

With the hip in abduction, ask the subject to perform rapid, consecutive internal rotations of the hip in order to mobilize the anterior fibers of the gluteus medius muscle more specifically. This movement also mobilizes the gluteus minimus muscle. In any event, this additional movement improves digital perception of the muscular body.

Comment: The hand creating the resistance should be placed against the lateral and inferior portion of the thigh, just above the knee (in order to prevent prompting of the knee).

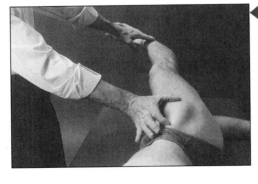

◀ **FIGURE 18-16**
TECHNIQUE TO DISTINGUISH THE GLUTEUS MEDIUS MUSCLE FROM THE TENSOR MUSCLE OF THE FASCIA LATA

From the same position, the subject should be asked to flex the hip slightly (with some guidance), keeping it in abduction, so that you may demonstrate the muscular body of the tensor muscle of the fascia lata between your fingers.

Comment: The vertical imaginary line drawn from the anterosuperior iliac spine to the greater trochanter, which delimits the gluteal region (Fig. 18-11) anteriorly, represents the posterior border of the tensor muscle of the fascia lata, which extends inferiorly onto the anterior part of the thigh (see also Fig. 18-14).

DEEP PLANE

The deep plane of the gluteal region includes

- The gluteus minimus muscle (Fig. 18-18)
- The piriformis muscle (Figs. 18-19 through 18-22)
- The inferior and superior gemellus muscles (Fig. 18-23)
- The obturator medialis muscle (Fig. 18-23)
- The quadratus femoris muscle (Fig. 18-24)
- The obturator lateralis muscle (Fig. 18-25)

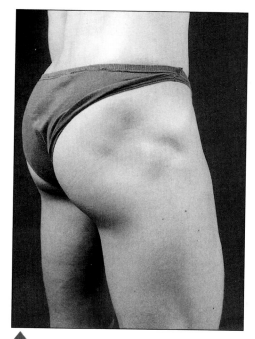

▲

FIGURE 18-17
POSTEROLATERAL VIEW OF THE HIP

Comment: The gluteus minimus muscle can be approached only through the muscular body of the gluteus medius muscle (Fig. 18-14). The other muscles of the deep plane can be approached only through the gluteus maximus muscle (1) (Fig. 18-17).

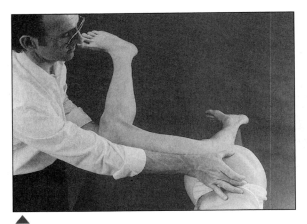

▲
FIGURE 18-18
THE GLUTEUS MINIMUS MUSCLE

Place your proximal palpating hand between the superior border of the greater trochanter and the most anterior part of the iliac crest, between the tubercle of the gluteus medius muscle and the anterosuperior iliac spine.

In this position, your thumb, opposed by the other fingers of your hand, straddles the gluteus minimus muscle, which is located under the gluteus medius muscle. Your distal hand supports the medial aspect of the knee and leg.

From this original position (hip and knee flexed at 90°), the subject is asked to perform an internal rotation of the hip. Practically speaking, the leg will be mobilized upward. A muscular mass corresponding to the gluteus medius and gluteus minimus muscles will move beneath your fingers.

Comment: Only the muscle's contraction is perceptible beneath your fingers. Direct access to the muscle is not possible, since it is covered by the anterior fibers of the gluteus medius muscle, which have the same actions as those of the gluteus minimus muscle.

The piriformis muscle is approached in three steps:

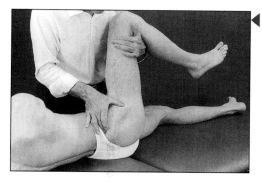

◀ **FIGURE 18-19**
**STEP 1 — LOCATE THE GLUTEUS MEDIUS MUSCLE
AND THE DEPRESSION AT THE BOTTOM OF IT,
FROM WHICH THE PIRIFORMIS MUSCLE IS APPROACHED**

The subject is placed on his or her side. With one support-ing hand, bring the limb to be examined against your shoul-der or chest. From this position, ask the subject to abduct against resistance horizontally. This muscular action allows the gluteus medius muscle to protrude.

Comment: Interestingly, this step demonstrates both the poste-rior border of this muscle as well as the depression that follows posteriorly, at the bottom of which is the piriformis muscle.

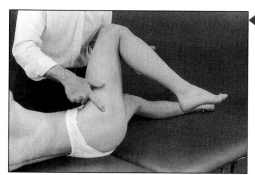

◀ **FIGURE 18-20**
STEP 2 — LOCATE THE GREATER TROCHANTER

The subject is placed on his or her side. With the subject's knee flexed, your distal hand grabs the medial aspect of the leg and knee in order to mobilize the hip in all planes, there-by demonstrating the greater trochanter. Refer also to Chapter 1, "Osteology," for more details about this structure.

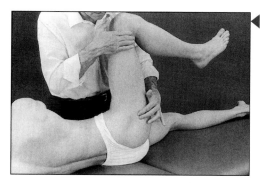

◀ **FIGURE 18-21**
**STEP 3 — LOCATE THE SUPEROLATERAL BORDER
OF THE GREATER TROCHANTER, THE INSERTION POINT
OF THE PIRIFORMIS MUSCLE**

While your one hand resists a horizontal abduction of the hip, your other hand is placed in the distal part of the demonstrated depression, in contact with the greater trochanter.

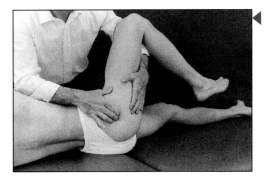

FIGURE 18-22
THE PIRIFORMIS MUSCLE

The subject's hip is flexed at 45° and the knee at 90°. Your proximal hand is placed on the upper part of the posterior border of the greater trochanter, at its junction with the superior border and in contact with the posterior border of the gluteus medius muscle. To appreciate the latter, ask the subject to rotate the hip internally or abduct it horizontally. Better yet, these two movements can be combined or alternated. A depression originating from the posterosuperior angle of the greater trochanter and extending toward the iliac crest will take shape under the skin and indicate the posterior border of the gluteus medius muscle through the anterior fibers of the gluteus maximus muscle.

The limb should be palpated through a perfectly relaxed gluteus maximus muscle, toward the greater sciatic notch and the lateral border of the sacrum, by following the posterior border of the gluteus medius muscle, as demonstrated previously.

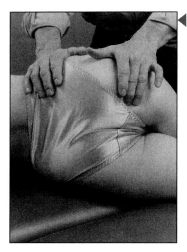

FIGURE 18-23
THE INFERIOR AND SUPERIOR GEMELLUS MUSCLES AND THE OBTURATOR MEDIALIS MUSCLE

A bidigital grip at the level of the lesser sciatic notch makes it possible to palpate these muscles through the mass of the gluteus maximus muscle.

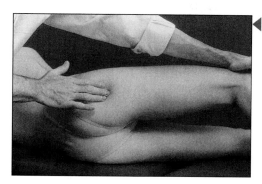

FIGURE 18-24
THE QUADRATUS FEMORIS MUSCLE

Direct examination of this muscle is not possible, since it is located under the gluteus maximus muscle.

The essential bony landmarks are the ischial tuberosity medially and the greater trochanter laterally.

The essential muscular landmark is the inferior border of the gluteus maximus muscle.

With the subject lying on his or her side and the hip slightly flexed, resistance is applied to the lateral aspect of the knee against an external rotation and abduction of the hip. The body of the muscle will tighten beneath your fingers through the mass of the gluteus maximus muscle (which should be perfectly relaxed) over its inferior aspect and between the bony landmarks described previously. The palpation is difficult in the normal subject.

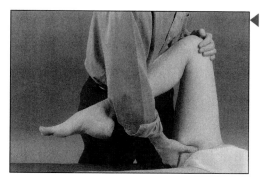

FIGURE 18-25
THE OBTURATOR LATERALIS MUSCLE

The subject's knee and hip are flexed at 90°. The thumb of your palpating hand is placed between the adductor longus and gracilis muscles (see Fig. 17-19). Your right arm applies resistance against an external rotation of the hip while you ask the subject to perform a sequence of contractions and relaxations. This muscular action tenses the muscle of interest, as perceived beneath your thumb. The other hand also supports the limb.

NERVES
AND VESSLES

THE MEDIAL INGUINOFEMORAL REGION
OR SCARPA'S TRIANGLE

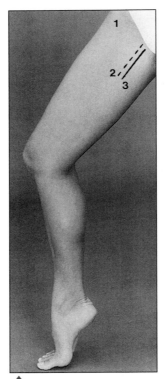

▲

FIGURE 19-1
MEDIAL VIEW OF THE THIGH

(1) Sartorius muscle
(2) Femoral nerve
(3) Femoral artery

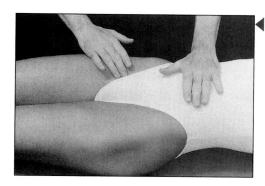

FIGURE 19-2
THE FEMORAL ARTERY

Perform a bidigital palpation with slight compression along the artery, in the middle of an imaginary line drawn between the anterosuperior iliac spine and the pubic tubercle. The arterial pulse will be better perceived with the hip in a neutral position or slight extension.

Note: Over the medial aspect of the artery, you may perceive superficial small round structures. These represent superficial inguinal lymph nodes.

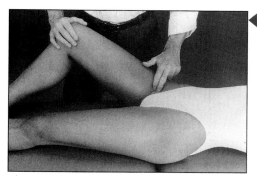

FIGURE 19-3
THE FEMORAL NERVE — STEP 1

As for the examination of the femoral pulse, the first maneuver is to perform a bidigital palpation in the middle of an imaginary line drawn between the anterosuperior iliac spine and the pubic tubercle.

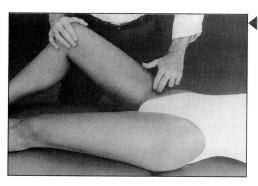

FIGURE 19-4
THE FEMORAL NERVE — STEP 2

In this step, your grip should be moved laterally by one finger's breadth toward the sartorius muscle so that it is positioned on top of the investigated structure. This should be approached carefully with a digital "claw type" grip, as shown in the figure, and with the caution required for this type of structure. The nerve is palpated beneath your fingers as a full cylindrical cord.

THE GLUTEAL REGION

THE GREATER SCIATIC NERVE

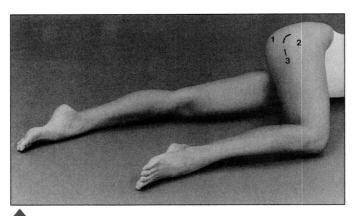

▲
FIGURE 19-5
LATERAL VIEW OF THE GLUTEAL REGION

(1) Ischial tuberosity
(2) Greater trochanter
(3) Sciatic nerve

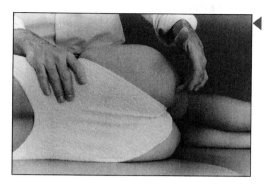

FIGURE 19-6
LOCATING THE GREATER SCIATIC NERVE: STEP 1 —
DEMONSTRATE THE ISCHIAL TUBEROSITY

In this position, where the hip is flexed, the ischial tuberosity is normally cleared from the gluteus maximus muscle. A bidigital grip (middle and ring fingers) should be placed over it.

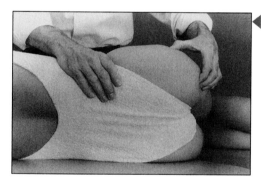

FIGURE 19-7
LOCATING THE GREATER SCIATIC NERVE: STEP 2 —
DEMONSTRATE THE GREATER TROCHANTER

While you maintain the previous grip (Fig. 19-6), your thumb is positioned over the greater trochanter.

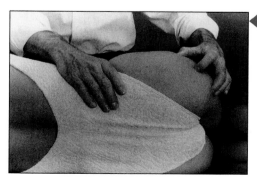

FIGURE 19-8
LOCATING THE GREATER SCIATIC NERVE — STEP 3

Imagine a line drawn between the two demonstrated bony structures. Place your index finger approximately in the middle. This is where the greater sciatic nerve normally lies.

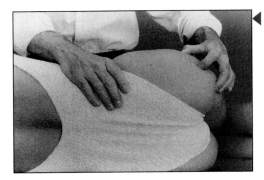

FIGURE 19-9
THE GREATER SCIATIC NERVE — STEP 4

At this level, the nerve's diameter is approximately one fingerbreadth. It should be approached transversely and cautiously with a bidigital grip.

Comment: The nerve is accessible only if the subject's morphology will allow for it and only through a perfectly relaxed gluteus maximus muscle. In that case, a full cylindrical cord is palpated under the fingers.

THE
THIGH

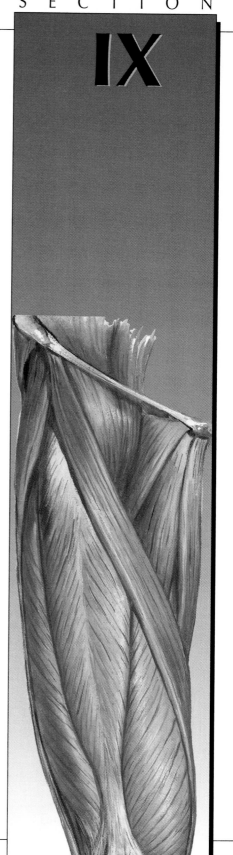

MUSCLES OF THE THIGH: ANTERIOR VIEW

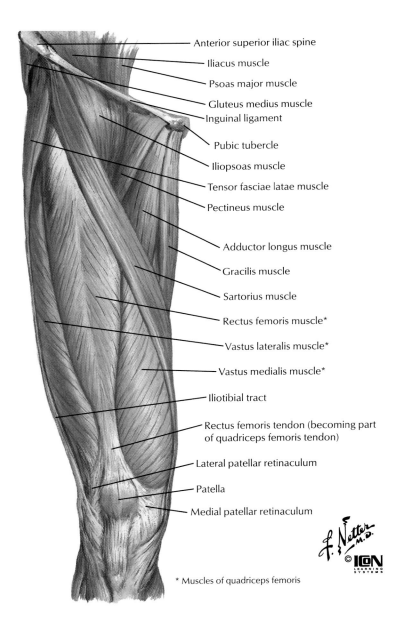

Anterior superior iliac spine

Iliacus muscle

Psoas major muscle

Gluteus medius muscle

Inguinal ligament

Pubic tubercle

Iliopsoas muscle

Tensor fasciae latae muscle

Pectineus muscle

Adductor longus muscle

Gracilis muscle

Sartorius muscle

Rectus femoris muscle*

Vastus lateralis muscle*

Vastus medialis muscle*

Iliotibial tract

Rectus femoris tendon (becoming part of quadriceps femoris tendon)

Lateral patellar retinaculum

Patella

Medial patellar retinaculum

* Muscles of quadriceps femoris

MUSCLES OF THE THIGH: ANTERIOR VIEW (DEEP DISSECTION)

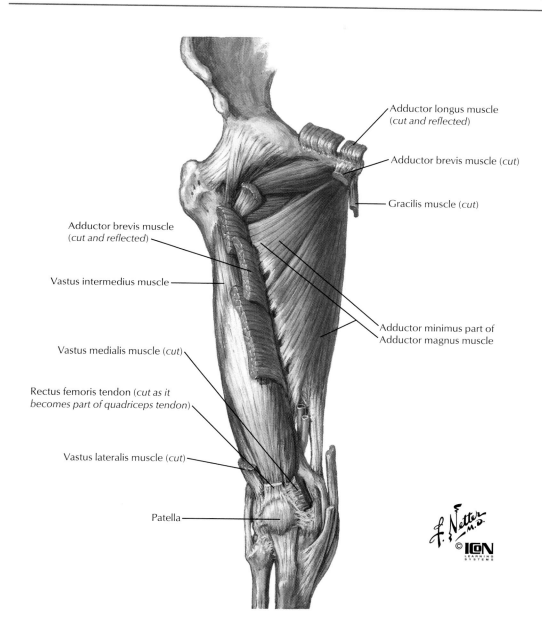

Adductor longus muscle
(*cut and reflected*)

Adductor brevis muscle (*cut*)

Gracilis muscle (*cut*)

Adductor brevis muscle
(*cut and reflected*)

Vastus intermedius muscle

Adductor minimus part of
Adductor magnus muscle

Vastus medialis muscle (*cut*)

Rectus femoris tendon (*cut as it
becomes part of quadriceps tendon*)

Vastus lateralis muscle (*cut*)

Patella

MUSCLES OF THE THIGH: POSTERIOR VIEW

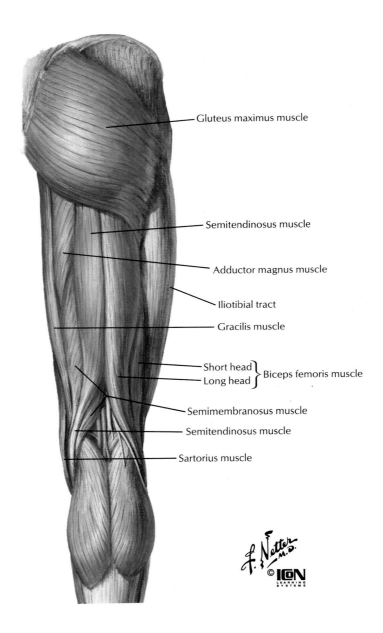

Gluteus maximus muscle

Semitendinosus muscle

Adductor magnus muscle

Iliotibial tract

Gracilis muscle

Short head
Long head } Biceps femoris muscle

Semimembranosus muscle

Semitendinosus muscle

Sartorius muscle

MUSCLES OF THE THIGH: LATERAL VIEW

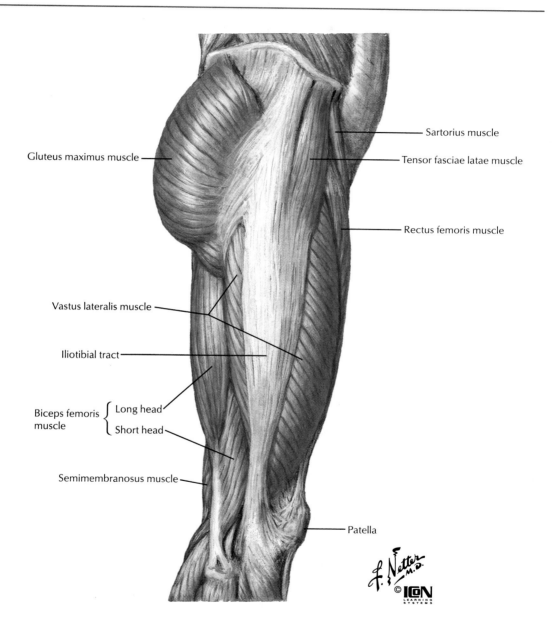

Gluteus maximus muscle

Sartorius muscle

Tensor fasciae latae muscle

Rectus femoris muscle

Vastus lateralis muscle

Iliotibial tract

Biceps femoris muscle { Long head

Short head

Semimembranosus muscle

Patella

TOPOGRAPHIC PRESENTATION OF THE THIGH (FEMUR)

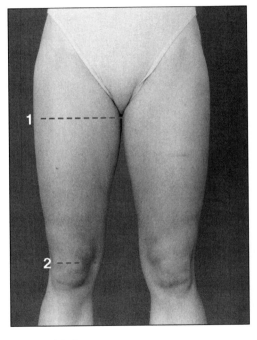

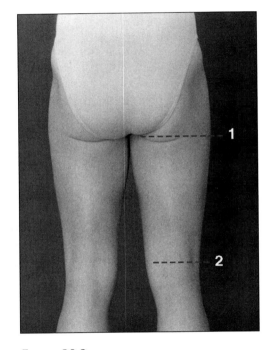

FIGURE 20-1
ANTERIOR VIEW

(1) Superior border

FIGURE 20-2
POSTERIOR VIEW

(2) Inferior border

C H A P T E R
T w e n t y

MYOLOGY

THE ANTEROFEMORAL REGION:
THE ANTERIOR MUSCULAR GROUP

This region is formed by the anterior muscular group, which includes

• The sartorius muscle (Figs. 20-5, 20-6, and 20-7)
• The quadriceps extensor muscle, which includes
  — the vastus medialis muscle (Fig. 20-10)
  — the vastus lateralis muscle (Fig. 20-11)

  — the rectus femoris muscle (Figs. 20-12 and 20-13)
  — the vastus intermedius muscle, which is not discussed in this book
• The tensor muscle of the fascia lata and the iliotibial tract (Figs. 20-15, 20-16, and 20-17)

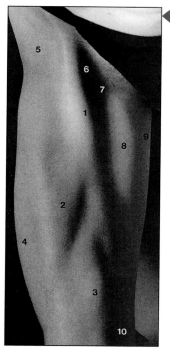

◄ **FIGURE 20-3**
ANTEROMEDIAL VIEW OF THE THIGH

(1) Sartorius muscle

(2) Rectus femoris muscle

(3) Vastus medialis muscle

(4) Vastus lateralis muscle

(5) Tensor muscle of the fascia lata

(6) Iliopsoas muscle

(7) Pectineus muscle

(8) Adductor longus muscle

(9) Gracilis muscle

(10) Distal tendon of insertion of the adductor magnus muscle: insertion into the adductor tubercle on the medial condyle of the femur

THE SARTORIUS MUSCLE

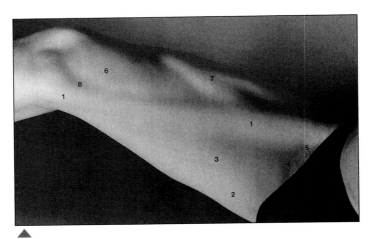

▲

FIGURE 20-4
**MEDIAL VIEW OF THE SARTORIUS MUSCLE AND DEMONSTRATION OF
ITS RELATIONSHIPS WITH THE OTHER THIGH MUSCLES**

(1) Sartorius muscle

(2) Gracilis muscle

(3) Adductor longus muscle

(4) Pectineus muscle

(5) Iliopsoas muscle

(6) Vastus medialis muscle

(7) Rectus femoris muscle

(8) Distal tendon of insertion of the adductor magnus muscle: insertion into the adductor tubercle on the medial condyle of the femur

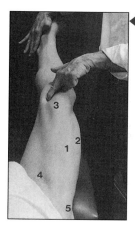

FIGURE 20-5
THE SARTORIUS MUSCLE IN ITS DISTAL ASPECT

Ask the subject to maintain an almost complete isometric extension of the knee and a slight flexion of the hip.

In order to resist its adduction isometrically, the hip should be rotated externally and a resistance should be applied on the inferomedial aspect of the leg.

Comment: The proximal hand pulls the sartorius muscle away from the vastus medialis muscle (3).

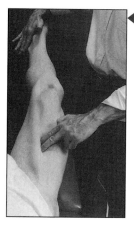

FIGURE 20-6
THE SARTORIUS MUSCLE AT THE THIGH LEVEL

The technique of placing the muscle under tension is the same as that described above. When it is not under tension, it is a flat muscle, which creates a depression at the junction of the anterior and medial compartments of the thigh. The adductor muscles adjoin its medial aspect, while the vastus medialis muscle (3) distally and the rectus femoris muscle (1) proximally adjoin its lateral aspect.

FIGURES 20-5, 20-6, AND 20-7

(1) Rectus femoris muscle

(2) Vastus lateralis muscle

(3) Vastus medialis muscle

(4) Pectineus muscle

(5) Tensor muscle of the fascia lata

(6) Adductor muscles

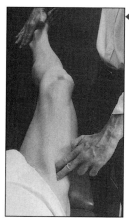

FIGURE 20-7
THE SARTORIUS MUSCLE IN ITS PROXIMAL ASPECT

The technique of putting the muscle under tension is the same as that described in Figure 20-5.

The proximal portion appears near the anterosuperior iliac spine (see also the region of the hip).

To push the sartorius muscle medially, position your grip in the depression between the sartorius muscle and the tensor muscle of the fascia lata (5). The iliopsoas muscle, not shown in this picture, and the pectineus muscle (4) adjoin its medial aspect.

THE QUADRICEPS EXTENSOR MUSCLE

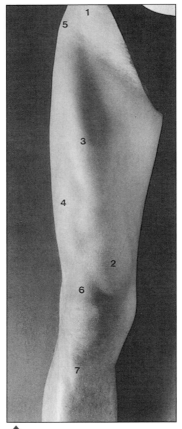

▲
FIGURE 20-8
ANTERIOR VIEW OF THE THIGH

(1) Sartorius muscle

(2) Vastus medialis muscle

(3) Rectus femoris muscle

(4) Vastus lateralis muscle

(5) Tensor muscle of the fascia lata

(6) Tendon of the quadriceps extensor muscle

(7) Patellar ligament

Comment: The crureus muscle, which forms the deep portion of the quadriceps extensor muscle, is not visible.

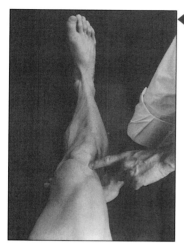

FIGURE 20-9
THE TENDON OF THE QUADRICEPS EXTENSOR MUSCLE

Your distal hand is placed under the knee to ensure that the contraction is performed properly. The subject is asked to carry out sequences of contraction-relaxation of the quadriceps extensor muscle. Note that your hand should be pressed against the table. The examination of the tendon proceeds above the level of the patella and between the vastus medialis and vastus lateralis muscles (figure below).

Comment: For the patellar ligament, see Figure 22-15.

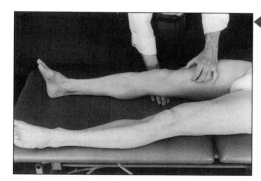

FIGURE 20-10
THE VASTUS MEDIALIS MUSCLE

To demonstrate this muscle, the subject must perform a knee extension. With the dorsum of your hand under the subject's knee at the level of the popliteal fossa, ask the subject to press your hand against the table. Your other hand palpates the vastus medialis muscle, which appears over the inferomedial aspect of the thigh.

Comment: The topographic characteristic of the vastus medialis muscle is that its distal end extends more distally than that of the vastus lateralis muscle (approximately four fingerbreadths).

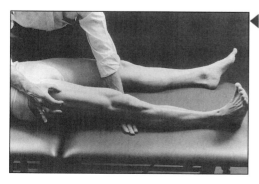

FIGURE 20-11
THE VASTUS LATERALIS MUSCLE

This muscle is located over the lateral surface of the thigh, lateral to the vastus intermedius muscle; its lateral surface is covered by the iliotibial tract or Maissiat's band (see Figs. 20-15 and 20-16).

The technique to put the muscle under tension is the same as that described for the vastus medialis muscle (Fig. 20-10).

Comment: Remember that this muscle extends posteriorly slightly beyond the iliotibial tract or Maissiat's band.

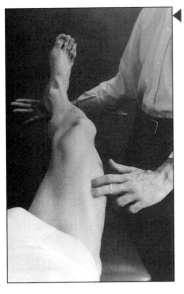

FIGURE 20-12
THE RECTUS FEMORIS MUSCLE AT THE THIGH LEVEL

The hip is in slight flexion and the knee in partial extension. Your hand is placed under the heel in order to modulate this position. Ask the subject to maintain an isometric contraction of the quadriceps extensor muscle. In most subjects, this muscle appears over the medial aspect of the thigh between the vastus medialis muscle medially and the vastus lateralis muscle laterally. In the others, one must look for the muscular mass in contraction through a varying thickness of adipose tissue.

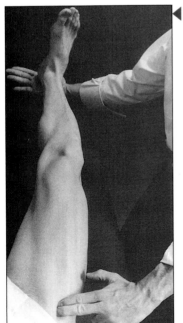

FIGURE 20-13
THE RECTUS FEMORIS MUSCLE IN ITS PROXIMAL PORTION

The hip is flexed and the knee is in partial extension in order to demonstrate the muscular body.

Your distal hand is placed under the subject's heel in order to control the requested movements.

Ask the subject to lift the heel slightly off your supporting hand, creating a contraction of the muscular body between the sartorius muscle medially and the tensor muscle of the fascia lata laterally (see also the region of the hip).

Comment: At this level, the muscular body slides between the two previously mentioned muscles and forms the floor of the lateral inguinal femoral region.

TENSOR MUSCLE OF THE FASCIA LATA

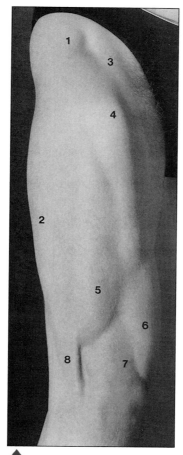

▲
FIGURE 20-14
ANTEROLATERAL VIEW
OF THE THIGH

(1) Tensor muscle of the fascia lata
(2) Iliotibial band
(3) Sartorius muscle
(4) Rectus femoris muscle
(5) Vastus lateralis muscle
(6) Vastus medialis muscle
(7) Tendon of the quadriceps extensor muscle
(8) Tendon of the iliotibial band

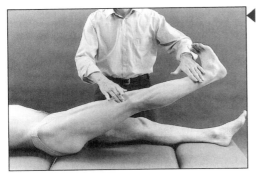

FIGURE 20-15
THE ILIOTIBIAL BAND IN ITS DISTAL PORTION

With the knee extended and the hip slightly flexed, create a resistance to the abduction of the hip by placing your hand over the lateral aspect of the limb just above the lateral malleolus (this technique opens up the lateral femorotibial interspace). The band is therefore under tension, since it inserts distal to the interspace mentioned previously.

In proximity to the knee, the band constitutes a strong tendon that acquires an identity of its own, particularly in male subjects.

Comment: The addition of an internal rotation of the hip to the movement described above will reinforce the perception of the band in some subjects.

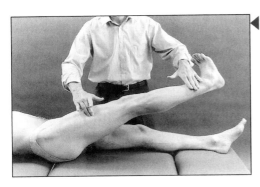

FIGURE 20-16
THE ILIOTIBIAL BAND AT THE LEVEL OF THE THIGH

The technical step here is the same as that described above.

It is important to remember that the band is located over the lateral aspect of the thigh and that the vastus lateralis muscle extends beyond it anteriorly and posteriorly.

Comment: The resistance applied by your distal hand on the subject's leg allows a better definition of this structure.

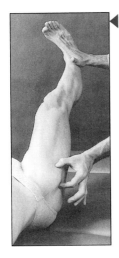

FIGURE 20-17
THE TENSOR MUSCLE OF THE FASCIA LATA

As shown above, with the hip in slight flexion and in internal rotation, resist, in an isometric fashion, an abduction of the hip through pressure applied against the distal aspect of the limb, just above the lateral malleolus.

In this position, the strength of the muscle is preferentially mobilized in its components of abduction and flexion of the hip; the third components (internal rotation), which the subject is asked to perform in an alternate and repetitive manner, allows a better localization of the muscular body.

In front of the gluteus medius muscle, the latter is perceived between the anterosuperior iliac spine and the anterior border of the greater trochanter.

Comment: One must be careful not to confuse the tensor muscle of the fascia lata with the gluteus medius muscle. See the region of the hip. In this picture, the grip straddles the most distal portion of the muscle which is located under the gluteus medius muscle.

THE POSTEROFEMORAL REGION

This region includes the medial and posterior muscular groups.

The medial muscular group consists of

• The four adductor muscles

— the pectineus muscle (Fig. 20-20)
— the adductor longus muscle (Fig. 20-21)
— the adductor brevis muscle (Fig. 20-22)
— the adductor magnus muscle (Figs. 20-23, 20-24, and 20-25)

• The gracilis muscle (Figs. 20-27, 20-28, and 20-29)

The posterior muscular group consists of

• The two medial hamstring muscles

— the semitendinosus muscle (Figs. 20-33, 20-34, and 20-40)
— the semimembranosus muscle (Figs. 20-35, 20-36, and 20-40)

• The lateral hamstring muscle

— the biceps femoris muscle: the long head and the short head (Figs. 20-38, 20-39, and 20-40)

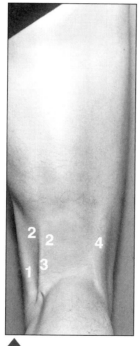

▲
FIGURE 20-18
POSTERIOR VIEW OF THE THIGH

(1) Gracilis muscle

(2) Semimembranosus muscle

(3) Tendon of the semi-tendinosus muscle

(4) Tendon of the biceps femoris muscle

THE MEDIAL MUSCULAR GROUP

Located in the posterofemoral region, this group includes

- The adductor muscles, composed of four muscles laid in three planes:
  - the superficial plane, formed by the pectineus muscle (Fig. 20-20) and the adductor longus muscle (Fig. 20-21)

  - the intermediate plane, formed by the adductor brevis muscle (Fig. 20-22)
  - the deep plane, formed by the adductor magnus muscle (Figs. 4-23 through 20-25)
- The gracilis muscle (Figs. 20-27 through 20-29)

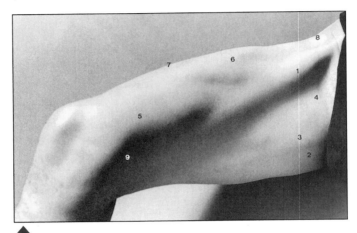

▲
FIGURE 20-19
MEDIAL VIEW OF THE THIGH

(1) Sartorius muscle

(2) Gracilis muscle

(3) Adductor longus muscle

(4) Pectineus muscle

(5) Vastus medialis muscle

(6) Rectus femoris muscle

(7) Vastus lateralis muscle

(8) Tensor muscle of the fascia lata

(9) Distal tendon of insertion of the adductor magnus muscle: insertion into the adductor tubercle on the medial condyle of the femur

The Adductor Muscles

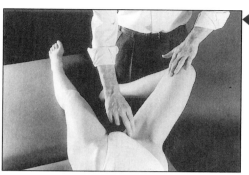

◀ FIGURE 20-20
THE PECTINEUS MUSCLE

This muscle is located in front of the adductor brevis muscle, between the iliopsoas muscle laterally and the adductor longus muscle medially.

With the hip and the knee in flexion, a slight isometric resistance is opposed to an adduction of the hip. The triangular depression (with its base at the top) appearing in the proximal aspect of the thigh corresponds to the investigated muscle.

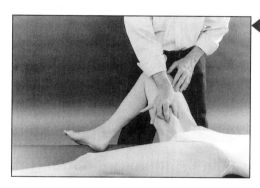

◀ FIGURE 20-21
THE ADDUCTOR LONGUS MUSCLE

The hip and the knee are in flexion. The hip is also positioned in horizontal abduction. Your distal grip is placed on the medial aspect of the thigh in order to oppose resistance, through your forearm, to a horizontal adduction requested of the subject.

This double maneuver demonstrates well an important muscular mass over the medial aspect of the thigh, representing the palpated structure.

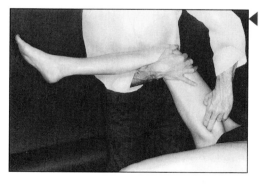

◀ FIGURE 20-22
THE ADDUCTOR BREVIS MUSCLE

With one hand supporting the knee, gradually bring the hip into abduction and ask the subject to oppose a slight resistance. The gracilis muscle then appears as a cord along the medial aspect of the thigh. It is then necessary to slide your fingers between this muscle and the adductor longus muscle in the most proximal aspect of the thigh in order to come into contact with the adductor brevis muscle, particularly with its inferior bundle.

Comment: In the female subject, the adipose tissue usually covers this muscular landmark formed by the gracilis muscle. The technique of examination remains identical, simply bringing the limb in maximal abduction and then, in this extreme position, opposing a resistance to the adduction of the hip. This modification allows a better localization of the gracilis muscle in order to slide the fingers between the latter muscle and the adductor longus muscle.

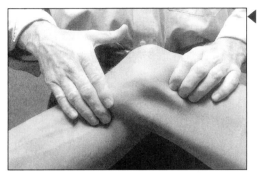

FIGURE 20-23

THE ADDUCTOR MAGNUS MUSCLE — MEDIAL PORTION, INFERIOR BUNDLE, OR VERTICAL BUNDLE (IN ITS DISTAL PART)

The bony landmark is the adductor tubercle (see Fig. 21-21). The notable muscular element is the vastus medialis muscle (Fig. 20-10).

After localizing the posterior portion of the latter muscle, look for the tendon of the adductor magnus muscle, which is palpated under your fingers as a full cylindrical cord.

Comment: It is possible to increase the tension of this tendon by opposing an isometric resistance to an adduction of the hip while the knee and hip are in flexion.

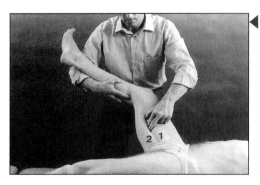

FIGURE 20-24

THE ADDUCTOR MAGNUS MUSCLE — LATERAL PORTION OR INTERMEDIATE BUNDLE

With one hand supporting the limb, bring the hip into abduction in order to tighten the involved adductor muscles and, more particularly, the adductor longus muscle (1) and the gracilis muscle (2). Your palpating hand slides between these two muscles as shown in this picture; it faces the lateral portion (intermediate bundle) of the adductor magnus muscle, which extends distally beyond the adductor longus muscle, and joins the middle aspect of the medial portion (or inferior bundle or vertical bundle) of the adductor magnus muscle.

FIGURES 20-24 AND 20-25

(1) Adductor longus muscle
(2) Gracilis muscle

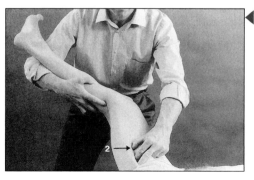

FIGURE 20-25

THE ADDUCTOR MAGNUS MUSCLE — MEDIAL PORTION OR VERTICAL BUNDLE AND INTERMEDIATE BUNDLE (IN ITS PROXIMAL ASPECT), POSTERIOR APPROACH

The technique of tightening the muscular landmarks is the same as that described above. With the proximal hand sliding between the adductor longus muscle (see Fig. 20-24) and the gracilis muscle (2), explore beyond the medial aspect of the thigh posteriorly in order to face the investigated structure.

Comment: Remember the proximal insertion points of the involved muscular bundle, the adductor magnus muscle, into the ischial tuberosity — a very posterior structure.

The Gracilis Muscle

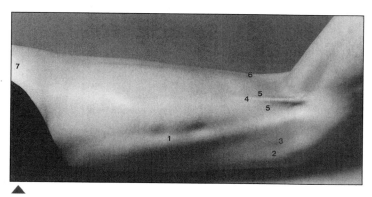

▲
FIGURE 20-26
POSTEROMEDIAL ASPECT OF THE THIGH

(1) Gracilis muscle

(2) Vastus medialis muscle

(3) Distal tendon of insertion of the adductor magnus muscle — insertion into the adductor tubercle on the medial condyle of the femur

(4) Semitendinosus muscle

(5) Semimembranosus muscle

(6) Biceps femoris muscle

(7) Gluteus maximus muscle

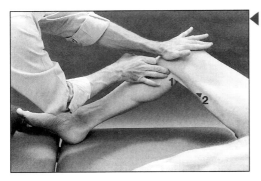

► **FIGURE 20-27**
THE GRACILIS MUSCLE IN ITS DISTAL PORTION OVER THE MEDIAL BORDER OF THE TIBIA

The subject is supine with the hip and knee in flexion. Ask the subject to perform a medial rotation as well as an isometric flexion of the knee (by pushing the heel against the table and toward the buttock). Your grip is placed over the medial border of the tibia, your middle finger is placed against the investigated tendon, and your ring finger faces the semitendinosus muscle (1). The semimembranosus muscle (2) appears in the distal half of the thigh between these two tendons.

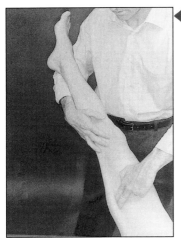

► **FIGURE 20-28**
THE GRACILIS MUSCLE AT THE THIGH LEVEL

Your distal hand supports the limb and brings the hip into abduction. Ask the subject to perform an adduction of the hip while resisting this movement in order to protrude the muscular body, which is more or less visible depending on the individual subject.

As shown in this figure, this muscle may be lifted off the underlying muscular planes with a bidigital grip.

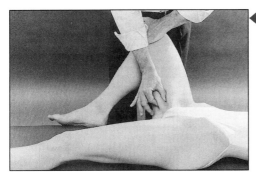

► **FIGURE 20-29**
THE GRACILIS MUSCLE IN ITS PROXIMAL ASPECT

The subject's knee is in flexion while the hip is positioned in flexion and in external rotation. Your distal hand is positioned against the medial aspect of the knee in order to resist a horizontal adduction of the hip. Your proximal hand grabs the examined muscle over the medial aspect of the thigh.

Comment: In the female subject, the amount of adipose tissue in this region may hamper the examination.

THE POSTERIOR MUSCULAR GROUP

Located in the posterofemoral region, this group includes

- The medial hamstring muscles, composed of two muscles:
  - the semitendinosus muscle (Figs. 20-33, 20-34, and 20-40)
  - the semimembranosus muscle (Figs. 20-35, 20-36, and 20-40)

- The lateral hamstring muscle, composed of
  - the biceps femoris muscle:
- Long head
- Short head (Figs. 20-38 through 20-40)

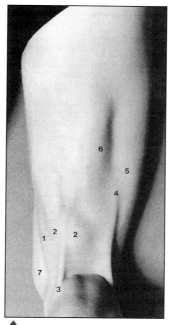

▲
FIGURE 20-30
POSTERIOR VIEW OF THE THIGH

(1) Gracilis muscle

(2) Semimembranosus muscle

(3) Semitendinosus muscle

(4) Tendon of the biceps femoris muscle

(5) Short head of the biceps

(6) Long head of the biceps

(7) Vastus medialis muscle

The Medial Hamstring Muscles

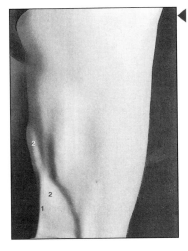

◄ FIGURE 20-31
POSTEROLATERAL VIEW OF THE THIGH

(1) Semitendinosus muscle

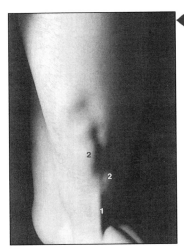

◄ FIGURE 20-32
POSTEROMEDIAL VIEW OF THE THIGH

(2) Semimembranosus muscle

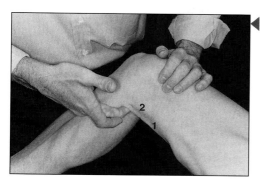

FIGURE 20-33
THE TENDON OF THE SEMITENDINOSUS MUSCLE
OVER THE MEDIAL BORDER OF THE TIBIA

In this figure, a digital grip is placed against the medial border of the tibia and your middle finger hooks up the tendon of the semitendinosus muscle (1). In this position (knee in flexion), the tendon of the gracilis muscle (2) is located in front of the tendon of the semitendinosus muscle.

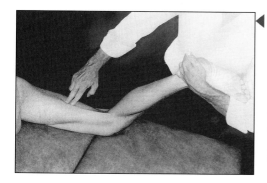

FIGURE 20-34
THE SEMITENDINOSUS MUSCLE OVER
THE POSTERIOR ASPECT OF THE THIGH

Your distal hand covers the heel and leans over the medial aspect of the foot in order to resist a simultaneous flexion and internal rotation of the knee. The body of the muscle is found in the extension of its tendon (Fig. 20-33).

The muscle is located in the posterior part of the thigh, medial to the biceps femoris muscle and behind the semi-membranosus muscle.

Comment: A particular aspect of this muscle is that its tendon extends proximally over the posterior aspect of the thigh, as clearly shown in this figure.

With regard to its proximal insertion into the ischial tuberosity, see Figure 20-40.

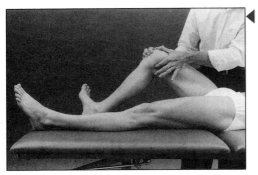

FIGURE 20-35
THE SEMIMEMBRANOSUS MUSCLE
IN ITS DISTAL ASPECT — MEDIAL VIEW

Your distal hand brings the leg into external rotation in order to isolate the distal end of the tendon. The latter is palpated as a large, cylindrical cord near its insertion into the posteromedial aspect of the proximal end of the medial condyle of the tibia.

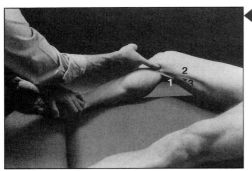

FIGURE 20-36
THE SEMIMEMBRANOSUS MUSCLE IN ITS DISTAL ASPECT —
POSTEROMEDIAL VIEW

In addition to the technique described above, you may ask the subject to perform a flexion and internal rotation of the knee while he or she opposes some resistance in order to better feel the tendon under the finger.

Comment: With your index finger placed against the semi-membranosus muscle at its insertion into the tibia, note that the gracilis muscle (2) runs across it posteriorly to position itself above the semitendinosus muscle (1), over the medial border of the tibia.

The Lateral Hamstring Muscle

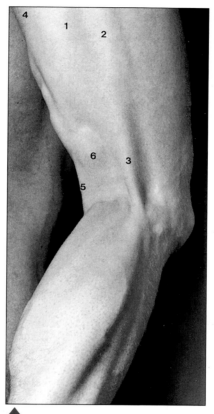

▲
FIGURE 20-37
POSTEROLATERAL VIEW OF THE THIGH

(1) Biceps femoris muscle — long head
(2) Biceps femoris muscle — short head
(3) Tendon of the biceps femoris muscle
(4) Semitendinosus muscle
(5) Tendon of the semitendinosus muscle
(6) Semimembranosus muscle

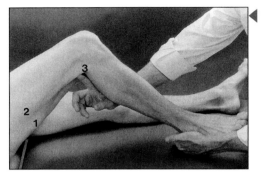

◀ FIGURE 20-38
THE BICEPS FEMORIS MUSCLE IN ITS DISTAL ASPECT

Your hand, covering the heel, resists a flexion of the knee, while you apply the anterior aspect of your forearm against the lateral border of the foot, resisting an external rotation of the knee.

The tendon is demonstrated over the lateral aspect of the knee, just proximal to its insertion into the head of the fibula.

Comment: The fibers of the long head of the biceps femoris muscle (1) end in the anterior portion of the tendon (3), while the fibers of the short head (2) also end in the anterior surface of this tendon (3), but over its lateral border.

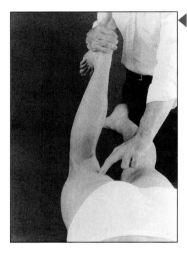

◀ FIGURE 20-39
THE BICEPS FEMORIS MUSCLE OVER THE POSTERIOR ASPECT OF THE THIGH

With the subject in prone position, your distal hand covers the heel and is placed against the lateral border of the foot in order to resist the flexion and external rotation of the knee. Over the posterior aspect of the thigh, the long and short heads of the biceps femoris muscle join the medial hamstring muscles.

FIGURES 20-38 AND 20-40

(1) Biceps femoris muscle — long head

(2) Biceps femoris muscle — short head

(3) Tendon of the biceps femoris muscle

(4) Gluteal fold

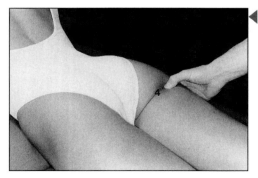

◀ FIGURE 20-40
TENDONS OF THE HAMSTRING MUSCLES INSERTING INTO THE ISCHIAL TUBEROSITY

The subject is in prone position and the essential landmark is the gluteal fold (4).

You can palpate muscular insertions into the ischial tuberosity through this fold.

For more details, refer to the pages dedicated to the involved muscles: the semitendinosus muscle (page 261), the semimembranosus muscle (page 262), and the biceps femoris muscle (this page). It might be interesting to offer resistance to the flexion of the knee for a better perception by the thumb of the tightening of these tendons.

THE KNEE

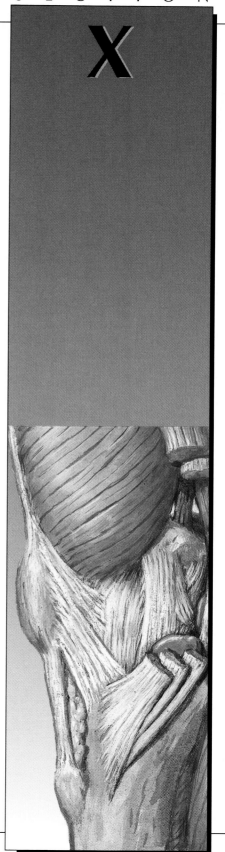

KNEE: ANTERIOR VIEW (RIGHT KNEE IN EXTENSION)

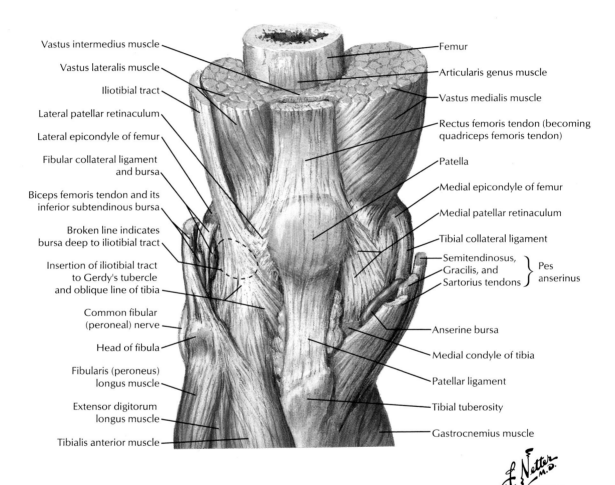

Vastus intermedius muscle

Vastus lateralis muscle

Iliotibial tract

Lateral patellar retinaculum

Lateral epicondyle of femur

Fibular collateral ligament and bursa

Biceps femoris tendon and its inferior subtendinous bursa

Broken line indicates bursa deep to iliotibial tract

Insertion of iliotibial tract to Gerdy's tubercle and oblique line of tibia

Common fibular (peroneal) nerve

Head of fibula

Fibularis (peroneus) longus muscle

Extensor digitorum longus muscle

Tibialis anterior muscle

Femur

Articularis genus muscle

Vastus medialis muscle

Rectus femoris tendon (becoming quadriceps femoris tendon)

Patella

Medial epicondyle of femur

Medial patellar retinaculum

Tibial collateral ligament

Semitendinosus, Gracilis, and Sartorius tendons } Pes anserinus

Anserine bursa

Medial condyle of tibia

Patellar ligament

Tibial tuberosity

Gastrocnemius muscle

KNEE: POSTERIOR VIEW (SUPERFICIAL DISSECTION)

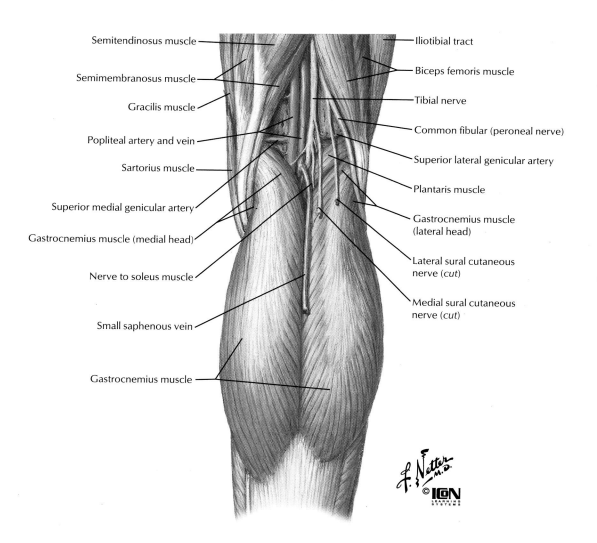

Semitendinosus muscle

Semimembranosus muscle

Gracilis muscle

Popliteal artery and vein

Sartorius muscle

Superior medial genicular artery

Gastrocnemius muscle (medial head)

Nerve to soleus muscle

Small saphenous vein

Gastrocnemius muscle

Iliotibial tract

Biceps femoris muscle

Tibial nerve

Common fibular (peroneal nerve)

Superior lateral genicular artery

Plantaris muscle

Gastrocnemius muscle (lateral head)

Lateral sural cutaneous nerve (*cut*)

Medial sural cutaneous nerve (*cut*)

KNEE: LATERAL VIEW

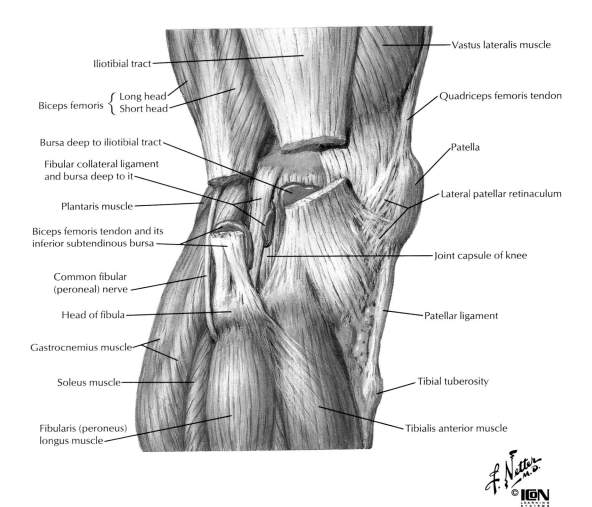

Iliotibial tract

Biceps femoris { Long head / Short head

Bursa deep to iliotibial tract

Fibular collateral ligament and bursa deep to it

Plantaris muscle

Biceps femoris tendon and its inferior subtendinous bursa

Common fibular (peroneal) nerve

Head of fibula

Gastrocnemius muscle

Soleus muscle

Fibularis (peroneus) longus muscle

Vastus lateralis muscle

Quadriceps femoris tendon

Patella

Lateral patellar retinaculum

Joint capsule of knee

Patellar ligament

Tibial tuberosity

Tibialis anterior muscle

F. Netter M.D.

© ICON
LEARNING
SYSTEMS

KNEE: MEDIAL VIEW

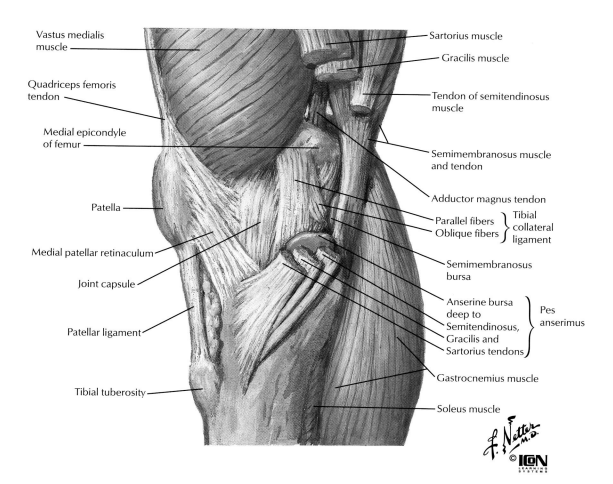

Vastus medialis muscle

Quadriceps femoris tendon

Medial epicondyle of femur

Patella

Medial patellar retinaculum

Joint capsule

Patellar ligament

Tibial tuberosity

Sartorius muscle

Gracilis muscle

Tendon of semitendinosus muscle

Semimembranosus muscle and tendon

Adductor magnus tendon

Parallel fibers
Oblique fibers
} Tibial collateral ligament

Semimembranosus bursa

Anserine bursa deep to Semitendinosus, Gracilis and Sartorius tendons
} Pes anserimus

Gastrocnemius muscle

Soleus muscle

TOPOGRAPHIC PRESENTATION OF THE KNEE

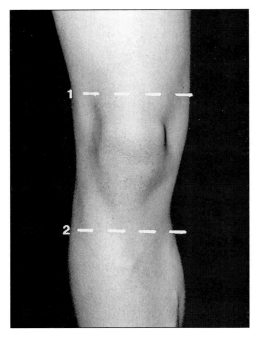

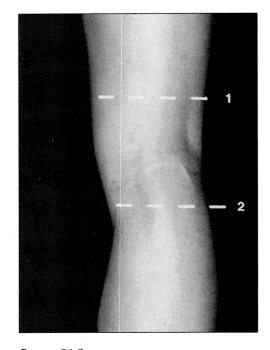

FIGURE 21-1
ANTERIOR VIEW

(1) Superior border

FIGURE 21-2
POSTERIOR VIEW

(2) Inferior border

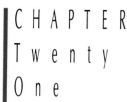

C H A P T E R
T w e n t y
O n e

OSTEOLOGY

THE ANTERIOR COMPARTMENT

The bony structures accessible by palpation are

• The suprapatellar fossa (Fig. 21-4)
• The patella
  — the base of the patella (Fig. 21-5)
  — the anterior surface (Fig. 21-6)
  — the apex (Fig. 21-7)
  — the lateral borders (Fig. 21-8)
  — the lateral approach to the posterior surface (Fig. 21-9)
  — the medial approach to the posterior surface (Fig. 21-10)

• The tibia
  — the anterior tuberosity of the tibia (Fig. 21-11)
  — the tibial plateau and the femorotibial articular interspace (Fig. 21-12)
• The femur
  — the articular surfaces of the medial and lateral condyles (Fig. 21-13)
  — the trochleocondylar grooves (Figs. 21-14 and 21-15)

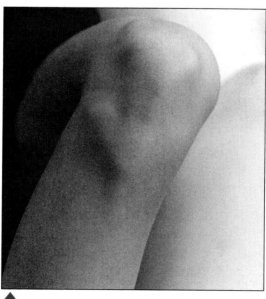

▲
FIGURE 21-3
FRONTAL VIEW — KNEE IN FLEXION

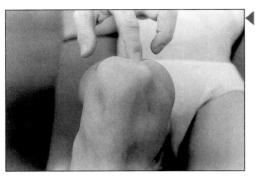

◀ **FIGURE 21-4**
THE SUPRAPATELLAR FOSSA OF THE FEMUR

Located above the condyles, at the level of the anterior aspect of the lower extremity of the femur, this area is triangular in shape and accepts the upper part of the patella during extension.

The knee must be maximally flexed in order to facilitate its palpation, starting at the base of the patella, which is easily found (see Fig. 21-5, below).

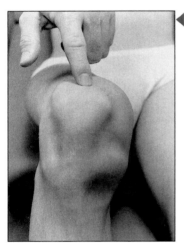

◀ **FIGURE 21-5**
THE BASE OF THE PATELLA

This triangular area, with a large anterior base and a posterior apex, is palpated as a sloped surface.

Comment: The base of the patella is a site of insertion of the tendon of the quadriceps extensor muscle anteriorly and of the articular capsule posteriorly, near its articular surface.

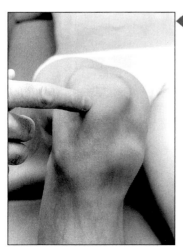

◀ **FIGURE 21-6**
THE ANTERIOR SURFACE OF THE PATELLA

Convex and perforated by numerous vascular apertures, this surface is rough; it consists of vertical striae formed by the tendon of the quadriceps extensor muscle.

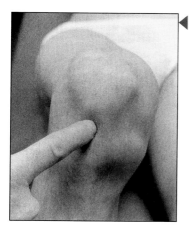

FIGURE 21-7
THE APEX OF THE PATELLA

This area is pointed toward the distal aspect of the limb; the patellar ligament is attached to it. It is possible to approach it with the knee in flexion or in extension.

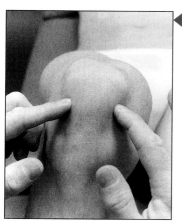

FIGURE 21-8
THE LATERAL BORDERS OF THE PATELLA

The medial and lateral borders are directed from above downward and medially if one refers to the median axis of the patella. They are directly accessible by palpation.

Comment: It is at the level of the junction of these borders with the base of the patella that the attachment of the corresponding patellar retinaculum is found.

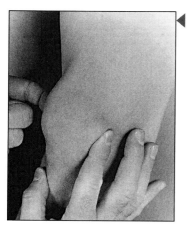

FIGURE 21-9
LATERAL APPROACH TO THE POSTERIOR SURFACE OF THE PATELLA

Only the lateralmost aspect of this facet is accessible. With the knee in hyperextension and the quadriceps extensor muscle completely relaxed, the patella should be pushed laterally.

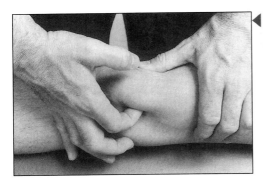

FIGURE 21-10
MEDIAL APPROACH TO THE POSTERIOR SURFACE
OF THE PATELLA

With the knee in hyperextension and the quadriceps extensor muscle completely relaxed, the patella should be pushed medially.

Comment: Less concave than the lateral facet, the medial facet is in contact with the medial condyle of the femur. It is, in fact, composed of two articular surfaces.

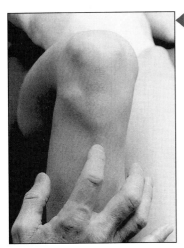

FIGURE 21-11
THE ANTERIOR TUBEROSITY OF THE TIBIA

This triangular surface, with a distal apex, separates the medial and lateral condyles of the tibia anteriorly.

It is easy to delineate and is the site of insertion of the patellar ligament.

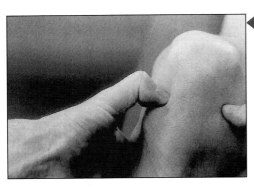

FIGURE 21-12
THE TIBIAL PLATEAU

With the knee flexed at 90°, your thumbs should be positioned on each side of the patellar ligament and the femorotibial articular interspace. The thumbs should be brought downward in order to be in contact with the nonarticular anterior border of this plateau (palpate its border up to its junction with the femur).

Comment: This grip also permits examination of the femorotibial articular interspace.

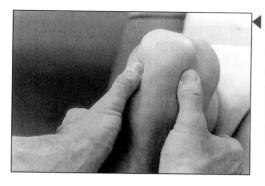

FIGURE 21-13

THE ARTICULAR SURFACES OF THE MEDIAL AND LATERAL CONDYLES OF THE FEMUR

With the knee flexed at 90°, your thumbs should be positioned on each side of the patellar ligament in the femorotibial articular interspace. The thumbs should be lifted upward in order to contact the investigated structures. If any difficulty is encountered, an increased degree of flexion of the knee will facilitate this examination.

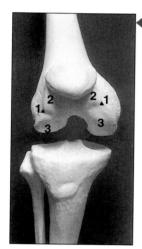

FIGURE 21-14

VISUALIZATION OF THE TROCHLEOCONDYLAR GROOVES OF THE FEMUR

These grooves are shaped by the articular surface of the inferior extremity of the femur, which is covered by cartilage in two parts. The articular surfaces located anteriorly above these grooves are part of the trochlea. The articular surfaces located posteriorly and under these grooves are called the articular surfaces of the condyles.

(1) Trochleocondylar grooves

(2) Trochlea of the femur

(3) Articular surfaces of the medial and lateral condyles

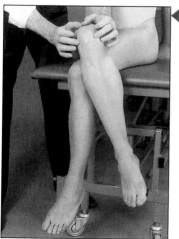

FIGURE 21-15

APPROACH TO THE TROCHLEOCONDYLAR GROOVES

The ideal position is a knee flexed at slightly more than 90°. Using a digital grip, follow the articular surface between the patella and the articular surfaces of the condyles in order to perceive these two grooves or depressions, called the trochleo-condylar grooves (see Fig. 21-14) (1).

Comment: The medial trochleocondylar groove is often palpated much more easily.

THE MEDIAL COMPARTMENT

The bony structures accessible by palpation are

• The femur

— the tuberosity of the medial condyle (Figs. 21-17 and 21-18)
— the medial border of the medial aspect of the articular surface of the medial condyle (Fig. 21-19)
— the medial supracondylar groove (Fig. 21-19)
— the medial trochleocondylar articular surface (Fig. 21-20)

— the adductor tubercle (Fig. 21-21)
• The tibia

— the medial tibial plateau (Fig. 21-22)
— the inferior border of the medial condyle of the tibia (Fig. 21-23)
— the superior portion of the medial border of the tibia [structure notable for the localization of the pes anserinus muscles (Fig. 21-24)]

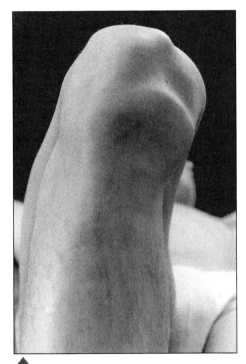

▲
FIGURE 21-16
ANTEROMEDIAL VIEW — KNEE IN FLEXION

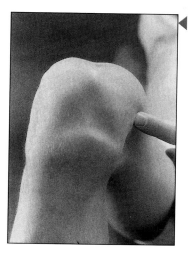

FIGURE 21-17
THE MEDIAL EPICONDYLE OF THE FEMUR — ANTERIOR VIEW

This subcutaneous structure, which is directly accessible by palpation, is the most prominent bony structure of the rough medial surface of the medial condyle.

Comment: On its posterior aspect is a depression for the insertion of the tibial collateral ligament of the knee.

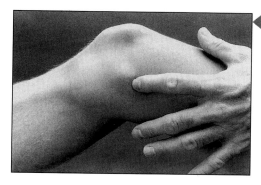

FIGURE 21-18
THE MEDIAL EPICONDYLE OF THE FEMUR — MEDIAL VIEW

This medial view of the medial epicondyle allows better visualization and localization of the investigated structure.

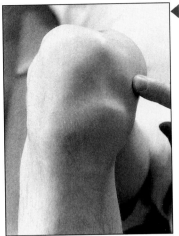

◀ **FIGURE 21-19**
THE MEDIAL BORDER OF THE MEDIAL ASPECT OF THE MEDIAL TROCHLEO-CONDYLAR ARTICULAR SURFACE OF THE FEMUR

This border is the medial boundary for the femoral condyle and the articular surface of the medial condyle. A maximal flexion of the knee facilitates its access.

The Medial Supracondylar Groove

Inferiorly, this structure lines the rough lateral surface of the medial condyle of the femur. Its depth is more pronounced in the back than in the front.

Position the knee in flexion to free it from the musculotendinous structures.

Comment: Do not forget that when the knee is flexed, a large portion of the inferior articular surface of the femur is exposed.

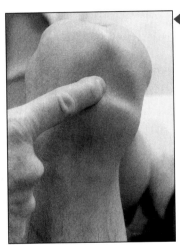

◀ **FIGURE 21-20**
THE MEDIAL TROCHLEOCONDYLAR ARTICULAR SURFACE OF THE FEMUR

With your thumb and index finger, locate the medial femorotibial articular interspace.

From this landmark, follow the articular surface, which is palpated as a smooth surface under your finger. This articular surface is limited by the medial border of the medial trochleocondylar articular surface.

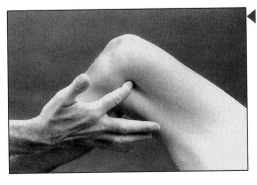

◀ **FIGURE 21-21**
THE ADDUCTOR TUBERCLE

Although the investigation of this structure is in itself somewhat difficult, it is possible to locate it by first finding the vertical tendon of the adductor magnus muscle (see Fig. 23-18) and following this tendon to its distal end, where a bony prominence represents the investigated structure.

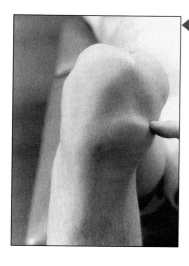

FIGURE 21-22
THE MEDIAL TIBIAL PLATEAU

With the knee flexed at 90°, this area is easy to locate. From an anterior view, the medial aspect of the plateau is interesting to visualize, since the tibial collateral ligament is approached from it.

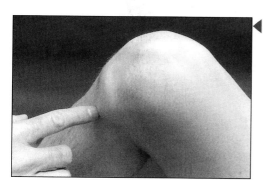

FIGURE 21-23
THE INFERIOR BORDER OF THE MEDIAL CONDYLE OF THE TIBIA

With the knee in flexion, the medial border of the tibia should be located and followed to its upper extremity. The medial tuberosity can then be easily palpated by a hook type of digital grip.

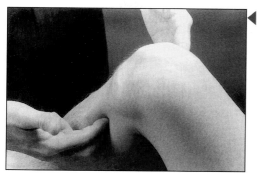

FIGURE 21-24
THE PROXIMAL ASPECT OF THE MEDIAL BORDER OF THE TIBIA

This bony structure is noteworthy because it is where the pes anserinus muscles (the semitendinosus, gracilis, and sartorius muscles) are located.

THE EXTERNAL COMPARTMENT

The accessible bony structures by palpation are

• The femur
   — the lateral border of the suprapatellar fossa (Fig. 21-26)
   — the lateral border of the lateral aspect of the lateral trochleocondylar articular surface (Fig. 21-27)
   — the lateral epicondyle of the femur (Fig. 21-28)
   — the lateral supracondylar groove (Fig. 21-29)
   — the lateral trochleocondylar articular surface (Figs. 21-29 and 21-30)

• The tibia
   — the lateral tibial plateau (Fig. 21-31)
   — the lateral condyle (Figs. 21-32 and 21-33)
   — the oblique crest (Fig. 21-34)

• The fibula
   — the head (Fig. 21-35)
   — the neck (Fig. 21-36)

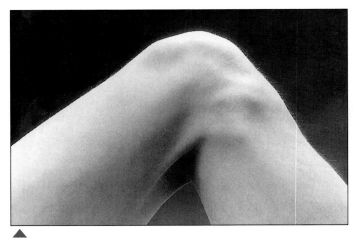

▲
FIGURE 21-25
LATERAL VIEW — KNEE IN FLEXION

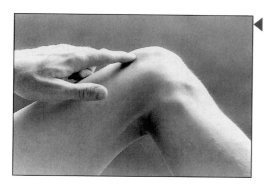

FIGURE 21-26
THE LATERAL BORDER OF THE SUPRAPATELLAR FOSSA

This is more pronounced than the medial border and becomes even more obvious as the knee is gradually brought into maximal flexion.

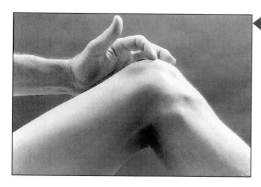

FIGURE 21-27
THE LATERAL BORDER OF THE LATERAL ASPECT OF THE LATERAL TROCHLEOCONDYLAR ARTICULAR SURFACE OF THE FEMUR

Its very lateral position reveals the off-center positioning of the patella when the knee is flexed.

Comment: Consequently, the trochleocondylar surface is more exposed on its medial than on its lateral aspect when the knee is flexed.

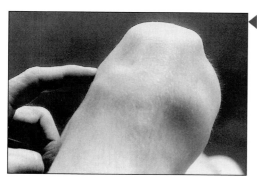

FIGURE 21-28
THE LATERAL EPICONDYLE OF THE FEMUR

Much less prominent than the medial tuberosity, this epicondyle is located over the middle aspect of the lateral surface of the condyle.

In case of difficulty in locating it, place the fibular collateral ligament under tension by opening the lateral femorotibial articular interspace with the subject's knee in flexion (see Fig. 22-3). The tuberosity is located above the point of insertion of the ligament mentioned above into the femur.

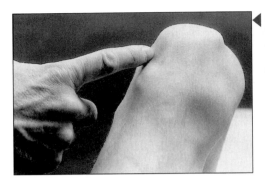

◀ **FIGURE 21-29**

THE LATERAL BORDER OF THE LATERAL ASPECT OF THE LATERAL TROCHLEOCONDYLAR ARTICULAR SURFACE OF THE FEMUR

This border delineates the femoral trochlea laterally and the articular surface of the lateral condyle. A maximal flexion of the knee facilitates its access.

The Lateral Supracondylar Groove

This area is lined inferiorly by the rough lateral surface of the lateral condyle. The depth of the groove is more pronounced in the back than in the front.

Position the knee in flexion in order to free it from the musculotendinous structures.

Comment: Do not forget that when the knee is flexed, the inferior extremity of the femur is exposed.

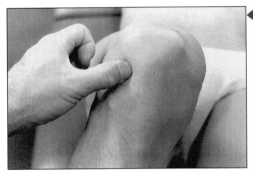

◀ **FIGURE 21-30**

THE LATERAL ASPECT OF THE LATERAL TROCHLEOCONDYLAR ARTICULAR SURFACE OF THE FEMUR

Using your thumb, locate the lateral femorotibial articular interspace. From this landmark, follow the articular surface, which is felt as a smooth surface. This articular surface is limited medially by the patellar ligament and the lateral border of the patella. It is limited laterally by the lateral border of the lateral trochleocondylar articular surface.

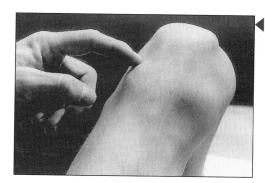

◀ **FIGURE 21-31**
THE LATERAL TIBIAL PLATEAU

With the knee in flexion at 90°, this plateau is located without difficulty. In an anterior view, it is interesting to visualize
the most lateral portion of the plateau, where the fibular
collateral ligament is approached at the level of the articular interspace.

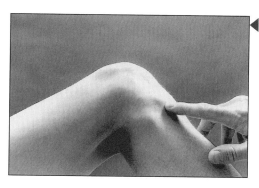

◀ **FIGURE 21-32**
**THE TUBERCLE OF THE LATERAL CONDYLE
OF THE TIBIA (GERDY) — LATERAL VIEW**

This is the most prominent structure of the lateral tuberosity of the tibia. With the knee in flexion at 90°, it is examined
just under the lateral aspect of the tibial plateau and lateral
to the tibial tuberosity.

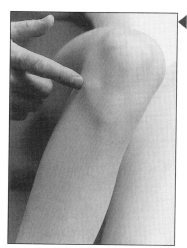

◀ **FIGURE 21-33**
**THE TUBERCLE OF THE LATERAL CONDYLE
OF THE TIBIA (GERDY) — ANTERIOR VIEW**

A complementary anterior view allows a more precise visualization and
localization of this structure. An additional bony landmark is offered by
the head of the fibula, which is located behind and distal to the investigated
structure.

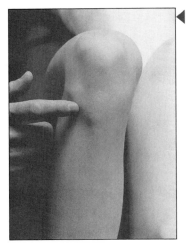

◀ **FIGURE 21-34**
"THE OBLIQUE CREST" OF THE TIBIA — FRONTAL VIEW

This is a bony crest extending from the tubercle of the lateral tuberosity of the tibia (Gerdy) (see Figs. 21-32 and 21-33) and the lateral border of the tibial tuberosity (see Fig. 21-13). It is oblique and directed downward and forward. It is directly accessible under the skin.

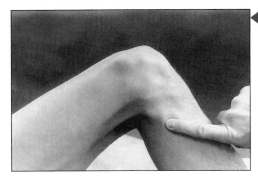

◀ **FIGURE 21-35**
THE HEAD OF THE FIBULA — LATERAL VIEW

Access to the head of the fibula is very easy. To make it more prominent, the leg may be rotated internally.

Comment: The styloid process is a bony prominence that projects behind and lateral to the articular surface of the head of the fibula.

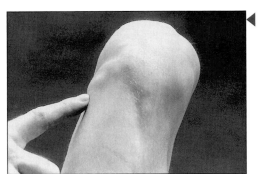

◀ **FIGURE 21-36**
THE NECK OF THE FIBULA — FRONTAL VIEW

This structure, which is interposed between the head and the shaft of the fibula, is noteworthy, since the common peroneal nerve passes around it before entering the leg.

CHAPTER
Twenty
Two

ARTHROLOGY

THE ARTICULATIONS

THE LIGAMENTS

The ligaments that are accessible by palpation are

- The fibular collateral ligament—visualization and placement under tension (Figs. 22-2 and 22-3)
- The lateral patellar retinaculum—placement under tension (Figs. 22-4, 22-5, and 22-6)
- The tibial collateral ligament—visualization and placement under tension (Figs. 22-7 through 22-10)

- The medial patellar retinaculum (Figs. 22-11, 22-12, and 22-13)
- The infrapatellar adipose tissue—visualization and approach (Fig. 22-14)
- The patellar ligament (Fig. 22-15)

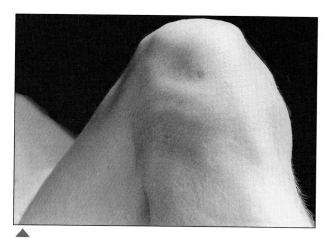

FIGURE 22-1
ANTERIOR VIEW OF THE KNEE

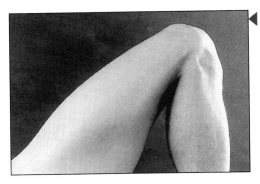

◀ **FIGURE 22-2**
VISUALIZATION OF THE FIBULAR COLLATERAL LIGAMENT

This ligament extends from the lateral tuberosity of the femur down the anterolateral aspect of the head of the fibula, in front of the styloid process.

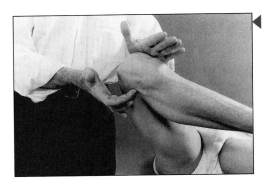

◀ **FIGURE 22-3**
PLACEMENT UNDER TENSION OF THE FIBULAR COLLATERAL LIGAMENT

For optimal localization, place the fibular collateral ligament under tension. Once it is located, its examination is facilitated in any position of the knee.

Position the subject as shown in this figure. Apply some pressure from inside out, using one hand positioned over the medial aspect of the knee in order to open up the lateral articular interspace, which places the ligament under tension. The other hand faces the lateral articular interspace, between the head of the fibula and the lateral tuberosity of the femur.

Comment: The ligament is palpated as a full cylindrical cord. Its thickness varies from person to person. Individuals with a varus deformity of the knee will obviously have a much stronger and thicker ligament, since it is constantly mobilized.

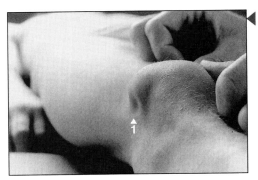

◀ **FIGURE 22-4**
VISUALIZATION OF THE LATERAL PATELLAR RETINACULUM — TRANSVERSE BUNDLE

The knee is in complete extension and the extensor quadriceps muscle is relaxed. The patella may either be pushed laterally, which places the investigated structure under tension (see figure), or be pushed medially, which has the same effect. The lateral patellar retinaculum is approached in a plane perpendicular to its course.

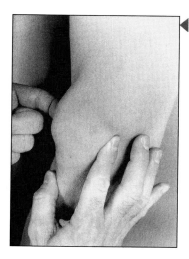

◀ FIGURE 22-5
PALPATION OF THE LATERAL PATELLAR RETINACULUM — TRANSVERSE BUNDLE

This maneuver brings the structure investigated and visualized in Figure 22-4 into a plane that is closer to the strict sagittal plane. It is a capsular reinforcement that is palpated as a fibrous band.

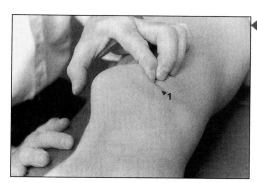

◀ FIGURE 22-6
VISUALIZATION OF THE PLACEMENT UNDER TENSION OF BOTH THE MEDIAL AND THE LATERAL PATELLAR RETINACULAE

An outward traction of the patella allows the examiner to create a projection of the medial patellar retinaculum (1) and, at the same time, to put under tension the lateral patellar retinaculum, not visible in this figure (see Fig. 22-4).

Comment: During this maneuver, the lateral patellar retinaculum is brought under tension in a plane that moves progressively closer to the strict sagittal plane, while the medial patellar retinaculum is brought under tension in a more and more horizontal plane. This figure presents an inferomedial view.

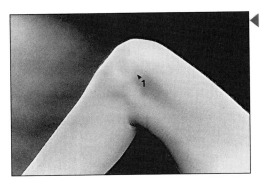

◀ FIGURE 22-7
VISUALIZATION OF THE TIBIAL COLLATERAL LIGAMENT

This ligament (1) extends from the superior aspect of the medial tuberosity of the femur. It is also inserted into a depression located just behind this tuberosity down to the superior portion of the internal border of the tibia and to the adjacent portion of the anteromedial surface of the same bone.

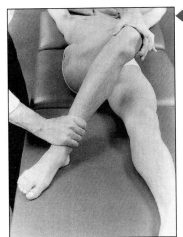

◀ FIGURE 22-8
PLACEMENT UNDER TENSION OF THE TIBIAL COLLATERAL LIGAMENT

The optimal placement of this ligament under tension is carried out in two steps. With the subject's knee flexed at 90°, the leg is first brought into external rotation, which puts the ligament under tension.

As a second step, push the knee medially (while the foot is immobilized on the table) with one hand. This opens up the medial articular interspace and increases the tension on the investigated structure.

Comment: The fingers of the same hand facing the articular interspace perceive the ligament as a relatively flat fibrous band.

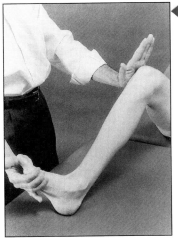

◀ FIGURE 22-9
ALTERNATIVE TECHNIQUE TO PLACE THE TIBIAL COLLATERAL LIGAMENT UNDER TENSION

With the heel leaning on the table, grab the medial aspect of the foot in order to bring the leg into external rotation.

As a second step, the other hand applies pressure against the lateral aspect of the knee and moves the knee medially, opening up the medial articular interspace and therefore putting the ligament under tension.

Comment: The ligament is clearly demonstrated at the level of the medial articular interspace (see Fig. 22-10).

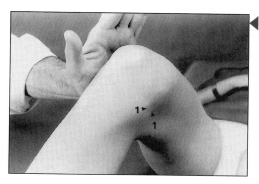

FIGURE 22-10
AS AN ALTERNATIVE TECHNIQUE TO PLACE THE TIBIAL COLLATERAL LIGAMENT UNDER TENSION, MANEUVER AS IN THE PREVIOUS FIGURE — CLOSE-UP VIEW

This picture demonstrates an anteromedial closeup view of the knee, clearly showing the placement of the tibial collateral ligament under tension.

Comment: The ligament is clearly demonstrated at the level of the medial articular interspace (1).

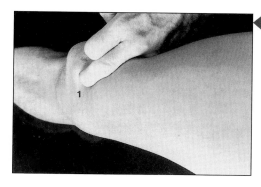

FIGURE 22-11
VISUALIZATION OF THE MEDIAL PATELLAR RETINACULUM: TRANSVERSE BUNDLE — MEDIAL VIEW WITH KNEE IN EXTENSION

With the knee in complete extension, the quadriceps extensor muscle is relaxed. The patella may be either pushed laterally, which puts the ligament under tension (see figure), or pushed medially (Fig. 22-12), which also puts the ligament under tension.

Palpation is the same in both cases. The medial patellar retinaculum is approached transversely.

(1) Medial patellar retinaculum

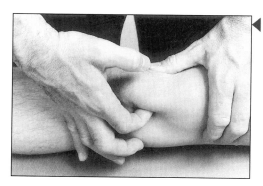

FIGURE 22-12
PALPATION OF THE MEDIAL PATELLAR RETINACULUM — TRANSVERSE BUNDLE

This maneuver puts the investigated structure under tension in a plane that is closer to the sagittal plane. It is a capsular reinforcement, which is palpated as a fibrous band.

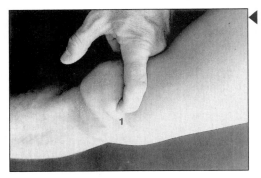

FIGURE 22-13

PLACEMENT UNDER TENSION OF THE MEDIAL PATELLAR RETINACULUM — TRANSVERSE BUNDLE — BY OUTWARD TRACTION OF THE PATELLA

This maneuver, the same as that described in Figure 22-6, tightens up the examined structure in a plane that is closer and closer to the horizontal plane. This is a capsular reinforcement which is palpated as a fibrous band.

(1) Medial patellar retinaculum

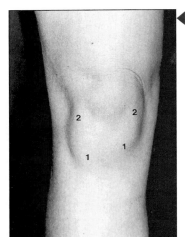

FIGURE 22-14

VISUALIZATION OF THE INFRAPATELLAR ADIPOSE TISSUE

Located between the patellar ligament and the nonarticular posterior aspect of the patella, this structure is found above the intercondylar aspect of the tibial plateau. This adipose tissue extends medially and laterally to the middle aspect of the lateral borders of the patella, forming rolls of fat also called plicae alares. They are seen more easily during extension of the knee, as shown in the figure.

(1) Infrapatellar adipose tissue

(2) Infrapatellar adipose tissue: plicae alares

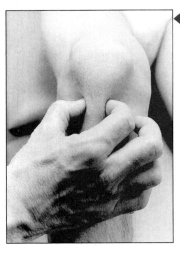

FIGURE 22-15

THE PATELLAR LIGAMENT

This ligament may be approached with the knee either flexed or in extension. Grab the medial and lateral borders of this ligament by a thumb–index finger grip. The ligament's slightly oblique downward and forward course is then better perceived.

CHAPTER
Twenty
Three

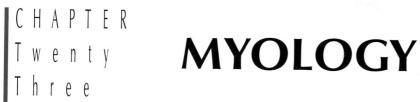

MYOLOGY

THE ANTEROLATERAL REGION

The muscular and tendinous structures accessible by palpation are

- The thigh
  - the vastus lateralis muscle (Fig. 23-2)
  - the iliotibial tract or Maissiat's band (Fig. 23-3)
  - the tendon of the biceps femoris muscle (Fig. 23-4)
- The leg
  - the anterior tibialis muscle (Figs. 23-5, 23-6, and 23-7)
  - the extensor digitorum longus muscle (Figs. 23-5, 23-6, and 23-8)

  - the peroneus longus muscle (Figs. 23-5, 23-6, and 23-9)

(The approach to the proximal aspect of the peroneus longus muscle is described as part of the examination of the lateral compartment.)

Comment: Since the patellar ligament is not an active structure, as indicated by its name, it is covered in the corresponding discussion (Fig. 22-15, page 290).

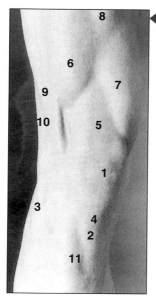

◀ **FIGURE 23-1**
ANTEROLATERAL VIEW OF THE KNEE

(1) Patella
(2) Tibial tuberosity
(3) Head of the fibula
(4) Patellar ligament
(5) Tendon of the quadriceps extensor muscle
(6) Vastus lateralis muscle
(7) Vastus medialis muscle
(8) Rectus femoris muscle
(9) Iliotibial band
(10) Tendon of the biceps femoris muscle
(11) Anterior tibialis muscle

THE THIGH

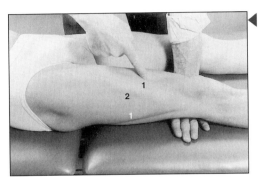

◀ FIGURE 23-2
THE VASTUS LATERALIS MUSCLE

Ask the subject to apply pressure on your hand, which is placed between the popliteal fossa and the table. The vastus lateralis muscle (1) appears over the anterolateral aspect of the thigh in front and behind the iliotibial band (2).

See also Figure 23-3.

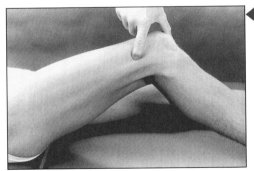

◀ FIGURE 23-3
THE TENDON OF THE ILIOTIBIAL TRACT OR MAISSIAT'S BAND

With the subject's knee flexed and foot resting on the table, the band appears or is felt under your fingers over the lateral aspect of the knee as the subject begins to extend the knee. An active internal rotation of the leg accentuates its demonstration. For a better perception of this structure, the subject may also perform a complete extension of the knee (see Figs. 20-15 and 20-16).

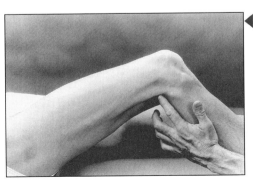

◀ FIGURE 23-4
THE DISTAL ASPECT OF THE TENDON OF THE BICEPS FEMORIS MUSCLE

The essential bony landmark is the head of the fibula.

With one hand, cover the heel and resist the flexion of the knee. The other hand, placed in the area of the head of the fibula, approaches the examined structure, which constitutes the superolateral border of the popliteal fossa (see also Figs. 23-24 and 23-25).

THE LEG

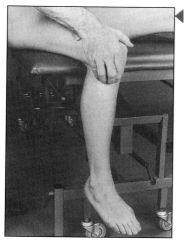

◀ FIGURE 23-5

LOCALIZATION OF THE ANTERIOR TIBIALIS, EXTENSOR DIGITORUM LONGUS, AND PERONEUS LONGUS MUSCLES

The subject is sitting on the side of the table, possibly with legs crossed. The foot is in a dependent, normally relaxed position.
The subject may also be placed in supine position, but with the trunk elevated so that he or she has visual control over the movements of the foot.

Your palpating hand is positioned with a digital grip over the superolateral aspect of the leg, between the head of the fibula and the anterior tuberosity of the tibia.

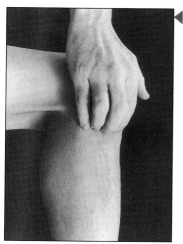

◀ FIGURE 23-6

CLOSE-UP ON THE LOCALIZATION DESCRIBED IN FIGURE 23-5

More precisely, your fifth and fourth fingers are placed against the anterior portion of the head of the fibula while the third and second fingers are positioned over the lateral border of the lateral tuberosity of the tibia, just below the oblique tibial crest and the tubercle of Gerdy (infracondylar tubercle).

With your hand in this position, your fifth finger faces the peroneus longus muscle. The fourth finger faces the extensor digitorum longus muscle, while the third and second fingers face the anterior tibialis muscle.

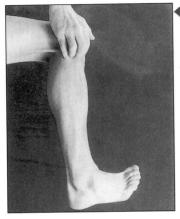

◀ **FIGURE 23-7**

LOCALIZATION OF THE PROXIMAL ASPECT OF THE ANTERIOR TIBIALIS MUSCLE

From the starting position described in Figs. 23-5 and 23-6, the subject is asked to bring the foot into adduction, supination, and dorsiflexion — the actions of the anterior tibialis muscle.

The muscular contraction is felt beneath the fingers, more precisely under the second and third fingers.

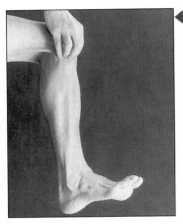

◀ **FIGURE 23-8**

LOCALIZATION OF THE PROXIMAL ASPECT OF THE EXTENSOR DIGITORUM LONGUS MUSCLE

From the starting position described in Figs. 23-5 and 23-6, the subject is asked to bring the foot into abduction, pronation, and dorsiflexion — the actions of the extensor digitorum longus muscle.

The muscular contraction is perceived beneath the fingers, more precisely under the fourth finger.

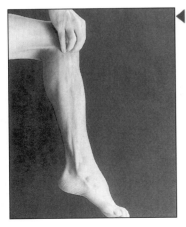

◀ **FIGURE 23-9**

LOCALIZATION OF THE PROXIMAL ASPECT OF THE PERONEUS LONGUS MUSCLE

From the position described above, the subject is asked to bring the foot into abduction, pronation, and plantarflexion — the actions of the peroneus longus muscle.

The muscular contraction is perceived beneath the fingers, more precisely under the fourth and fifth fingers.

THE ANTEROMEDIAL REGION

With the knee flexed at 90°, the muscular and tendinous structures accessible by palpation are, from below upward

- The tendon of the semitendinosus muscle (Figs. 23-11 through 23-14)
- The tendon of the gracilis muscle (Figs. 23-11, 23-12, 23-13, and 23-15)
- The semimembranosus muscle (Fig. 23-17)
- The sartorius muscle (Figs. 23-11, 23-12, 23-13, and 23-16)

- The distal tendon of the vertical bundle of the adductor magnus muscle (Fig. 23-18)
- The muscular body of the vastus medialis muscle (Fig. 23-19)

Comment: The semitendinosus, gracilis, and sartorius muscles constitute the muscles of the pes anserinus. Their approach is discussed on the next page.

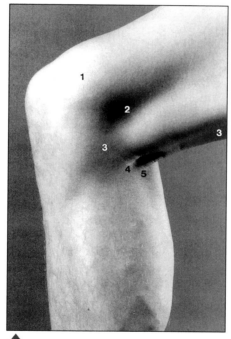

▲
FIGURE 23-10
MEDIAL VIEW OF THE KNEE

(1) Vastus medialis muscle
(2) Tendon of the adductor magnus muscle
(3) Semimembranosus muscle
(4) Tendon of the gracilis muscle
(5) Tendon of the semitendinosus muscle

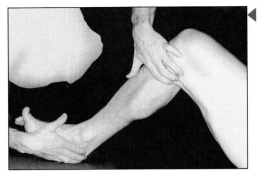

FIGURE 23-11

LOCALIZATION OF THE MUSCLES OF THE PES ANSERINUS OVER THE MEDIAL BORDER OF THE TIBIA

First localize the upper end of the medial border of the tibia and position your fingers as shown in the figure. With the other hand, offer resistance to a flexion and an isometric internal rotation of the knee. The subject then proceeds with movements in a contraction-relaxation sequence to permit better perception of the tendons and their topography.

• The tendon of the semitendinosus is the most posterior and is well perceived under the index finger

• The tendon of the gracilis muscle is located just above the previous tendon and is perceived under the middle finger

• The distal aspect of the sartorius muscle overlies that of the gracilis muscle. The placement under tension of this muscle is perceived under the ring finger (see also Fig. 23-16).

Comment: If the perception of the tendons over the medial border of the tibia is difficult, a more proximal palpation should be done by moving the fingers slightly backward.

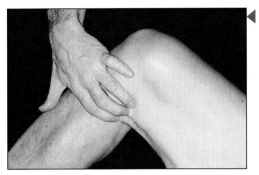

FIGURE 23-12

CLOSE-UP OF THE LOCALIZATION DESCRIBED IN FIGURE 23-11

This figure is interesting since it clearly shows the respective positions of the different tendons and muscular bodies. The index finger faces the tendon of the semitendinosus muscle. The middle finger, which is not visualized in this picture, faces the tendon of the gracilis muscle and the ring finger faces the sartorius muscle.

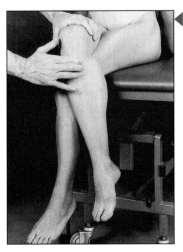

FIGURE 23-13

LOCALIZATION OF THE PLACEMENT UNDER TENSION OF THE MUSCLES OF THE PES ANSERINUS OVER THE ANTERIOR AND MEDIAL ASPECTS OF THE TIBIA

With a wide grip, position your fingers below the medial condyle of the tibia, covering the anterior tuberosity of the tibia in the extension of the examined tendons (Figs. 23-11 and 23-12).

The muscular action is the same as that demonstrated in Figure 23-11. A flexion of the subject's knee, which may be carried out isometrically against the contralateral lower extremity, is associated with an internal rotation of the leg (performed by bringing the forefoot medially), since these muscles of the pes anserinus are also internal rotators of the leg. One then perceives through the skin the placement of the pes anserinus muscles under tension.

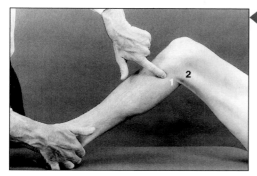

◄ **FIGURE 23-14**
THE DISTAL TENDON OF THE SEMITENDINOSUS MUSCLE

The essential bony landmark is the superior end of the medial border of the tibia.

With the knee flexed at approximately 90°, your one hand, positioned against the medial aspect of the foot, offers resistance to the flexion and internal rotation of the knee, while the other hand slides up along the medial border of the tibia until it meets the investigated tendon (1).

The subject may also be asked to press his or her heel against the table, thereby performing an isometric contraction of the knee flexion, and to carry out rapid, consecutive internal rotations of the leg. Your two hands are then free for the examination.

Difficulty of approach: The localization of this tendon is reasonably easy in the male subject but much more difficult in the female in view of the presence of adipose tissue. In this case, if any difficulty is encountered, it should be investigated more posteriorly in the soft tissues of the upper calf or at the level of the popliteal fossa (see Fig. 23-21).

FIGURES 23-14 AND 23-15

(1) Semitendinosus muscle
(2) Gracilis muscle

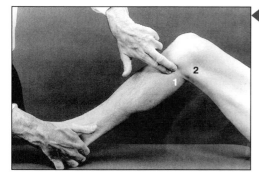

◄ **FIGURE 23-15**
THE DISTAL TENDON OF THE GRACILIS MUSCLE

The bony landmark — the medial border of the tibia — remains the same, and this is where your fingers should be placed. Your other hand offers resistance to the flexion and internal rotation of the knee by covering the heel and applying the forearm against the medial border of the foot.

The investigated tendon (2) (see also Fig. 23-22) is perceived above the tendon of the semitendinosus muscle and below the sartorius muscle (see also Fig. 23-16), which may cover it partially.

Difficulty of approach: The comment is the same as that made for the tendon of the semitendinosus muscle (Fig. 23-14).

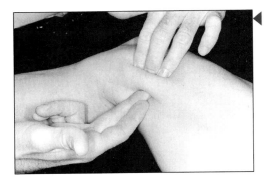

◀ FIGURE 23-16
DISTAL ASPECT OF THE SARTORIUS MUSCLE — MEDIAL VIEW,
KNEE SEMIFLEXED

The subject's knee should be placed in almost complete
extension and the hip in slight external rotation in order to
have the muscular body appear over the medial aspect of
the knee.

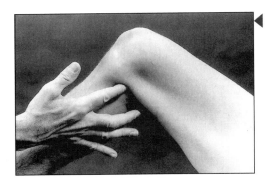

◀ FIGURE 23-17
THE TENDON OF THE SEMIMEMBRANOSUS MUSCLE

The essential bony landmark is formed by the junction of
the medial and posterior surfaces of the medial condyle of
the tibia. Position the leg in external rotation in order to
demonstrate this bony structure. Your hand offers resistance to the flexion and internal rotation of the knee. The
other hand looks for the tendon presenting under the fingers as a full, relatively thick cylindrical cord.

More anteriorly, the reflected tendon of this muscle slides
under the horizontal tibial ligament of the tibia's internal
tuberosity.

Difficulty of approach: There is none if one remembers to
position the leg properly in external rotation, thereby clearing out this tendon.

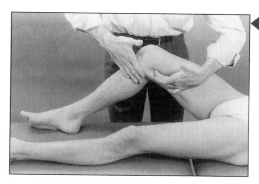

◀ FIGURE 23-18

THE DISTAL TENDON OF THE VERTICAL BUNDLE OF THE ADDUCTOR MAGNUS MUSCLE — ALSO CALLED INFERIOR BUNDLE OR INTERNAL PORTION OF THE ADDUCTOR MAGNUS MUSCLE

The essential bony landmark is the adductor tubercle (see also Fig. 21-21).

The essential muscular landmark is the vastus medialis muscle (see Fig. 23-19).

The investigated tendon is located behind this muscle. It presents beneath the fingers as a full and relatively thick cylindrical cord (see also Fig. 20-23).

Comment: Your distal hand may be placed against the medial aspect of the knee, pushing laterally in the direction of the abduction of the hip, while the subject is asked to resist this movement. The tendon will be better perceived under the fingers.

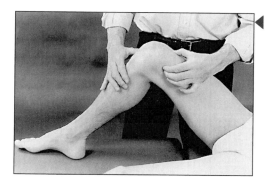

◀ FIGURE 23-19

THE MUSCULAR BODY OF THE VASTUS MEDIALIS MUSCLE

To make this muscle prominent if the knee is flexed, ask the subject to press his or her heel against the ground or the table.

If the knee is in extension, ask for a contraction of the quadriceps extensor muscle.

In relation to the patella, the muscular body is demonstrated superiorly and medially.

Comment: Note the lower position of this muscle as compared with that of the vastus lateralis muscle (Fig. 23-1) (see Fig. 20-10).

THE POSTERIOR REGION

The muscular and tendinous structures accessible by palpation are

At the level of the thigh:
- The tendon of the semitendinosus muscle (Fig. 23-21)
- The tendon of the gracilis muscle (Fig. 23-22)
- The semimembranosus muscle (Fig. 23-23)
- The tendon of the biceps femoris muscle (Fig. 23-24)
- The biceps femoris muscle — short head (see Fig. 23-25)

At the level of the leg:
- The medial head of the gastrocnemius muscle (see Fig. 26-25)
- The lateral head of the gastrocnemius muscle (see Fig. 26-26 and 26-28)

Comment: In this part, we discuss only the muscles located at the level of the thigh as well as the tendon of the popliteus muscle. For the other muscles, refer to Section XI, "The Leg."

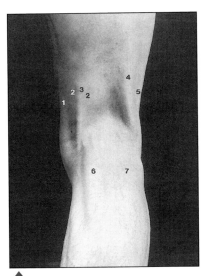

▲
FIGURE 23-20
POSTERIOR VIEW OF THE KNEE

(1) Gracilis muscle

(2) Semimembranosus muscle

(3) Semitendinosus muscle

(4) Biceps femoris muscle

(5) Iliotibial band

(6) Medial head of the gastrocnemius muscle

(7) Lateral head of the gastrocnemius muscle

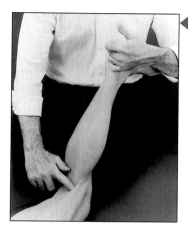

FIGURE 23-21
TENDON OF THE SEMITENDINOSUS MUSCLE

With the subject prone, wrap your distal hand around the heel and offer resistance to the flexion of the knee. Resistance may also be offered to the internal rotation of the knee (then your forearm is placed against the medial border of the foot).

The tendon of the semitendinosus muscle is the most posterior and lateral of the musculotendinous structures demonstrated over the posteromedial aspect of the thigh.

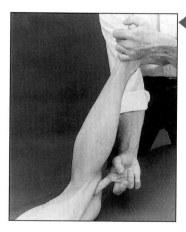

FIGURE 23-22
THE TENDON OF THE GRACILIS MUSCLE

The subject's position and the resistance offered are the same as described in Figure 23-21.

The tendon of the gracilis muscle is demonstrated anterior and medial to the tendon of the semitendinosus muscle.

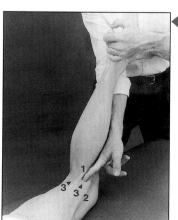

FIGURE 23-23
THE SEMIMEMBRANOSUS MUSCLE

The subject's position as well as the resistance offered are the same as those described in Figure 23-21.

The semimembranosus muscle (3) is a muscular body perceived beneath the fingers between the tendons of the semitendinosus (1) and gracilis (2) muscles. It is also palpated lateral to the tendon of the semitendinosus muscle (1).

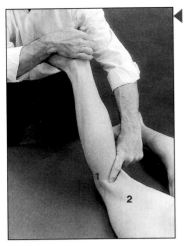

◀ **FIGURE 23-24**
LOCALIZATION OF THE TENDON OF THE BICEPS FEMORIS MUSCLE IN THE POPLITEAL FOSSA

With the subject prone, cover the heel with one hand and place your forearm against the lateral border of the foot in order to resist a flexion and an external rotation of the knee simultaneously. The tendon is demonstrated (see figure) (1) in the posterolateral portion of the popliteal fossa. The muscular body (2) of the biceps femoris muscle is also visible (see figure).

(1) Tendon of the biceps femoris muscle inserting into the head of the fibula

(2) Muscular body of the long head of the biceps femoris muscle

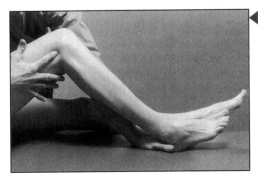

◀ **FIGURE 23-25**
THE TENDON OF THE POPLITEUS MUSCLE

While your one hand offers resistance to the flexion of the knee, the other is placed behind the fibular collateral ligament (see also Figs. 22-2 and 22-3).

The investigated tendon is palpated just behind the latter structure. Its palpation is not obvious in all subjects.

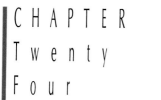

CHAPTER
Twenty
Four

NERVES
AND VESSELS

THE POPLITEAL FOSSA

The neurovascular structures accessible by palpation are

• The tibial nerve (Figs. 24-3 and 24-5)
• The common peroneal nerve (Fig. 24-7)

• The sural nerve (or sural) (Fig. 24-8)
• The popliteal artery (Figs. 24-10, 24-11, and 24-12)

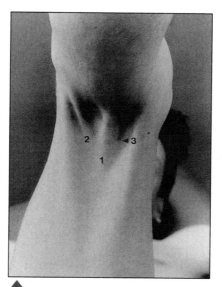

▲
FIGURE 24-1
POSTERIOR VIEW OF THE POPLITEAL
FOSSA: POSITION OF THE SUBJECT —
DORSAL DECUBITUS, HIP AND KNEE
FLEXED

(1) Tibial nerve
(2) Common peroneal nerve
(3) Popliteal artery

Comment: The arrowhead indicates the landmark for an optimal approach to the popliteal artery.

THE TIBIAL NERVE

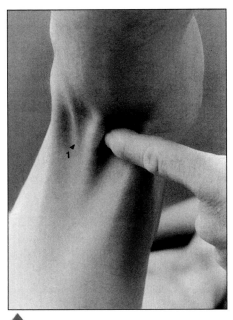

▲
FIGURE 24-2
POSTERIOR VIEW OF THE POPLITEAL FOSSA:
POSITION OF THE SUBJECT — SUPINE, HIP
AND KNEE FLEXED

The index finger indicates the tibial nerve.

(1) Common peroneal nerve

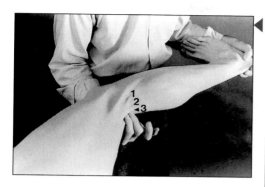

FIGURE 24-3
DEMONSTRATION OF THE TIBIAL NERVE IN "SIDE-LYING"

The subject is in a side-lying position. The hip is flexed beyond 90°, the knee is slightly flexed, and the ankle is also placed in dorsiflexion.

The index finger indicates the investigated structure.

FIGURES 24-3 AND 24-4

(1) Common peroneal nerve

(2) Sural nerve

(3) Tibial nerve

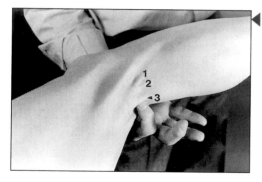

FIGURE 24-4
CLOSE-UP VIEW OF THE POPLITEAL FOSSA

The technique of demonstration is the same as that described above. The subject is placed in side-lying position, the ankle is brought into complete dorsiflexion, the knee is slightly flexed, and the hip is progressively brought in more or less complete flexion.

If this is not sufficient to demonstrate the nerve in the middle of the popliteal fossa, the subject should be asked to flex the upper body (Fig. 24-5).

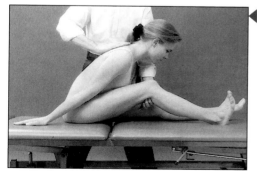

FIGURE 24-5
DEMONSTRATION OF THE TIBIAL NERVE

With the knee in flexion between 90 and 45°, the subject brings the ankle into maximal dorsiflexion. The palpating hand should be positioned in the center of the popliteal fossa. The other hand, placed on the subject's back, supports a flexion of the upper body in order to place the sciatic nerve and its terminal branches, including the tibial nerve, under more tension and to make them more accessible to examination.

The investigated nerve is palpated as a full cylindrical cord.

THE PERONEAL NERVE

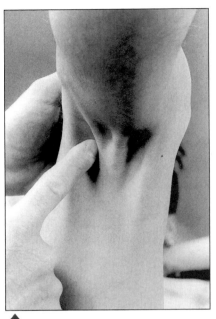

▲
FIGURE 24-6
POSTERIOR VIEW OF THE POPLITEAL
FOSSA: SUBJECT'S POSITION — SUPINE,
HIP AND KNEE FLEXED

The index finger indicates the peroneal nerve.

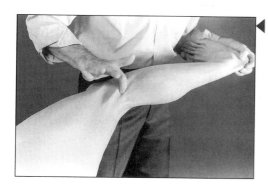

FIGURE 24-7
DEMONSTRATION OF THE PERONEAL NERVE

The technique of demonstration is the same as that described for the tibial nerve.

The index finger indicates the investigated structure.

THE SURAL NERVE

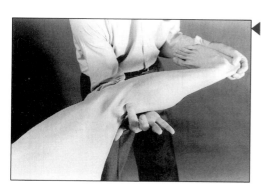

FIGURE 24-8
DEMONSTRATION OF THE ACCESSORY/SUBORDINATE EXTERNAL SURAL NERVE

The technique of demonstration is the same as that described for the tibial nerve.

The index finger indicates the investigated structure.

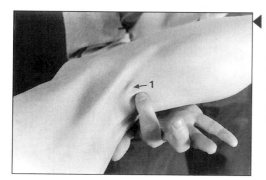

FIGURE 24-9
CLOSE-UP ON THE POPLITEAL FOSSA

With regard to the technique of demonstration, see Figures 24-2 and 24-4.

The index finger indicates the investigated structure, i.e., the external saphenous or sural nerve. Laterally, the peroneal nerve (1) is seen as it passes toward the neck of the fibula.

THE POPLITEAL ARTERY

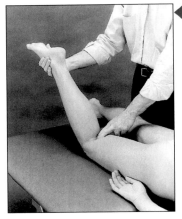

◀ **FIGURE 24-10**
PULSE EXAMINATION IN THE POPLITEAL FOSSA — STEP 1

The knee is brought into more or less complete extension. By leaning on the tendon of the semitendinosus muscle, you can apply a two- or three-finger grip in the superomedial aspect of the popliteal fossa.

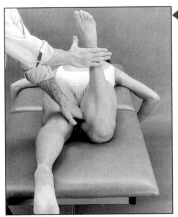

◀ **FIGURE 24-11**
PULSE EXAMINATION IN THE POPLITEAL FOSSA — STEP 2

As you look for the popliteal pulse, which is found in proximity to the tibial nerve, the subject's knee is progressively brought into flexion and your digital grip is directed toward the central portion of the popliteal fossa.

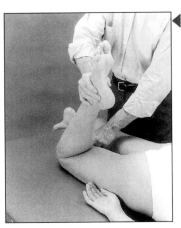

◀ **FIGURE 24-12**
PULSE EXAMINATION IN THE POPLITEAL FOSSA — STEP 3

Knee positioning in more or less maximal flexion allows an optimal relaxation of the posterior fibrous plane of the knee. Access to the popliteal artery is facilitated, and it is palpated over the medial aspect of the tibial nerve.

THE LEG

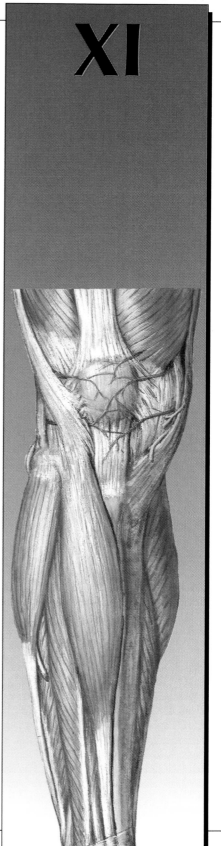

MUSCLES OF LEG (SUPERFICIAL DISSECTION): ANTERIOR VIEW

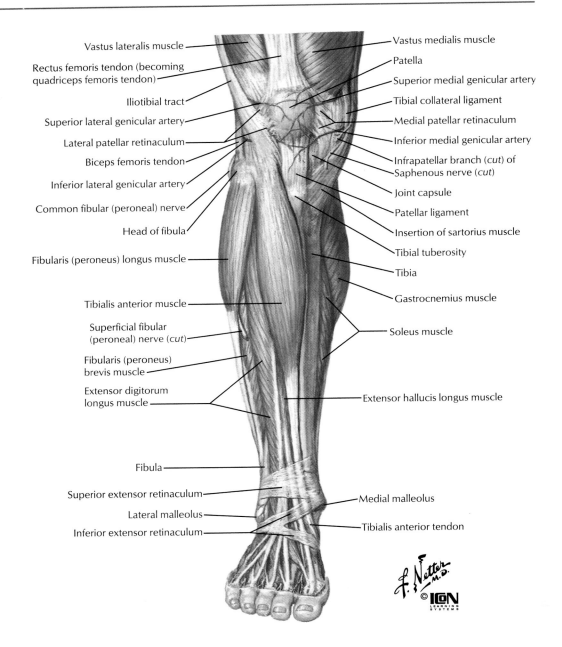

Vastus lateralis muscle

Rectus femoris tendon (becoming quadriceps femoris tendon)

Iliotibial tract

Superior lateral genicular artery

Lateral patellar retinaculum

Biceps femoris tendon

Inferior lateral genicular artery

Common fibular (peroneal) nerve

Head of fibula

Fibularis (peroneus) longus muscle

Tibialis anterior muscle

Superficial fibular (peroneal) nerve (cut)

Fibularis (peroneus) brevis muscle

Extensor digitorum longus muscle

Fibula

Superior extensor retinaculum

Lateral malleolus

Inferior extensor retinaculum

Vastus medialis muscle

Patella

Superior medial genicular artery

Tibial collateral ligament

Medial patellar retinaculum

Inferior medial genicular artery

Infrapatellar branch (cut) of Saphenous nerve (cut)

Joint capsule

Patellar ligament

Insertion of sartorius muscle

Tibial tuberosity

Tibia

Gastrocnemius muscle

Soleus muscle

Extensor hallucis longus muscle

Medial malleolus

Tibialis anterior tendon

MUSCLES OF LEG (DEEP DISSECTION): ANTERIOR VIEW

Superior lateral genicular artery

Fibular collateral ligament

Lateral patellar retinaculum

Iliotibial tract (*cut*)

Biceps femoris tendon (*cut*)

Inferior lateral genicular artery

Common fibular (peroneal) nerve

Head of fibula

Fibularis (peroneal) longus muscle (*cut*)

Anterior tibial artery

Extensor digitorum longus muscle (*cut*)

Superficial fibular (peroneal) nerve

Deep fibular (peroneal) nerve

Fibularis (peroneus) longus muscle

Extensor digitorum longus muscle

Fibularis (peroneus) brevis muscle and tendon

Fibularis (peroneus) longus tendon

Perforating branch of fibular (peroneal) artery

Anterior lateral malleolar artery

Lateral malleolus and arterial network

Lateral tarsal artery and lateral branch of deep fibular (peroneal) nerve

Extensor digitorum brevis and extensor hallucis brevis muscles (*cut*)

Fibularis (peroneus) brevis tendon

Posterior perforating branches from deep planter arch

Extensor digitorum longus tendons (*cut*)

Extensor digitorum brevis tendons (*cut*)

Dorsal digital arteries

Branches of proper plantar digital arteries and nerves

Superior medial genicular artery

Quadriceps femoris tendon

Tibial collateral ligament

Medial patellar retinaculum

Infrapatellar branch of saphenous nerve (*cut*)

Inferior medial genicular artery

Saphenous nerve (*cut*)

Patellar ligament

Insertion of sartorius tendon

Anterior tibial recurrent artery and recurrent branch of deep peroneal nerve

Interosseous membrane

Tibialis anterior muscle (*cut*)

Gastrocnemius muscle

Soleus muscle

Tibia

Superficial fibular (peroneal) nerve (*cut*)

Extensor hallucis longus muscle and tendon (*cut*)

Interosseous membrane

Anterior medial malleolar artery

Medial malleolus and arterial network

Dorsalis pedis artery

Tibialis anterior tendon

Medial tarsal artery

Medial branch of deep fibular (peroneal) nerve

Arcuate artery

Deep plantar artery

Dorsal metatarsal arteries

Extensor hallucis longus tendon (*cut*)

Extensor hallucis brevis tendon (*cut*)

Dorsal digital branches of deep fibular (peroneal) nerve

MUSCLES OF LEG (SUPERFICIAL DISSECTION): POSTERIOR VIEW

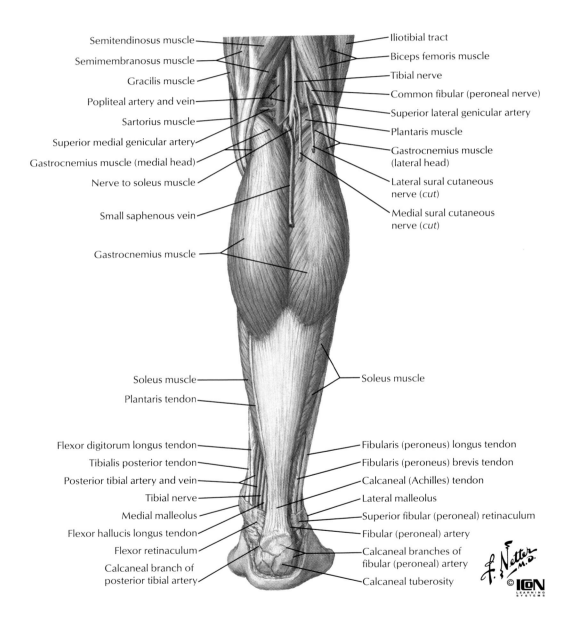

Semitendinosus muscle

Semimembranosus muscle

Gracilis muscle

Popliteal artery and vein

Sartorius muscle

Superior medial genicular artery

Gastrocnemius muscle (medial head)

Nerve to soleus muscle

Small saphenous vein

Gastrocnemius muscle

Iliotibial tract

Biceps femoris muscle

Tibial nerve

Common fibular (peroneal nerve)

Superior lateral genicular artery

Plantaris muscle

Gastrocnemius muscle (lateral head)

Lateral sural cutaneous nerve (*cut*)

Medial sural cutaneous nerve (*cut*)

Soleus muscle

Plantaris tendon

Soleus muscle

Flexor digitorum longus tendon

Tibialis posterior tendon

Posterior tibial artery and vein

Tibial nerve

Medial malleolus

Flexor hallucis longus tendon

Flexor retinaculum

Calcaneal branch of posterior tibial artery

Fibularis (peroneus) longus tendon

Fibularis (peroneus) brevis tendon

Calcaneal (Achilles) tendon

Lateral malleolus

Superior fibular (peroneal) retinaculum

Fibular (peroneal) artery

Calcaneal branches of fibular (peroneal) artery

Calcaneal tuberosity

MUSCLES OF LEG: LATERAL VIEW

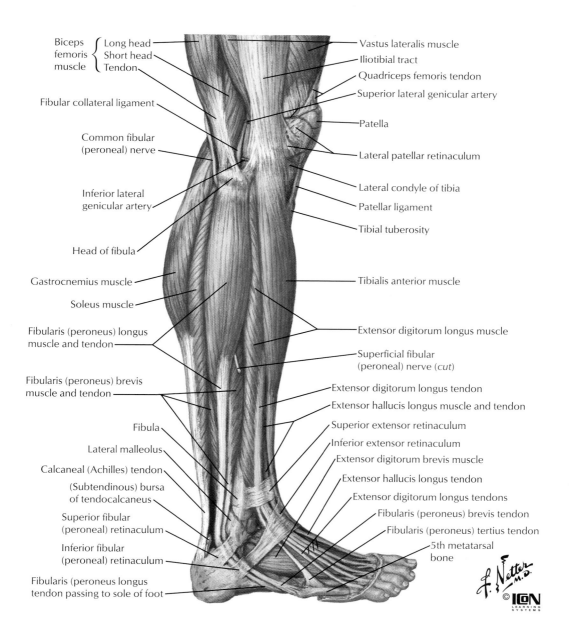

Biceps femoris muscle { Long head — Short head — Tendon —

Fibular collateral ligament

Common fibular (peroneal) nerve

Inferior lateral genicular artery

Head of fibula

Gastrocnemius muscle

Soleus muscle

Fibularis (peroneus) longus muscle and tendon

Fibularis (peroneus) brevis muscle and tendon

Fibula

Lateral malleolus

Calcaneal (Achilles) tendon

(Subtendinous) bursa of tendocalcaneus

Superior fibular (peroneal) retinaculum

Inferior fibular (peroneal) retinaculum

Fibularis (peroneus longus tendon passing to sole of foot

Vastus lateralis muscle

Iliotibial tract

Quadriceps femoris tendon

Superior lateral genicular artery

Patella

Lateral patellar retinaculum

Lateral condyle of tibia

Patellar ligament

Tibial tuberosity

Tibialis anterior muscle

Extensor digitorum longus muscle

Superficial fibular (peroneal) nerve (cut)

Extensor digitorum longus tendon

Extensor hallucis longus muscle and tendon

Superior extensor retinaculum

Inferior extensor retinaculum

Extensor digitorum brevis muscle

Extensor hallucis longus tendon

Extensor digitorum longus tendons

Fibularis (peroneus) brevis tendon

Fibularis (peroneus) tertius tendon

5th metatarsal bone

TOPOGRAPHIC PRESENTATION OF THE LEG

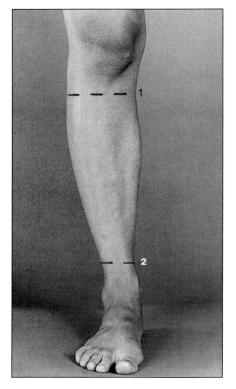

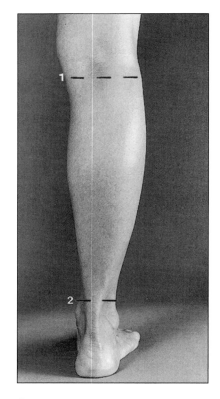

FIGURE 25-1
ANTERIOR VIEW

FIGURE 25-2
POSTERIOR VIEW

(1) Superior border

(2) Inferior border

CHAPTER
Twenty
Five

OSTEOLOGY

LEG

The bony structures accessible by palpation are

• The tibia
  — the anterior border (Fig. 25-3)
  — the medial border (Fig. 25-4)
  — the medial surface (Fig. 25-5)

  — the posterior surface (Fig. 25-6)
• The fibula
  — the lateral surface (Fig. 25-7)

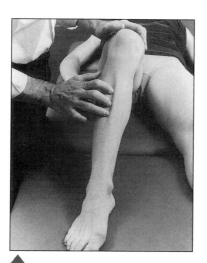

▲
FIGURE 25-3
THE ANTERIOR BORDER OF THE TIBIA

This border extends from the tibial tuberosity down to the medial malleolus.

In its superior three-quarters, it has the shape of a fish bone and it is called the crest of the tibia.

In its inferior quarter, the border deviates medially toward the medial malleolus and becomes rounded.

Directly under the skin, the anterior border is entirely accessible.

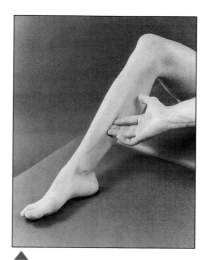

▲
FIGURE 25-4
THE MEDIAL BORDER OF THE TIBIA

Extending from the medial condyle of the tibia down to the medial malleolus, this structure borders medially the medial surface of the tibial shaft. It is also entirely accessible for investigation.

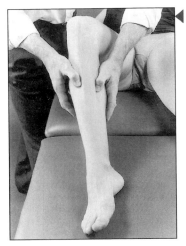

◀ FIGURE 25-5
THE MEDIAL SURFACE OF THE TIBIA

This area has a smooth, flat surface which is in direct contact with the skin throughout its length.

Very close to the anterior tuberosity of the tibia, the muscles of the pes anserinus insert into the proximal portion of this surface.

Located between the anterior border (Fig. 25-3) and the medial border (Fig. 25-4), it is entirely accessible for investigation.

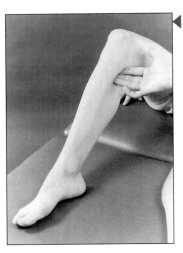

◀ FIGURE 25-6
THE POSTERIOR SURFACE OF THE TIBIA

This area is partially accessible for investigation, behind the medial border of the tibia, particularly at the proximal and distal ends of the tibial shaft. In this figure, the leg is positioned in external rotation in order to expose the posterior surface of the tibia, palpated behind the proximal aspect of its medial border (see also Fig. 25-4). Care must be taken to relax the posterior muscles of the leg significantly.

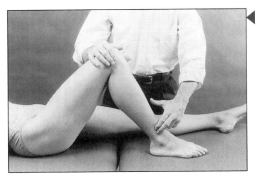

◀ FIGURE 25-7
THE LATERAL SURFACE OF THE FIBULA

This surface is directly accessible in its distal part. The distal end is covered by an oblique crest extending downward and backward, dividing it in two parts:

· An anterior part, triangular in shape, directly subcutaneous and accessible without difficulty
· A posterior part, over which the tendons of the lateral peroneal muscles (peroneus longus and peroneus brevis muscles) slide

C H A P T E R
T w e n t y
S i x

MYOLOGY

THE ANTERIOR MUSCULAR GROUP

The anterior muscular group includes these four muscles:

- The anterior tibialis muscle (Figs. 26-2 through 26-5)

- The extensor hallucis longus muscle (Figs. 26-8, 26-9, and 26-10)

- The extensor digitorum longus muscle (Figs. 26-11 and 26-12)

- The peroneus tertius muscle (Fig. 26-13)

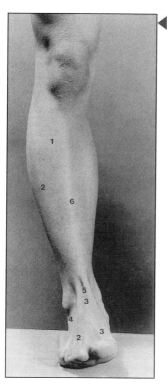

◀ **FIGURE 26-1**
ANTERIOR VIEW OF THE LEG

(1) Anterior tibialis muscle
(2) Extensor digitorum longus muscle
(3) Extensor hallucis longus muscle
(4) Peroneus tertius muscle
(5) Extensor retinaculum
(6) Anterior border of the tibia

THE ANTERIOR TIBIALIS MUSCLE

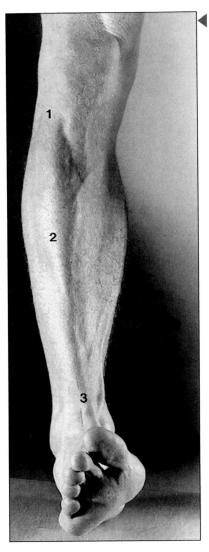

◀ **FIGURE 26-2**
ANTERIOR VIEW OF THE LEG

(1) Anterior tibialis muscle — proximal insertion
(2) Anterior tibialis muscle — muscular body
(3) Anterior tibialis muscle — distal tendon

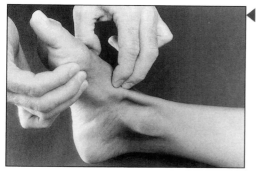

FIGURE 26-3

THE DISTAL PORTION OF THE TENDON OF THE ANTERIOR TIBIALIS MUSCLE

After bringing the foot into adduction, supination, and dorsiflexion, resist this muscular action by placing a digital grip positioned over the medial border of the foot in order to demonstrate the tendon. This tendon is the most medial of the tendons of the proximal foot and is located just in front of the medial malleolus.

In this figure, the digital grip faces the tendon, close to its distal insertion into the anteroinferior aspect of the medial surface of the medial cuneiform bone. This insertion extends into the inferomedial aspect of the base of the first metatarsal bone.

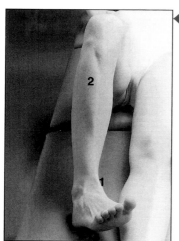

FIGURE 26-4

THE ANTERIOR TIBIALIS MUSCLE IN THE LEG

The tendon (1) follows the lateral aspect of the tibial crest or of the anterior border of the tibia. It extends as a muscular body (2), which is also lateral to the tibial crest and medial to the extensor digitorum longus muscle. The requested muscular action is the same as that described above.

Comment: In this photograph, the muscle is easily demonstrated.

(1) Tendon of the anterior tibialis muscle
(2) Muscular body of the anterior tibialis muscle.

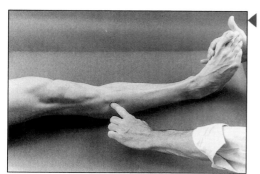

FIGURE 26-5

PROXIMAL INSERTION OF THE ANTERIOR TIBIALIS MUSCLE

Also see Section X, "The Knee," (Figs. 23-5, 23-6, and 23-7.)

Obtain the same foot positioning as that described in Figure 26-3. The resistance is also applied against the medial border of the foot in order to clearly note the muscular body as it tightens under the fingers.

THE EXTRINSIC EXTENSOR MUSCLES OF THE TOES
AND THE PERONEUS TERTIUS MUSCLE

This group includes three muscles:

• The extensor hallucis longus muscle (Figs. 26-8, 26-9, and 26-10)
• The extensor digitorum longus muscle (Figs. 26-11 and 26-12)
• The peroneus tertius muscle (Fig. 26-13)

This last muscle, which is not consistent, extends from the inferior third of the fibula to the fifth metatarsal bone.

Comment: The extensor digitorum brevis muscle also participates in the extension of the toes, but it is an intrinsic muscle of the foot; see Figure 29-7.

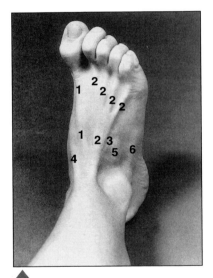

▲
FIGURE 26-6
DORSAL VIEW OF THE FOOT

(1) Extensor hallucis longus muscle
(2) Extensor digitorum longus muscle
(3) Peroneus tertius muscle
(4) Anterior tibialis muscle
(5) Extensor hallucis brevis muscle
(6) Peroneus brevis muscle

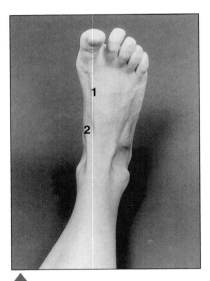

▲
FIGURE 26-7
ANTERIOR VIEW OF THE ANKLE

(1) Extensor hallucis longus muscle
(2) Anterior tibialis muscle

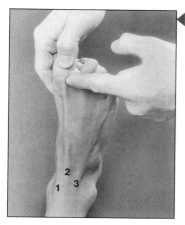

FIGURE 26-8
THE TENDON OF THE EXTENSOR HALLUCIS LONGUS MUSCLE NEAR ITS DISTAL INSERTION

The subject is asked to perform a complete extension of the first toe. A resistance is applied by the examiner's thumb against the dorsal aspect of the distal phalanx of the first toe, attempting to bring it in flexion.

The index finger shows the tendon near its distal sites of insertion into the base of the dorsal aspect of the distal phalanx of the first toe as well as into the medial and lateral aspects of the base of the proximal phalanx.

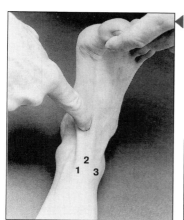

FIGURE 26-9
THE TENDON OF THE EXTENSOR HALLUCIS LONGUS MUSCLE IN THE PROXIMAL FOOT (OR "HINDFOOT")

The requested muscular action is the same as that described above.

The index finger shows the tendon as it passes through the proximal aspect of the foot.

FIGURES 26-8, 26-9, AND 26-10

(1) Anterior tibialis muscle
(2) Extensor hallucis longus muscle
(3) Extensor digitorum longus muscle

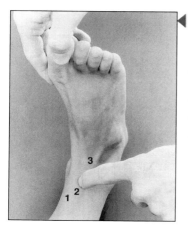

FIGURE 26-10
THE MUSCULAR BODY OF THE EXTENSOR HALLUCIS LONGUS MUSCLE OVER THE DISTAL ASPECT OF THE LEG

The tendon slides behind the extensor retinaculum and joins a muscular body located proximally between the anterior tibialis muscle medially and the extensor digitorum longus muscle laterally.

To better visualize the position of the investigated muscle, consult the figures demonstrating these two muscles (pages 319 and 322, respectively).

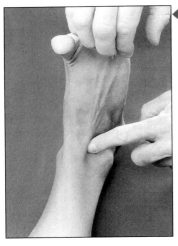

FIGURE 26-11
THE TENDONS OF THE EXTENSOR DIGITORUM LONGUS MUSCLE

The distal hand is positioned as shown here in order to resist an extension of the toes. It is useful to ask the subject to maintain an active dorsiflexion, abduction, and pronation of the foot (these last two movements are not demonstrated in this figure).

Each of the tendons leading to the four toes must be followed from its distal end up to the proximal foot. In this picture, the tendon is approached at the level of the proximal foot.

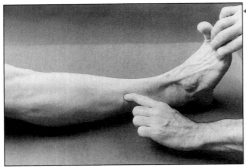

FIGURE 26-12
THE EXTENSOR DIGITORUM LONGUS MUSCLE AT THE LEVEL OF THE DISTAL LEG

The muscular body, which follows the tendon, lies throughout the length of the leg and is located, from above downward, between the peroneus longus and peroneus brevis muscles laterally, and the anterior tibialis muscle medially. The latter muscles are located through their actions. This allows a better localization of the investigated muscular body (see also Fig. 26-15).

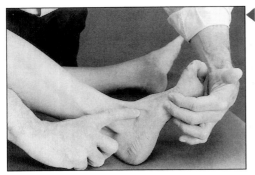

FIGURE 26-13
THE PERONEUS TERTIUS MUSCLE

This structure appears as a tendon over the lateral aspect of the tendon of the extensor digitorum longus muscle, leading to the fifth toe.

To make this muscle prominent, the subject is asked to invert the foot with or without resistance. The tendon extends toward the dorsal surface of the base of the fifth metatarsal bone.

THE LATERAL MUSCULAR GROUP

This group includes two muscles:

• The peroneus longus muscle (Figs. 26-16, 26-17, and 26-18)

• The peroneus brevis muscle (Figs. 26-20, 26-21, and 26-22)

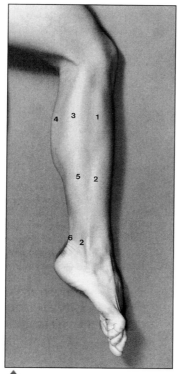

▲

FIGURE 26-14
LATERAL VIEW OF THE LEG

(1) Peroneus longus muscle

(2) Peroneus brevis muscle

(3) Lateral head of the gastrocnemius muscle

(4) Medial head of the gastrocnemius muscle

(5) Soleus muscle

(6) Achilles tendon

THE PERONEUS LONGUS MUSCLE

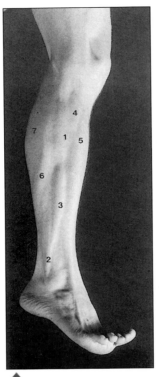

▲
FIGURE 26-15
LATERAL VIEW OF THE LEG

(1) Peroneus longus muscle

(2) Tendon of the peroneus longus muscle

(3) Peroneus brevis muscle

(4) Extensor digitorum longus muscle

(5) Anterior tibialis muscle

(6) Soleus muscle

(7) Lateral head of the gastrocnemius muscle

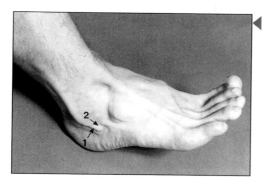

◀ **FIGURE 26-16**

THE TENDON OF THE PERONEUS LONGUS MUSCLE AT THE LATERAL BORDER OF THE FOOT

The subject is asked to position the foot in abduction. After passing around the lateral malleolus, the tendon (1) slides against the lateral surface of the calcaneum, passes behind the peroneal tubercle (2), and enters the lateral border of the foot in the peroneal groove of the cuboid bone.

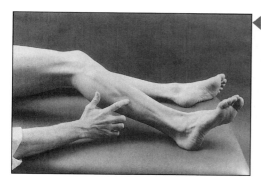

◀ **FIGURE 26-17**

TENDON OF THE PERONEUS LONGUS MUSCLE AT THE LEVEL OF THE LEG

The muscular action is identical to that described above. At this level, the tendon is located at approximately the middle aspect of the lateral surface of the leg. It lies against the muscular body of the peroneus brevis muscle, which extends beyond it anteriorly and posteriorly (see Fig. 26-22).

FIGURES 26-17 AND 26-18

(1) Peroneus longus muscle	(3) Extensor digitorum longus muscle
(2) Peroneus brevis muscle	(4) Soleus muscle

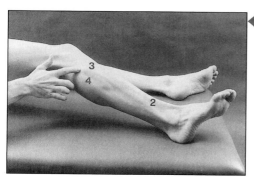

◀ **FIGURE 26-18**

THE MUSCULAR BODY OF THE PERONEUS LONGUS MUSCLE

The muscular action is the same as that described above (Fig. 26-16).

The muscular body is located in the superior portion of the lateral surface of the leg, between the extensor digitorum longus muscle (3) anteriorly and the soleus muscle (4) posteriorly.

THE PERONEUS BREVIS MUSCLE

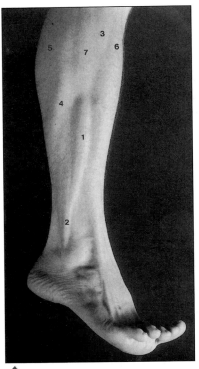

▲
FIGURE 26-19
LATERAL VIEW OF THE INFERIOR
TWO THIRDS OF THE LEG

(1) Peroneus brevis muscle

(2) Tendon of the peroneus longus
muscle

(3) Extensor digitorum longus muscle

(4) Soleus muscle

(5) Lateral head of the gastrocnemius
muscle

(6) Anterior tibialis muscle

(7) Peroneus longus muscle

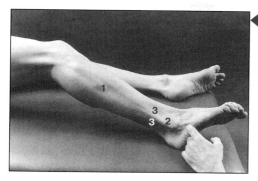

◄ FIGURE 26-20
THE TENDON OF THE PERONEUS BREVIS MUSCLE IN ITS MOST DISTAL COURSE OVER THE LATERAL BORDER OF THE FOOT

A movement of pure abduction at the level of the foot is sufficient to make this tendon prominent. Its course should be followed over the lateral border of the foot down to its insertion into the tuberosity of the fifth metatarsal.

Comment: To visualize its passage over the lateral surface of the calcaneum, above and in front of the peroneal tubercle, see Section XII, "The Ankle and Foot."

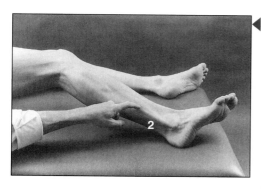

◄ FIGURE 26-21
THE PERONEUS BREVIS MUSCLE AT THE LEVEL OF THE DISTAL LEG

The movement requested is the same as that described above. The muscular body appears in front of the tendon of the peroneus longus muscle. Movements in a contraction–relaxation sequence can improve perception of the position of the relaxed muscle.

FIGURES 26-20, 26-21, AND 26-22

(1) Peroneus longus muscle

(2) Tendon of the peroneus longus muscle

(3) Peroneus brevis muscle

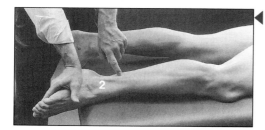

◄ FIGURE 26-22
THE PERONEUS BREVIS MUSCLE AT THE LEG LEVEL

The movement requested is the same as that described above. A plantarflexion of the foot may be added to improve perception of the contraction.

The muscular body is also perceived behind the tendon of the peroneus longus muscle.

THE POSTERIOR MUSCULAR GROUP

This group includes

The superficial plane, composed of

• The triceps surae muscle, formed by

— the soleus muscle (Figs. 26-29, 26-30, and 26-31)

— the medial head of the gastrocnemius muscle (Figs. 26-25 and 26-26)

— the lateral head of the gastrocnemius muscle (Figs. 26-26 and 26-28)

• The plantaris muscle (Fig. 26-33)

The deep plane, composed of

• The popliteus muscle (Fig. 26-28)

• The posterior tibialis muscle (Figs. 26-35, 26-36, and 26-37)

• The flexor digitorum longus muscle (Figs. 26-39, 26-40, and 10-41)

• The flexor hallucis longus muscle (Figs. 26-43, 26-44, and 10-45)

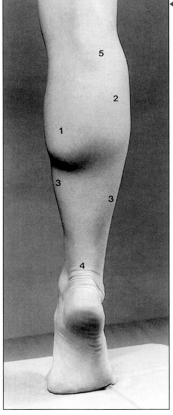

◀ **FIGURE 26-23**
POSTERIOR VIEW OF THE LEG

(1) Medial head of the gastrocnemius muscle

(2) Lateral head of the gastrocnemius muscle

(3) Soleus muscle

(4) Achilles tendon

(5) Plantaris muscle

THE SUPERFICIAL PLANE
The Triceps Surae Muscle and the Plantaris Muscle

• The triceps surae muscle is formed by three muscles:

— the medial head of the gastrocnemius muscle (Figs. 26-25 and 26-26)

— the lateral head of the gastrocnemius muscle (Figs. 26-27 and 26-28)

— the soleus muscle (Figs. 26-29, 26-30, and 26-31)

These three muscles insert distally into the calcaneum by a common tendon, the Achilles tendon (Fig. 26-32).

• The plantaris muscle (Fig. 26-33)

Comment: For didactic reasons, the gastrocnemius muscle, the soleus muscle, and the plantaris muscle are studied separately and in that order.

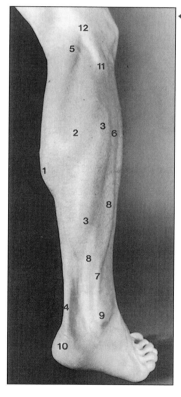

◀ FIGURE 26-24
POSTEROLATERAL VIEW OF THE LEG

(1) Medial head of the gastrocnemius muscle

(2) Lateral head of the gastrocnemius muscle

(3) Soleus muscle

(4) Achilles tendon

(5) Plantaris muscle

(6) Peroneus longus muscle

(7) Tendon of the peroneus longus muscle

(8) Peroneus brevis muscle

(9) Lateral malleolus

(10) Posterior surface of the calcaneum

(11) Head of the fibula

(12) Tendon of the biceps femoris muscle

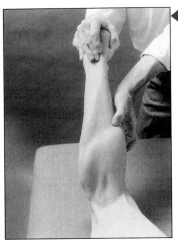

FIGURE 26-25
THE MEDIAL HEAD OF THE GASTROCNEMIUS MUSCLE AT THE LEG LEVEL

With your forearm leaning on the plantar aspect of the foot, the distal hand grip allows use of the "contraction–relaxation" technique by prompting plantarflexion of the ankle. With your hand covering the calcaneum, you may also offer resistance to the flexion of the knee. These two muscular actions are those of the examined muscle, which is found over the posteromedial aspect of the leg, behind the soleus muscle.

Comment: The muscular body of the medial head of the gastrocnemius muscle extends more inferiorly than the lateral head of the gastrocnemius muscle.

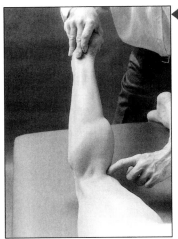

FIGURE 26-26
THE MEDIAL HEAD OF THE GASTROCNEMIUS MUSCLE AT THE KNEE LEVEL

The technique of placement under tension is the same as that described above.

Its proximal aspect is attached, among other structures, to the medial condylar capsule of the femur, which is only a reinforcement of the articular capsule of the knee over the posterior surface of the medial condyle of the femur. It is, therefore, approachable over the medial portion of the popliteal fossa, forming its inferomedial border.

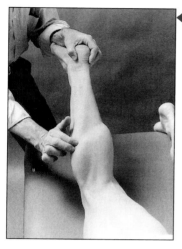

FIGURE 26-27

THE LATERAL HEAD OF THE GASTROCNEMIUS MUSCLE AT THE LEG LEVEL

Here again, the distal hand grip, with the hand covering the heel and the forearm leaning on the plantar surface of the foot, allows you to resist both plantarflexion of the ankle and flexion of the knee. These two combined muscular actions put the investigated muscle under tension.

It is always helpful to alternate between movements of contraction and relaxation in order to perceive the muscular tension clearly.

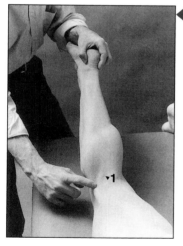

FIGURE 26-28

THE LATERAL HEAD OF THE GASTROCNEMIUS MUSCLE AT THE KNEE LEVEL AND THE POPLITEUS MUSCLE

The technique of placement under muscular tension is the same as that described above.

Like the medial head, the lateral head is attached, among other structures, to a reinforcement of the articular capsule on the posterior surface of the lateral condyle of the femur.

The proximal part of this muscle is a notable region in palpation anatomy, since it forms the inferolateral border of the popliteal fossa. This proximal muscular end is lined medially by the plantaris muscle (1), located in a deeper plane.

Comment: The muscular body of the popliteus muscle, located in the proximal and posterior portion of the leg, is approached indirectly through the muscular mass of the gastrocnemius muscle (palpation not demonstrated). Deep palpation of this region should be performed carefully in view of the presence of the tibial nerve. The tendon of this muscle is discussed in Fig. 23-25.

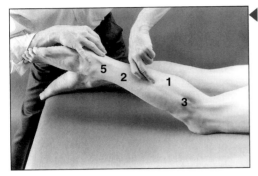

FIGURE 26-29

THE SOLEUS MUSCLE — THE PERONEAL HEAD IN ITS DISTAL PORTION

The distal end of the peroneal head of the soleus muscle (see comment) is located above the peroneus brevis muscle (2) and behind the tendon of the peroneus longus muscle (3). Your distal hand covers the heel while your forearm is placed against the plantar surface of the foot to offer resistance to a plantarflexion. A contraction–relaxation sequence is ideal to perceive this muscular head well. It should be searched for along the fibula between the lateral head of the gastrocnemius muscle, located behind, and the peroneus longus muscle (3), located in front.

Comment: The peroneal head of the soleus muscle is the part of the muscular body attaching to the fibula. It extends much more widely to the lateral surface of the leg than the tibial head to the medial aspect.

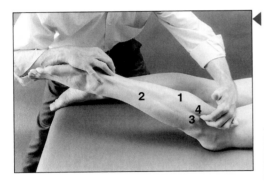

FIGURE 26-30

THE SOLEUS MUSCLE — THE PERONEAL HEAD IN ITS PROXIMAL PORTION

The proximal (see comment Fig. 26-29) and middle portions of the peroneal head of the soleus muscle (4) are located behind the peroneus longus muscle (3) and in front of the lateral head of the gastrocnemius muscle (1).

FIGURES 26-29 AND 26-30

(1) Lateral head of the gastrocnemius muscle

(2) Peroneus brevis muscle

(3) Peroneus longus muscle

(4) Soleus muscle — peroneal head and tibial head

(5) Tendon of the peroneus longus muscle

(6) Medial head of the gastrocnemius muscle

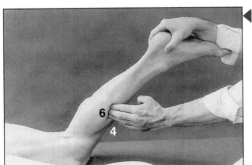

FIGURE 26-31

THE SOLEUS MUSCLE — THE TIBIAL HEAD

Your distal hand covers the calcaneum while your forearm is positioned against the plantar aspect of the foot in order to offer resistance to a plantarflexion of the ankle.
A contraction-relaxation sequence is ideal to perceive this muscular head well. It should be searched for along the medial border of the tibia up to its middle third, in front of the medial head of the gastrocnemius muscle (6).

Comment: The tibial head (4), which is the portion of the muscular body attaching to the tibia, extends much less widely to the medial surface of the leg than the peroneal head to the lateral surface.

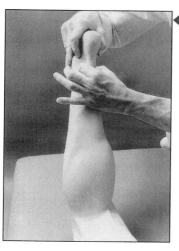

FIGURE 26-32
THE ACHILLES TENDON

The distal hand covers the heel and the forearm leans on the plantar surface of the foot, allowing the examiner to vary widely the degree of tension of the tendon.

The placement under tension may be done in two ways:

· by applying pressure on the plantar surface of the foot, bringing it in dorsiflexion and therefore stretching the tendon

· by using the technique of contraction-relaxation during plantarflexion of the foot

Comment: Once the tendon is located, the approach to it may also be carried out in the relaxed position and over its three surfaces (posterior, anterior, and lateral).

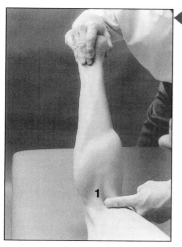

FIGURE 26-33
THE PLANTARIS MUSCLE IN THE POPLITEAL FOSSA

This muscle is located in front of the lateral head of the gastrocnemius muscle, beyond which it extends medially; it is not constant and is hardly accessible.

Your distal hand covers the heel while your forearm is applied against the plantar aspect of the foot, allowing a simultaneous resistance to plantarflexion of the foot and flexion of the knee.

The perception of the contraction of this muscle depends on the subject's morphology. The muscle (1) is perceived in the popliteal fossa, medial to the lateral head of the gastrocnemius muscle.

DEEP PLANE
The Posterior Tibialis Muscle

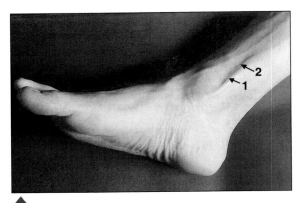

▲

FIGURE 26-34
MEDIAL VIEW OF THE INFERIOR THIRD OF THE LEG

(1) Tendon of the posterior tibialis muscle
(2) Muscular body of the posterior tibialis muscle

Comment: Refer to page 336 to visualize the relations of this structure with the two other tendons of the medial retromalleolar groove, also belonging to the muscles of the deep plane of the leg:

·   *The flexor digitorum longus muscle*
·   *The flexor hallucis longus muscle*

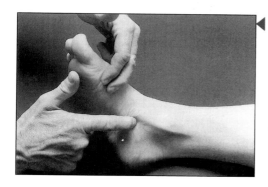

FIGURE 26-35
THE TENDON OF THE POSTERIOR TIBIALIS MUSCLE
BETWEEN THE TUBEROSITY OF THE NAVICULAR BONE
AND THE MEDIAL MALLEOLUS

Your distal hand guides and/or offers resistance to an adduction of the foot, positioned beforehand in plantarflexion. The tendon is perceived between the two structures mentioned above. It may be useful in certain cases to localize the tuberosity of the navicular bone. (See Figs. 27-37 and 27-38.)

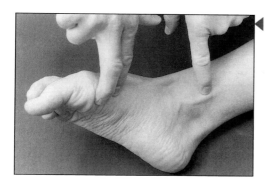

FIGURE 26-36
THE TENDON OF THE POSTERIOR TIBIALIS MUSCLE
AT THE ANKLE

Your distal hand guides and/or offers resistance to adduction of the foot, positioned beforehand in plantarflexion. The tendon appears behind the medial malleolus. It is palpated as a very hard cylindrical cord.

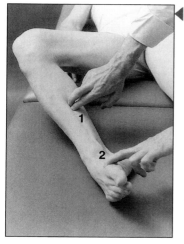

FIGURE 26-37
THE TENDON AND THE MUSCULAR BODY OF THE POSTERIOR
TIBIALIS MUSCLE IN THE LEG

The subject's leg lies on its lateral aspect. To perceive the muscular contraction well, the digital grip is moved along the medial border of the tibia (1). The contraction is better perceived if a contraction-relaxation sequence is used. From an initial positioning of the foot in plantarflexion, the subject is asked to perform consecutive adductions against resistance. The muscular body that extends from the tendon (2) of the posterior tibialis muscle is situated in front of the flexor digitorum longus muscle up to the arch of the latter muscle, which is attached to the tibia at approximately 10 cm above the medial malleolus. After passing under this arch, the muscular body is located lateral to the flexor digitorum longus muscle. At this level, it is not directly approachable. It is covered by the triceps surae muscle.

The Flexor Digitorum Longus Muscle

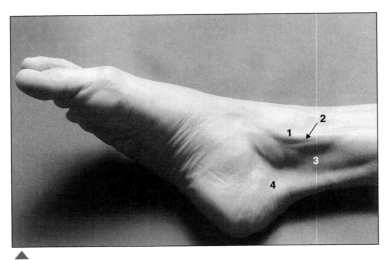

▲
FIGURE 26-38
MEDIAL VIEW OF THE LOWER THIRD OF THE LEG

(1) Posterior tibialis muscle
(2) Flexor digitorum longus muscle
(3) Flexor hallucis longus muscle
(4) Achilles tendon

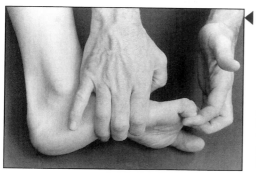

◀ **FIGURE 26-39**

THE TENDONS OF THE FLEXOR DIGITORUM LONGUS MUSCLE AT THE LEVEL OF THE SOLE OF THE FOOT

Your distal hand guides and/or offers light resistance to alternate and rapid flexions of the toes, the ankle having been placed in neutral position earlier. The other hand is applied against the plantar aspect of the foot by covering its lateral border. The grip is wide in order to perceive the contraction well. The tendons themselves cannot be palpated directly, since they are covered by those of the flexor digitorum brevis muscle.

Comment: The muscular contraction involving these two muscles will be better perceived under the fingers if the proximal phalanges of the toes are positioned in hyperextension beforehand.

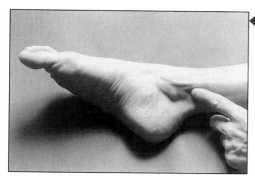

◀ **FIGURE 26-40**

THE FLEXOR DIGITORUM LONGUS MUSCLE IN THE MEDIAL RETROMALLEOLAR GROOVE

The subject performs alternate and rapid flexions of the toes while the foot lies on the heel or on its lateral border.

The tendon is perceived in the area of the medial malleolus, behind the tendon of the posterior tibialis muscle.

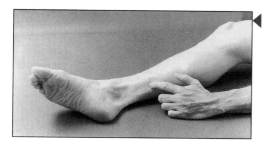

◀ **FIGURE 26-41**

THE MUSCULAR BODY OF THE FLEXOR DIGITORUM LONGUS MUSCLE IN THE LOWER THIRD OF THE LEG

The leg lies on its lateral aspect and the ankle is in a relaxed position.

The index finger indicates the muscular body, which is located behind the posterior tibialis muscle up to an arch formed by the investigated muscle, which inserts into the tibia at approximately 10 cm above the medial malleolus. Above this arch, the muscular body is located medial to the posterior tibialis muscle.

The muscular contraction is better perceived if a sequence of contraction-relaxation is used. The subject is asked to perform rapidly consecutive flexions of the toes.

The Flexor Hallucis Longus Muscle

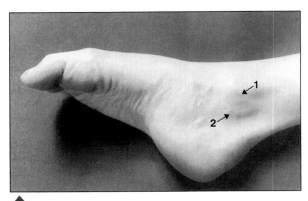

▲
FIGURE 26-42
MEDIAL VIEW OF THE LOWER THIRD OF THE LEG

(1) Tendon of the posterior tibialis muscle

(2) Tendon of the flexor hallucis longus muscle

Comment: Refer to page 336 to visualize the relations of this structure with the two other tendons of the medial retromalleolar groove also belonging to the muscles of the deep plane of the leg:

· *The posterior tibialis muscle*
· *The flexor digitorum longus muscle*

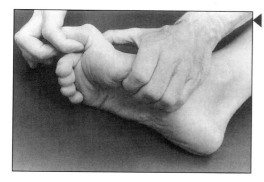

◀ **FIGURE 26-43**

THE FLEXOR HALLUCIS LONGUS MUSCLE AT THE LEVEL OF THE SOLE OF THE FOOT

With the subject's ankle placed in neutral position and the foot lying on the heel or on its lateral border, your distal hand guides and/or offers light resistance to alternate and rapid flexions of the first toe. The other hand is positioned against the plantar aspect of the first metatarsal bone through a wide grip for a better perception of the contraction. This allows a better approach to the tendon, which is perceived somewhat as a cord beneath the fingers.

Comment: This tendinous structure will be perceived much better if the proximal phalanx of the first toe is placed in hyperextension beforehand.

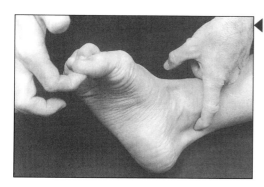

◀ **FIGURE 26-44**

THE FLEXOR HALLUCIS LONGUS MUSCLE IN THE MEDIAL RETROMALLEOLAR GROOVE

Your distal hand guides and/or offers resistance to alternate and rapid flexions of the subject's first toe, the ankle having been placed in neutral position with the leg lying on its posterolateral surface. The muscle is palpated in the medial retromalleolar groove, between the medial malleolus and the Achilles tendon, and behind the tendon of the flexor digitorum longus muscle. See also Figure 29-17.

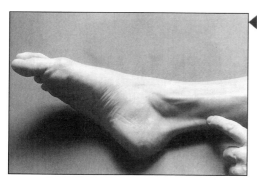

◀ **FIGURE 26-45**

THE FLEXOR HALLUCIS LONGUS MUSCLE IN THE MEDIAL RETROMALLEOLAR GROOVE — VISUALIZATION OF THE MUSCULAR BODY

This figure simply allows a better visualization of the muscular body (indicated by the index finger), already investigated in Figure 26-44 and located behind the flexor digitorum longus muscle (2) (see Fig. 26-38).

The contraction is better perceived if the subject is asked to perform consecutive flexions of the first toe.

THE
ANKLE
AND
FOOT

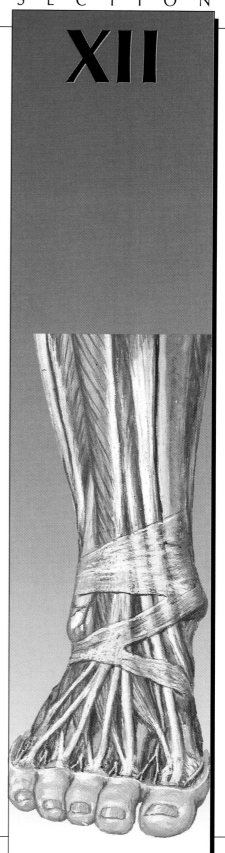

MUSCLES OF DORSUM OF THE FOOT: SUPERFICIAL DISSECTION

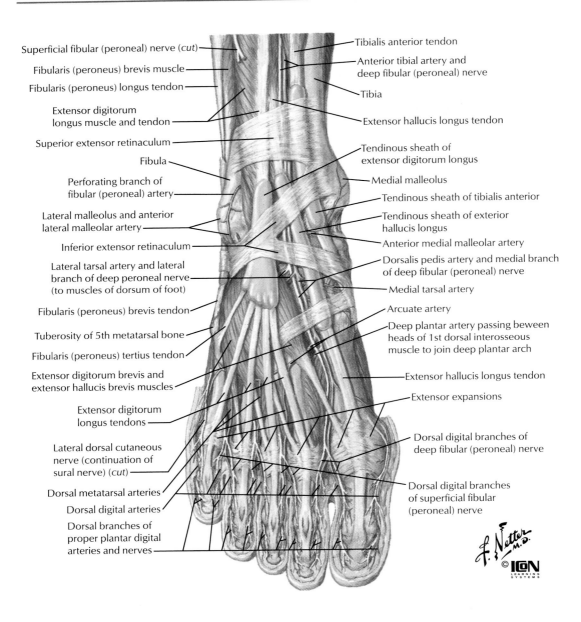

Superficial fibular (peroneal) nerve (*cut*)

Fibularis (peroneus) brevis muscle

Fibularis (peroneus) longus tendon

Extensor digitorum longus muscle and tendon

Superior extensor retinaculum

Fibula

Perforating branch of fibular (peroneal) artery

Lateral malleolus and anterior lateral malleolar artery

Inferior extensor retinaculum

Lateral tarsal artery and lateral branch of deep peroneal nerve (to muscles of dorsum of foot)

Fibularis (peroneus) brevis tendon

Tuberosity of 5th metatarsal bone

Fibularis (peroneus) tertius tendon

Extensor digitorum brevis and extensor hallucis brevis muscles

Extensor digitorum longus tendons

Lateral dorsal cutaneous nerve (continuation of sural nerve) (*cut*)

Dorsal metatarsal arteries

Dorsal digital arteries

Dorsal branches of proper plantar digital arteries and nerves

Tibialis anterior tendon

Anterior tibial artery and deep fibular (peroneal) nerve

Tibia

Extensor hallucis longus tendon

Tendinous sheath of extensor digitorum longus

Medial malleolus

Tendinous sheath of tibialis anterior

Tendinous sheath of exterior hallucis longus

Anterior medial malleolar artery

Dorsalis pedis artery and medial branch of deep fibular (peroneal) nerve

Medial tarsal artery

Arcuate artery

Deep plantar artery passing beween heads of 1st dorsal interosseous muscle to join deep plantar arch

Extensor hallucis longus tendon

Extensor expansions

Dorsal digital branches of deep fibular (peroneal) nerve

Dorsal digital branches of superficial fibular (peroneal) nerve

MUSCLES OF THE ANKLE AND THE FOOT: ANTERIOR VIEW

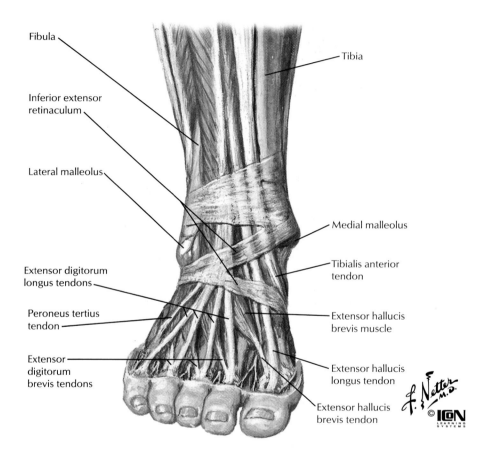

Fibula

Inferior extensor retinaculum

Lateral malleolus

Extensor digitorum longus tendons

Peroneus tertius tendon

Extensor digitorum brevis tendons

Tibia

Medial malleolus

Tibialis anterior tendon

Extensor hallucis brevis muscle

Extensor hallucis longus tendon

Extensor hallucis brevis tendon

TENDON SHEATHS OF THE ANKLE: LATERAL VIEW

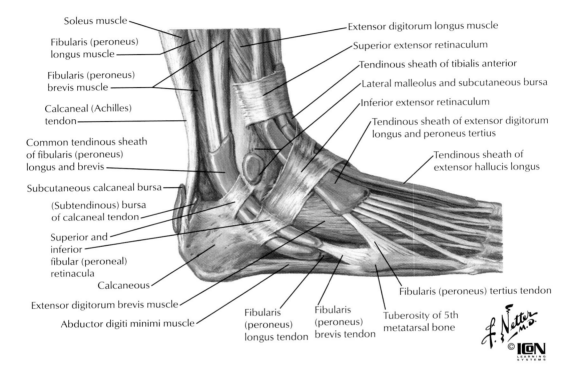

Soleus muscle

Fibularis (peroneus) longus muscle

Fibularis (peroneus) brevis muscle

Calcaneal (Achilles) tendon

Common tendinous sheath of fibularis (peroneus) longus and brevis

Subcutaneous calcaneal bursa

(Subtendinous) bursa of calcaneal tendon

Superior and inferior fibular (peroneal) retinacula

Calcaneous

Extensor digitorum brevis muscle

Abductor digiti minimi muscle

Fibularis (peroneus) longus tendon

Fibularis (peroneus) brevis tendon

Tuberosity of 5th metatarsal bone

Fibularis (peroneus) tertius tendon

Tendinous sheath of extensor hallucis longus

Tendinous sheath of extensor digitorum longus and peroneus tertius

Inferior extensor retinaculum

Lateral malleolus and subcutaneous bursa

Tendinous sheath of tibialis anterior

Superior extensor retinaculum

Extensor digitorum longus muscle

TENDON SHEATHS OF THE ANKLE: MEDIAL VIEW

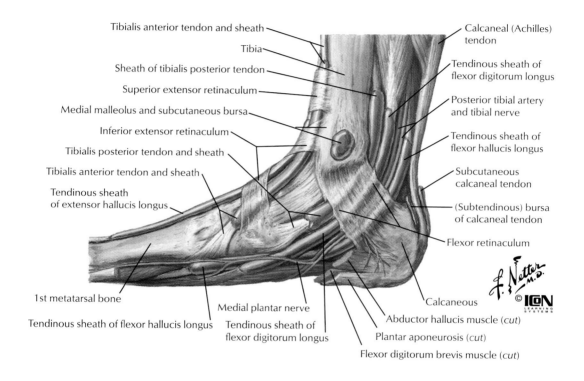

Tibialis anterior tendon and sheath

Tibia

Sheath of tibialis posterior tendon

Superior extensor retinaculum

Medial malleolus and subcutaneous bursa

Inferior extensor retinaculum

Tibialis posterior tendon and sheath

Tibialis anterior tendon and sheath

Tendinous sheath of extensor hallucis longus

1st metatarsal bone

Tendinous sheath of flexor hallucis longus

Medial plantar nerve

Tendinous sheath of flexor digitorum longus

Calcaneal (Achilles) tendon

Tendinous sheath of flexor digitorum longus

Posterior tibial artery and tibial nerve

Tendinous sheath of flexor hallucis longus

Subcutaneous calcaneal tendon

(Subtendinous) bursa of calcaneal tendon

Flexor retinaculum

Calcaneous

Abductor hallucis muscle (cut)

Plantar aponeurosis (cut)

Flexor digitorum brevis muscle (cut)

TOPOGRAPHIC PRESENTATION OF THE FOOT

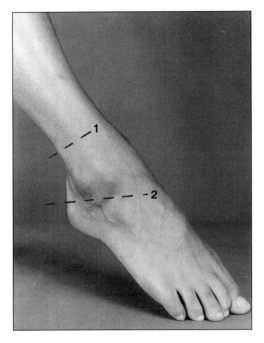

FIGURE 27-1
ANTEROLATERAL VIEW OF THE ANKLE AND FOOT

(1) Superior border of the region of the ankle

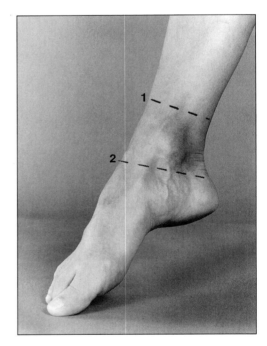

FIGURE 27-2
ANTEROMEDIAL VIEW OF THE ANKLE AND FOOT

(2) Inferior border of the region of the ankle

CHAPTER
Twenty
Seven

OSTEOLOGY

THE LATERAL BORDER

The bony structures accessible by palpation are

- The fifth metatarsal bone
  — the head (Fig. 27-4)
  — the lateral surface of the shaft (Fig. 27-5)
  — the inferior border of the shaft (Fig. 27-6)
  — the base of the fifth metatarsal bone — located by a global approach to the lateral border of the foot (Fig. 27-7)
  — the styloid process or tubercular eminence of the fifth metatarsal bone (Fig. 27-8)
- The cuboid bone
  — the lateral border (Fig. 27-9; also see Fig. 27-7)
  — the dorsal surface (Fig. 27-10)
  — the plantar surface (Fig. 27-11)
- The calcaneus
  — the lateral surface (Fig. 27-12)
  — the greater process (Fig. 27-13; also see Fig. 27-7)
  — the anterior surface or cuboid facet (Fig. 27-14)

  — the floor of the sinus tarsi (Fig. 27-15)
  — the peroneal trochlea (Fig. 27-16)
  — the tubercle of insertion of the calcaneofibular ligament (Fig. 27-17)
  — the posterior portion of the lateral surface (Fig. 27-18)
  — the lateral portion of the posterior segment — posterior surface (Fig. 27-19)
- The talus
  — the lateral surface of the neck (Fig. 27-20; also see Fig. 27-7)
  — the lateral process (Fig. 27-21)
- The lateral malleolus
  — the anterior border (Fig. 27-22)
  — the apex (Fig. 27-23)
  — the posterior border (Fig. 27-24).

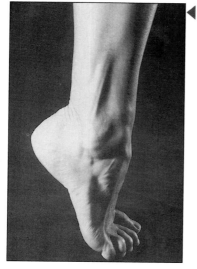

◀ **FIGURE 27-3**
THE LATERAL SURFACE OF THE ANKLE AND OF THE FOOT

THE FIFTH METATARSAL BONE

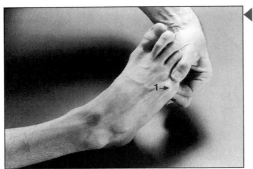

◄ **FIGURE 27-4**
THE HEAD OF THE FIFTH METATARSAL BONE

The fifth toe should be brought into plantarflexion in order to demonstrate the head (1) of the fifth metatarsal bone on the dorsal portion of the lateral border of the foot. This demonstration also allows the localization of the metatarsophalangeal joint.

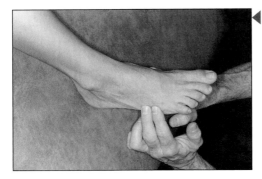

◄ **FIGURE 27-5**
THE LATERAL SURFACE OF THE SHAFT OF THE FIFTH METATARSAL BONE

The lateral surface is directly under the skin. There is no difficulty in following it since it is located just above the abductor muscle of the fifth toe (abductor digiti minimi).

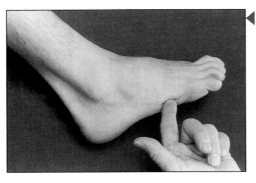

◄ **FIGURE 27-6**
THE INFERIOR BORDER OF THE SHAFT OF THE FIFTH METATARSAL BONE

The inferior border of the shaft is palpated by the index finger as a slightly curved structure with a plantar concavity, which is well perceived. In this picture, the index finger pushes away the abductor muscle of the fifth toe in order to be in contact with the investigated bony structure.

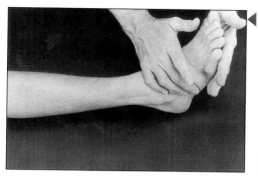

FIGURE 27-7
THE BASE OF THE FIFTH METATARSAL BONE, LOCALIZED BY A GLOBAL APPROACH TO THE LATERAL BORDER OF THE FOOT

The foot is in a relaxed position, with the subject lying on a table or with the foot resting on your knee. Your proximal hand is placed on the proximal aspect of the foot, gently covering the lateral border of the foot. The lateral border of the little finger is placed against the lateral malleolus.

In this case, the little finger is in contact with the greater process of the calcaneus. The ring finger faces the cuboid bone. The middle finger faces the base of the fifth metatarsal bone.

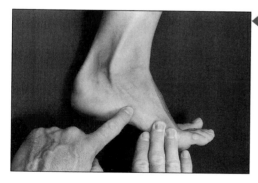

FIGURE 27-8
TUBEROSITY OF THE FIFTH METATARSAL BONE

Articulating its posterior extremity with the cuboid bone, the fifth metatarsal bone, peculiarity, presents a prominent process behind, below, and outside its base. It is into this tubercular eminence that the tendon of the peroneus brevis muscle is inserted. Posteriorly, this process partially overlooks the lateral border of the cuboid bone.

THE CUBOID BONE

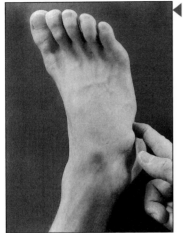

◄ FIGURE 27-9
THE LATERAL BORDER OF THE CUBOID BONE

In the posterior aspect of the foot the cuboid bone (see Fig. 27-7) is the bony structure immediately following the styloid process of the fifth metatarsal bone (Figs. 27-7 and 27-8). Once this process is located, your fingers should slide posteriorly into a depression over the lateral border of the foot, to be in contact with a ridge that represents the investigated structure.

Comment: The tendon of the peroneus brevis muscle, which runs along this ridge, hampers the investigation unless it is relaxed.

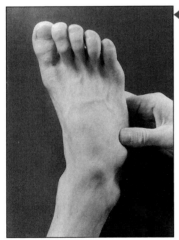

◄ FIGURE 27-10
THE DORSAL SURFACE OF THE CUBOID BONE

The two bony structures used for proper positioning on this surface are
· the tuberosity of the fifth metatarsal bone, already located (Figs. 27-7 and 27-8),
· the greater process of the calcaneus (Fig. 27-13). The dorsal surface of the cuboid bone is obviously located between these two structures, which represent its anterior and posterior borders.

Your thumb should first be placed on the lateral border of the cuboid bone (Fig. 27-9), then moved slightly toward the dorsal surface of the foot in order to be in contact with the investigated bony structure.

Comment: Rough, directed downward and laterally, it is directly under the skin and easy to palpate. The tendon of the peroneus brevis muscle runs along its lateral aspect and the extensor digitorum brevis muscle partially covers it.

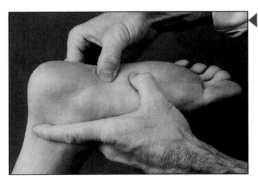

◄ FIGURE 27-11
THE PLANTAR SURFACE OF THE CUBOID BONE

After localizing the styloid process or tubercular eminence of the fifth metatarsal bone (Figs. 27-7 and 27-8) and the greater process of the calcaneus (Figs. 27-7 and 27-13), your thumb is placed between the two structures, and then moved around the lateral border of the foot and the lateral border of the cuboid bone to be positioned on the plantar surface of this bone.

THE CALCANEUS

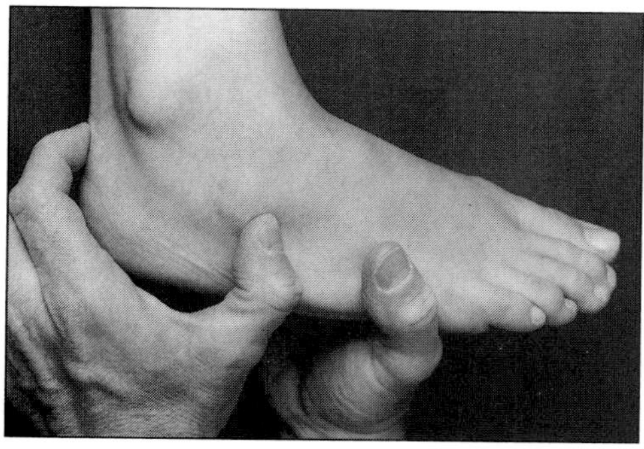

FIGURE 27-12
THE LATERAL SURFACE OF THE CALCANEUS

The forefoot is adducted and supinated in order to project the anterior articular surface of the calcaneus and to partially uncover it.

Your thumb is positioned on this surface and the index finger is positioned on the posterior surface of the calcaneus in order to clearly perceive the dimension of this bone among the bones of the foot.

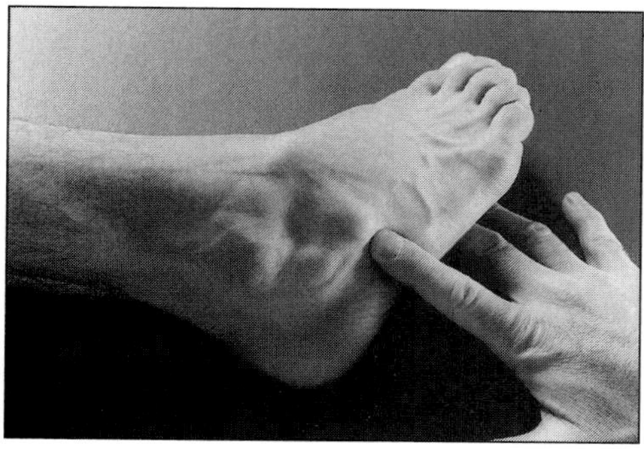

FIGURE 27-13
THE GREATER PROCESS OF THE CALCANEUS

The greater process of the calcaneus delimits the lateral calcaneocuboidal interspace posteriorly. A supination of the forefoot facilitates its access. It may be very prominent in certain subjects, as is the case in this figure. See also Figure 27-7.

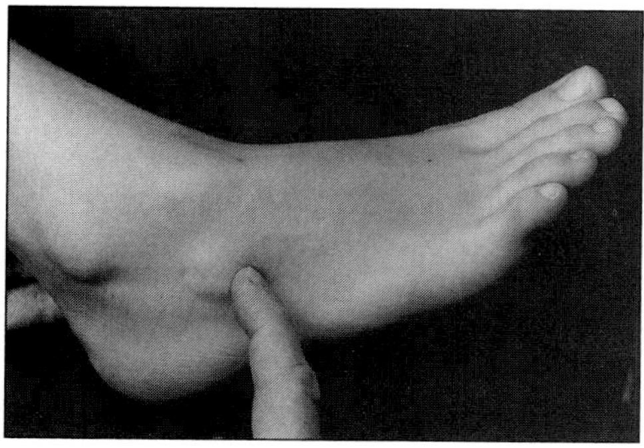

FIGURE 27-14
THE ANTERIOR (ARTICULAR) SURFACE OR CUBOID FACET OF THE CALCANEUS

In order to uncover the superior anterolateral portion of this facet, it is usually sufficient to ask the subject to adduct and supinate the forefoot placed in slight flexion.

If this is not sufficient, it is possible to perform this maneuver using a passive technique. One hand is used to stabilize the calcaneus while the other hand brings the forefoot into adduction, supination, and slight plantarflexion (also see Fig. 27-7).

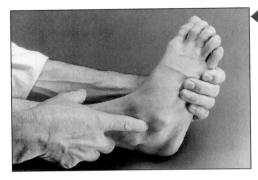

◄ FIGURE 27-15
THE FLOOR OF THE SINUS TARSI

Anatomic reminder: The sinus tarsi is formed by the inter-
locking of the calcaneus and of the talus. It becomes progressively wider as it runs outward and forward. Its floor is
the calcaneal sulcus, while its roof is the sulcus tali. The
superposition of these two grooves forms a conduit called
the sinus tarsi. The sinus itself is therefore not accessible,
but its floor is, exactly where it opens on the superior surface of the calcaneus at the level of its anterior segment.

*Comment: The posterior portion of the sinus tarsi is occupied
by the two or three bundles of the calcaneotalar ligament.*

Technique of approach: With the subject's foot in a neutral
position, place your index finger on the anterior border of
the lateral malleolus. As the finger is advanced slightly
toward the sole of the foot, the investigated structure is palpated as a depression. The extensor digitorum brevis muscle may hamper this approach (one should make sure it is
relaxed). The tendon of the extensor digitorum longus muscle and the lateral aspect of the neck of the talus are located medially.

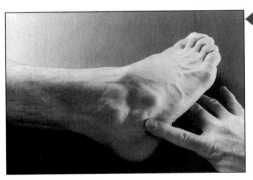

◄ FIGURE 27-16
THE PERONEAL TROCHLEA

This is a bony prominence located approximately one finger's breadth below the lateral malleolus. The peroneal
trochlea separates the underlying groove of the peroneus
longus muscle from the overlying groove of the peroneus
brevis muscle. It is palpated approximately one finger's
breadth from the apex of the lateral malleolus (also see Figs.
27-12 and 27-23).

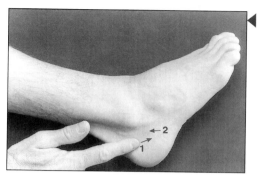

◀ FIGURE 27-17
TUBERCLE OF INSERTION OF THE CALCANEOFIBULAR LIGAMENT

This structure is not always well differentiated. It is the site of insertion for the middle fasciculus or calcaneofibular ligament of the lateral lateral ligament of the ankle. With the subject's foot in a neutral position (0°), the tubercle is located behind the peroneal tubercle (2) (Fig. 27-16) at approximately one finger's breadth below and one finger's breadth behind the lateral calcaneotalar articular interspace.

Comment: The tubercle is not constant. In its absence, the calcaneofibular ligament inserts directly into the lateral surface of the calcaneus.

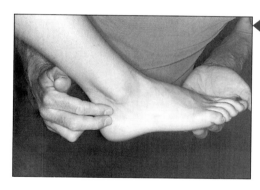

◀ FIGURE 27-18
THE POSTERIOR PORTION OF THE LATERAL SURFACE OF THE CALCANEUS

This structure is perceived beneath the fingers as flat and rough over essentially the entire lateral surface of the calcaneus, which is directly under the skin. In this figure, the grip is somewhat withdrawn in order to demonstrate as widely as possible the bony structure discussed.

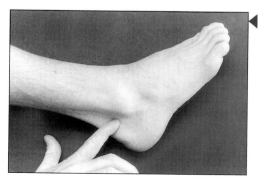

◀ FIGURE 27-19
THE LATERAL PORTION OF THE POSTERIOR SEGMENT OF THE CALCANEUS — POSTERIOR SURFACE

In this figure, the index finger lies on the bony structure mentioned above (Fig. 27-18), behind the talus and lateral to the Achilles tendon.

THE TALUS

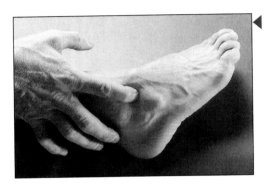

◀ **FIGURE 27-20**
THE LATERAL SURFACE OF THE NECK OF THE TALUS

The subject's foot is first placed in a neutral position. Your index finger is placed on the anterior border of the lateral malleolus. On being advanced slightly forward and inward, it faces the investigated structure. Tip the forefoot over in slight supination to make the lateral surface more accessible (see also Fig. 27-7).

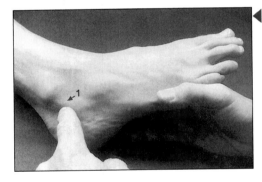

◀ **FIGURE 27-21**
THE LATERAL PROCESS OF THE TALUS

This structure is a tubercle located in front of the peroneal tubercle and under the lateral calcaneotalar interspace. With the subject's foot in neutral position (0°), apply your index finger against the posterior portion of the inferior or distal end of the fibula. This tubercle is palpated approximately one finger's breadth in front of the peroneal tubercle.

Comment: In this figure, the index finger is displaced backward, in order not to hamper visualization of the investigated structure (1).

THE LATERAL MALLEOLUS

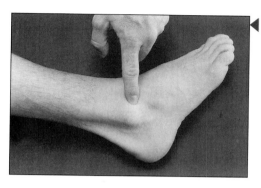

◀ **FIGURE 27-22**
THE ANTERIOR BORDER OF THE LATERAL MALLEOLUS

In its uppermost portion, this is the site of insertion of the anterior tibiofibular ligament. In its lowermost or distal portion, it is the site of insertion of the anterior talofibular fibular ligament and of the calcaneofibular ligament.

Comment: These last two ligaments are respectively the anterior and middle fasciculi of the lateral lateral ligament.

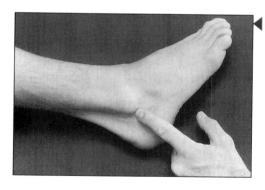

◀ **FIGURE 27-23**
THE APEX OF THE LATERAL MALLEOLUS

The apex presents, just in front of its most prominent point, a groove for the attachment of a part of the middle fasciculus (calcaneofibular ligament) of the lateral lateral ligament of the ankle. The other portion of this ligament is located on the lowermost portion of the apex's anterior border.
It is therefore an important landmark for localizing the fibular insertions of this ligament.

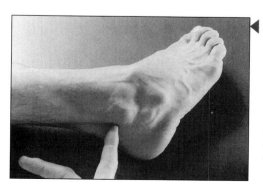

◀ **FIGURE 27-24**
THE POSTERIOR BORDER OF THE LATERAL MALLEOLUS

One must ensure that the peroneus muscles (peroneus longus and peroneus brevis) are relaxed to prevent their tendons, passing behind this border, from hampering its access.

Comment: This border is the site of attachment of the posterior tibiofibular ligament as well as the posterior fasciculus (posterior talofibular-fibular ligament) of the lateral ligament of the ankle.

THE MEDIAL BORDER

The bony structures accessible by palpation are

• The first metatarsal bone
  — the phalanges of the first toe and the head of the metatarsal bone — dorsal approach (Fig. 27-26)
  — the head and the sesamoid bones of the metatarsal bone — plantar approach (Fig. 27-27)
  — the shaft (Figs. 27-28 through 27-31)
  — the base—located by a global approach to the medial border of the foot (Fig. 27-32)
  — the posteromedial tubercle (Fig. 27-33)
  — the posterolateral tubercle (Fig. 27-34)

• The medial cuneiform bone
  — the medial surface — located by using the anterior tibialis muscle (Fig. 27-35; also see Fig. 27-32)
  — the superior surface (Fig. 27-36)

• The navicular bone
  — the tuberosity of the navicular bone — direct approach (Fig. 27-37; see also Fig. 27-32)

  — the tuberosity of the navicular bone—located by using the posterior tibialis muscle (Fig. 27-38)

• The talus
  — the ligamentous field or middle field of the head (Fig. 27-39; see also Fig. 27-32)
  — the neck (Figs. 27-40 and 27-41; see also Fig. 27-32)
  — the posteromedial tubercle (Fig. 27-42)
  — the posterolateral tubercle (Fig. 27-43)

• The calcaneus
  — the lesser process (Fig. 27-44)
  — the groove of the calcaneus (Fig. 27-45)

• The medial malleolus
  — the anterior border (Fig. 27-46)
  — the inferior extremity (Fig. 27-47)
  — the posterior border (Fig. 27-48)

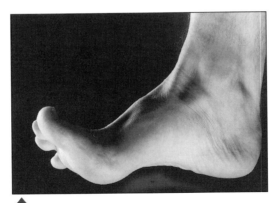

▲
FIGURE 27-25
THE MEDIAL BORDER OF THE FOOT

THE FIRST METATARSAL BONE

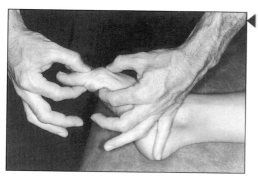

◀ FIGURE 27-26

THE PHALANGES OF THE FIRST TOE AND THE HEAD OF THE FIRST METATARSAL BONE — DORSAL APPROACH

The phalanges are not difficult to examine. Remember that each toe except for the first is composed of three phalanges, while the first toe has two.

A precise palpation allows the examiner to perceive the medial and lateral surfaces as well as the plantar and dorsal surfaces of the shaft of each phalanx of the first toe.

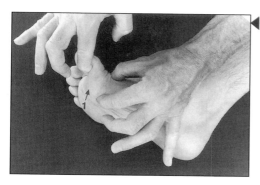

◀ FIGURE 27-27

THE HEAD AND THE SESAMOID BONES OF THE FIRST METATARSAL BONE — PLANTAR APPROACH

Placing your distal digital grip on the plantar aspect of the proximal phalanx, bring it into extension. You will then palpate the plantar base of this phalanx — the inferior or plantar articular surface of the head of the first metatarsal bone and the two sesamoid bones.

Comment: The anterior extremity or head of each metatarsal bone ends by a convex articular surface, which is much larger in its plantar (1) than its dorsal portion. This grip allows you to free up the articular surface.

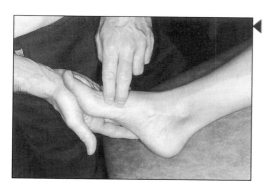

◀ FIGURE 27-28

THE MEDIAL BORDER OF THE FIRST METATARSAL BONE

This border is located over the medial aspect of the foot. Directly under the skin, it has the characteristic of being situated in the dorsal half of the medial border of the foot.

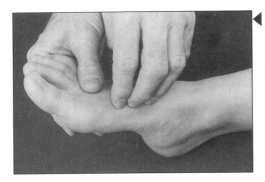

◀ **FIGURE 27-29**
THE DORSAL SURFACE OF THE FIRST METATARSAL BONE

The shaft of each metatarsal bone is prismoid and triangular in shape. This shaft presents a dorsal surface that is generally narrow but much wider in the back than in the front.

Comment: An anatomic characteristic of all metatarsal bones is the presence of two borders for each dorsal surface, medial and lateral.

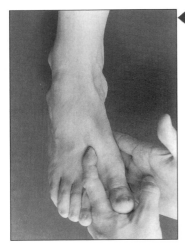

◀ **FIGURE 27-30**
THE LATERAL SURFACE OF THE FIRST METATARSAL BONE

The lateral facet of each metatarsal bone demarcates respectively with the medial facet of the adjacent metatarsal bone a particular space called the interosseus or metatarsal interspace.

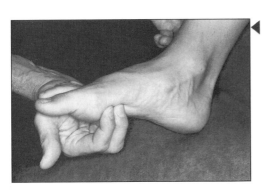

◀ **FIGURE 27-31**
THE INFERIOR BORDER OF THE SHAFT OF THE FIRST
METATARSAL BONE

The inferior or plantar border of the shaft of the first metatarsal bone is clearly palpated as a curved structure with plantar concavity (Figs. 27-4 and 27-7).

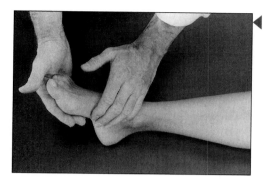

◀ FIGURE 27-32

THE BASE OF THE FIRST METATARSAL BONE — LOCATED
THROUGH A GLOBAL APPROACH TO THE MEDIAL BORDER
OF THE FOOT

The subject's foot is in a normal, relaxed position, with the
subject lying on a table or with the foot on the knee of the
examiner.

Your proximal hand is positioned on the proximal aspect of
the foot and gently covers its medial border. The ulnar side
of the small finger is placed on the anterior border of the
medial malleolus.

In this case:
· the small finger faces the medial surface of the neck of
  the talus
· the ring finger faces the navicular bone
· the middle finger faces the medial cuneiform bone
· the index finger faces the base of the first metatarsal bone

*Comment: This global approach of the bony structures of
the medial border of the foot may be considered to be reli-
able in most subjects.*

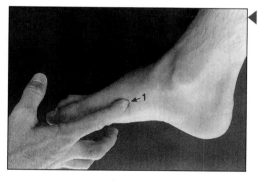

◀ FIGURE 27-33

THE POSTEROMEDIAL TUBERCLE OF THE BASE OF THE FIRST
METATARSAL BONE

The metatarsal extension of the anterior tibialis muscle
inserts into this tubercle. Its other site of distal insertion is the
inferior portion of the medial cuneiform bone (1) (Fig. 27-35).

Your index finger slides between the muscular body of the
abductor hallucis muscle and the plantar border of the first
metatarsal bone, which is palpated as a curved structure
(Fig. 27-31). This tubercle may be found near the base of the
metatarsal bone by following the medial border of its shaft.

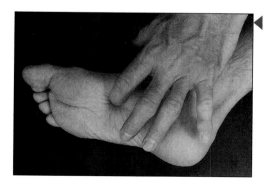

◀ FIGURE 27-34

THE POSTEROLATERAL TUBERCLE OF THE FIRST METATARSAL
BONE

Located below, outside, and behind the previous tubercle,
this tubercle receives the main distal extension of the peroneus longus muscle.

It is obvious that this bony prominence, covered by the soft
tissues, will be better perceived in a case of muscular wast-
ing, which occurs when a person is bedridden for a long
period. In the opposite case, the pressure applied must be
quite firm in order to perceive the investigated structure.

THE MEDIAL CUNEIFORM BONE

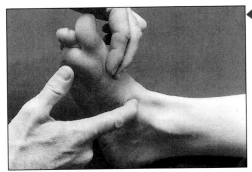

◀ **FIGURE 27-35**
THE MEDIAL CUNEIFORM BONE — THE MEDIAL SURFACE

An effective technique to localize this surface is to place the anterior tibialis muscle under tension, asking the subject to perform a supination and dorsiflexion of the foot with or without resistance. The investigated surface is then easy to locate, since this muscle attaches to its anteroinferior portion. See also Figure 27-32.

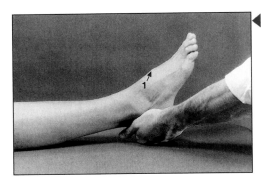

◀ **FIGURE 27-36**
LATERAL VIEW OF THE SUPERIOR BORDER OF THE MEDIAL CUNEIFORM BONE

Positioned on the medial border of the foot, between the navicular bone and the first metatarsal bone, the medial cuneiform bone presents a sharp superior or dorsal border (1) resembling a fish bone, particularly in its posterior aspect.

Comment: This characteristic is demonstrated in this picture by a lateral view.

THE NAVICULAR BONE

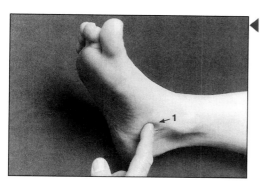

◀ FIGURE 27-37
**THE TUBEROSITY OF THE NAVICULAR BONE —
DIRECT APPROACH**

This tuberosity projects over the inferior portion of the medial surface of the navicular bone (1). It is the site of insertion of the posterior tibialis muscle.

It is accessible just behind and medial to the tendon of the anterior tibialis muscle (see Fig 27-59). In many subjects, this tuberosity is clearly visible, as in this picture.

See also Figure 27-32.

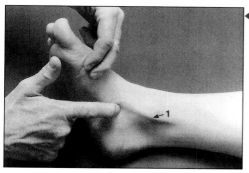

◀ FIGURE 27-38
**THE TUBEROSITY OF THE NAVICULAR BONE —
LOCALIZATION BY USING THE POSTERIOR TIBIALIS MUSCLE**

Placing the posterior tibialis muscle (1) under tension is an effective method of locating the tuberosity of the navicular bone when it is less apparent.

The foot is positioned in plantarflexion beforehand and the subject is asked to perform an adduction of the foot.
From the medial malleolus, follow the tendon of the muscle mentioned above downward to the investigated tuberosity.

THE TALUS

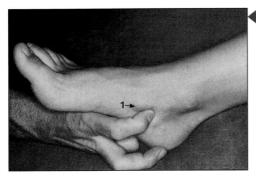

FIGURE 27-39
THE LIGAMENTOUS FIELD OR MIDDLE FIELD OF THE HEAD

As indicated by its name, this structure is in relation with the inferior or plantar calcaneonavicular ligament.
It is located behind the anterosuperior field of the head of the talus, which articulates with the navicular bone.

Position your finger behind the tuberosity of the navicular bone (1), over the medial border of the foot, to perceive this smooth surface under the finger.

Comment: Depending on the subject, it is sometimes useful to abduct and pronate the forefoot in order to better palpate this structure.

See also Figure 27-32.

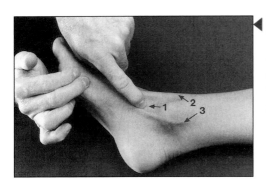

FIGURE 27-40
THE MEDIAL PORTION OF THE NECK OF THE TALUS

The medial aspect of the neck of the talus (1) is essentially examined between the tendons of the anterior tibialis muscle (2) laterally and of the posterior tibialis muscle (3) medially.

See also Figure 27-32.

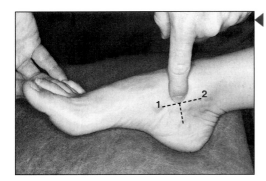

FIGURE 27-41
THE MEDIAL PORTION OF THE NECK OF THE TALUS
(SECOND METHOD)

In addition to a localization by using the tendons (figure above), it is also possible to locate this structure through an imaginary line drawn between the tuberosity of the navicular bone (1) and the medial malleolus (2).

From the middle of this line and toward the malleolus (2), you face the neck of the talus (rough surface under the fingers).

From the middle of this line and toward the tuberosity of the navicular bone (1), one faces the ligamentous field of the head of the talus (structure perceived as smooth under the fingers) (Fig. 27-39).

Comment: A rough ridge, more or less prominent depending on the subject, separates these two portions of the talus: the head and the neck.

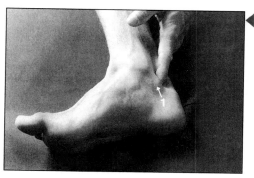

◀ FIGURE 27-42
THE MEDIAL TUBERCLE OF THE TALUS

It is important to remember that this bony structure (1) belongs to the posterior surface of the talus and that it is the site of insertion of the posterior talofibular fasciculus, the deep layer of the deltoid ligament.

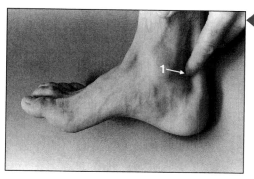

◀ FIGURE 27-43
THE LATERAL TUBERCLE OF THE TALUS

This tubercle (1) also belongs to the posterior surface of the talus. Your finger should be placed against the Achilles tendon, and, to investigate, the posterior border of the talus should be approached.

Comment: In most subjects, this structure is difficult to access, but it is a remarkable bony structure, since it is the site of insertion of the posterior talofibular-fibular ligament, posterior fasciculus of the lateral lateral ligament of the ankle.

THE CALCANEUS

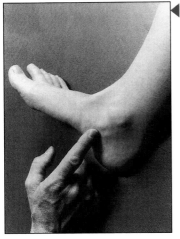

◀ FIGURE 27-44
SUSTENTACULUM TALI

This structure is located approximately one finger's breadth below the medial malleolus. Its superior portion supports the medial articular surface of the calcaneus, intended for the talus.

When this process is approached, the medial calcaneotalar interspace is very close.

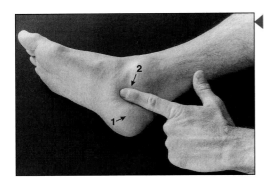

◀ FIGURE 27-45
THE GROOVE OF THE CALCANEUS

Directed downward and forward, it occupies the width of the medial surface. It is limited posteriorly and inferiorly by the posteromedial tuberosity of the calcaneus (1) and anteriorly and superiorly by a projection, the size of which depends on the subject: sustentaculum tali (2).

THE MEDIAL MALLEOLUS

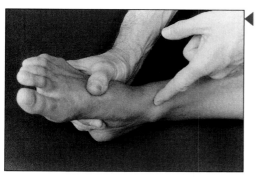

◄ FIGURE 27-46
THE ANTERIOR BORDER OF THE MEDIAL MALLEOLUS

Very thick and rough, this is the site of insertion of the superficial layer of the medial lateral ligament of the ankle.

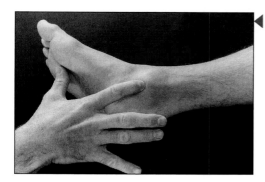

◄ FIGURE 27-47
THE INFERIOR EXTREMITY OF THE MEDIAL MALLEOLUS

This structure is formed by two tubercles (anterior and posterior) separated by a depression, which is the site of insertion of the superficial and deep layers of the medial lateral ligament of the ankle.

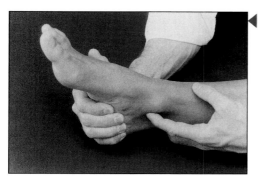

◄ FIGURE 27-48
THE POSTERIOR BORDER OF THE MEDIAL MALLEOLUS

This structure presents a malleolar sulcus directed downward and medially. It is accessible for examination if the tendons contained in it are maintained in a relaxed position. The tendon of the posterior tibialis muscle is the most anterior and that of the flexor digitorum longus muscle the most posterior.

Comment: In fact, these two tendons travel behind the medial malleolus in their respective osteofibrous sheaths.

THE ANTERIOR SURFACE OF THE ANKLE
AND THE DORSAL SURFACE OF THE FOOT

The structures accessible by palpation are

- The heads of the metatarsal bones in dorsal view (Fig. 27-50)
- The fifth metatarsal bone (Fig. 27-51)
- The fourth metatarsal bone (Fig. 27-52)
- The third metatarsal bone (Fig. 27-53)
- The second metatarsal bone (Fig. 27-54)
- The first metatarsal bone (Fig. 27-55)
- The neck of the talus (Fig. 27-56)
- The anterior border of the lower extremity of the tibia (Fig. 27-57)

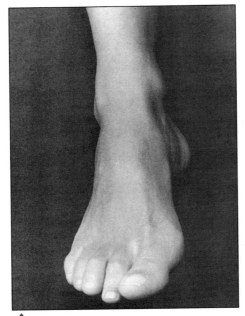

▲
FIGURE 27-49
ANTERIOR VIEW OF THE ANKLE AND DORSAL VIEW OF THE FOOT

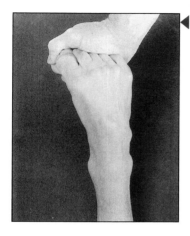

◄ **FIGURE 27-50**
THE HEADS OF THE METATARSAL BONES — DORSAL VIEW

By taking a global grip of all toes, carry out a plantarflexion that will be sufficient to project the metatarsal heads. This maneuver can obviously be performed for each metatarsal bone separately.

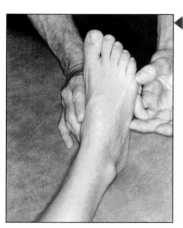

◄ **FIGURE 27-51**
THE FIFTH METATARSAL BONE

First the head (see Fig. 27-4) is located as well as the base (see Figs. 27-7 and 27-8). After positioning the head on the related articular interspace (Fig. 28-7), the fifth metatarsal bone may be grabbed between the thumb and the index finger.

It is interesting to note the position and the dimension of this bone relative to the other metatarsal bones. It faces the cuboid bone posteriorly and the fourth metatarsal bone medially. Its posterolateral aspect shows a styloid process also called the tuberosity of the fifth metatarsal bone.

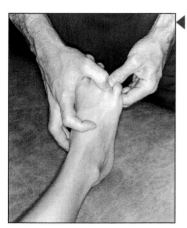

◄ **FIGURE 27-52**
THE FOURTH METATARSAL BONE

The head and the base are located after locating the related articular interspace (Fig. 28-8).

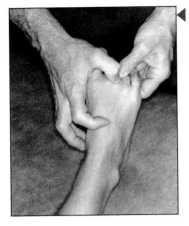

◀ **FIGURE 27-53**
THE THIRD METATARSAL BONE

The head and the base are located after locating the related articular inter-space (Fig. 28-9).

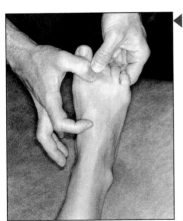

◀ **FIGURE 27-54**
THE SECOND METATARSAL BONE

The head and the base are located after locating the related articular inter-space (Fig. 28-10).

Comment: This is the longest of the metatarsal bones.

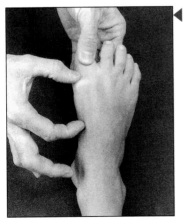

◀ **FIGURE 27-55**
THE FIRST METATARSAL BONE

The head (Fig. 27-26) and the base (Figs. 27-32 and 27-33) are located after locating the related articular interspace (Figs. 27-32 and 28-11).

Comment: This is the shortest and the broadest of the metatarsal bones.

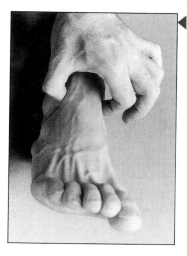

FIGURE 27-56
THE NECK OF THE TALUS

In this picture, the neck of the talus is grabbed through its medial and lateral surfaces. The thumb is positioned on the lateral surface and the index finger on the medial surface [these two portions of the neck were seen during the examination of the lateral (Figs. 27-7 and 27-20) and medial (Figs. 27-32, 27-40, and 27-41) borders of the foot, respectively].

The superior surface of the neck of the talus is located between the thumb and the index finger.

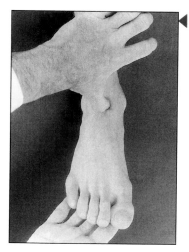

FIGURE 27-57
THE ANTERIOR BORDER OF THE LOWER EXTREMITY OF THE TIBIA

Comment: It is this border that is embedded in the transverse groove of the superior surface of the neck of the talus during dorsiflexion of the ankle.

THE POSTERIOR SURFACE OF THE ANKLE AND OF THE FOOT

The bony structures accessible by palpation are

• The medial malleolus (Fig. 27-59)
• The lesser process of the calcaneus (Fig. 27-60)
• The posterior surface of the calcaneus (Fig. 27-61)

• The posterior segment of the superior surface of the calcaneus (Fig. 27-62)
• The lateral malleolus (Fig. 27-63)
• The peroneal tubercle (Fig. 27-64)

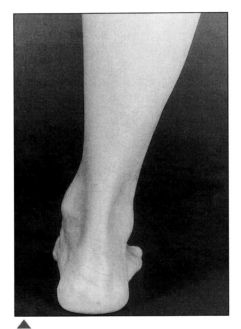

▲
FIGURE 27-58
POSTERIOR VIEW OF THE ANKLE AND OF THE FOOT

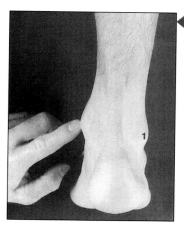

◀ **FIGURE 27-59**
THE MEDIAL MALLEOLUS

This structure, indicated by the index finger, was also located during the approach to the medial border of the foot. This is a different view, which underlines its topography in relation to the other anatomic structures of the region.

Comment: In this figure, the relatively high position of the medial malleolus in relation to the lateral malleolus (1) is clearly shown.

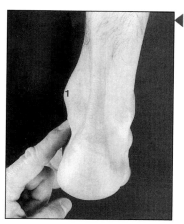

◀ **FIGURE 27-60**
THE SUSTENTACULUM TALI

This structure, indicated by the index finger, was also discussed during the examination of the medial border of the foot. This posterior view confirms its topography in relation to the medial malleolus (1), approximately one finger's breadth below.

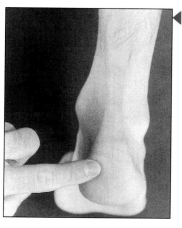

◀ **FIGURE 27-61**
THE POSTERIOR SURFACE OF THE CALCANEUS

Narrow and smooth in its upper portion, this structure is wide and rough in its lower portion, where the Achilles tendon is attached. It is globally perceived under the fingers as triangular in shape with a wide inferior base.

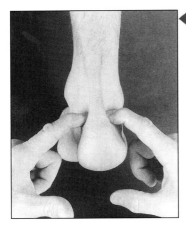

◀ FIGURE 27-62
THE POSTERIOR SEGMENT OF THE SUPERIOR SURFACE OF THE CALCANEUS

Concave in the sagittal plane and convex in the transverse plane, this segment is approached on each side of the Achilles tendon.

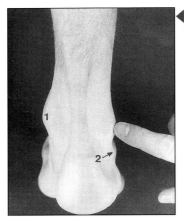

◀ FIGURE 27-63
THE LATERAL MALLEOLUS

Indicated by the index finger, this structure was discussed during the examination of the lateral border of the foot. This different view emphasizes its relatively low position in relation to the medial malleolus (1) as well as its position in relation to the peroneal trochlea (2) (see Fig. 27-64).

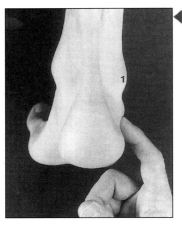

◀ FIGURE 27-64
THE PERONEAL TROCHLEA

This structure was also discussed during the examination of the lateral border of the foot. This view stresses its position in relation to the apex of the lateral malleolus (1), which is approximately one finger's breadth above.

THE PLANTAR SURFACE

The bony structures accessible by palpation are

- The heads of the five metatarsal bones—plantar view (Fig. 27-66)
- The plantar surface of the cuboid bone (Fig. 27-67)
- The medial and lateral sesamoid bones (Figs. 27-68 and 27-69)
- The posterolateral tubercle of the first metatarsal bone (Fig. 27-70)

- The anterior tubercle of the inferior surface of the calcaneus (plantar view) (Fig. 27-71)
- The posterior segment of the inferior surface of the calcaneus (Fig. 27-72)
- The posteromedial tubercle or tuberosity of the calcaneus (Fig. 27-73)
- The posterolateral tubercle or tuberosity of the calcaneus (Fig. 27-74)

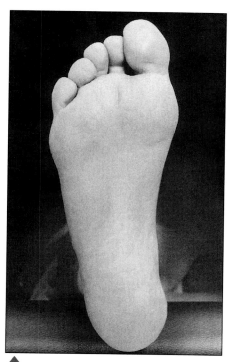

▲
FIGURE 27-65
PLANTAR VIEW OF THE FOOT

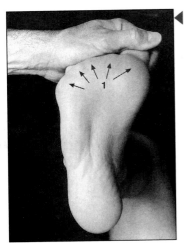

FIGURE 27-66
THE HEADS OF THE FIVE METATARSAL BONES — PLANTAR VIEW

A characteristic of each metatarsal bone is that the head is covered by a convex articular surface that extends more on the plantar side than on the dorsal side.

This characteristic is recognized during palpation by finding a wide convex and smooth surface under the fingers (1) just behind the metatarsophalangeal joint of each of the five metatarsal bones.

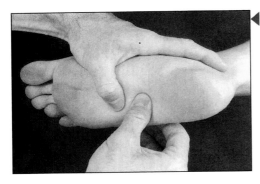

FIGURE 27-67
THE PLANTAR SURFACE OF THE CUBOID BONE

This bone was already studied during the examination of the lateral border of the foot. After locating the tuberosity of the fifth metatarsal bone (Figs. 27-7 and 27-8) and the greater process of the calcaneus (Figs. 27-7 and 27-13), the thumb is placed between the two structures mentioned and slides around the lateral border of the foot and the lateral border of the cuboid bone (Fig. 27-9). It is now positioned on the plantar surface of this bone.

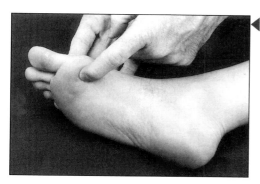

FIGURE 27-68
THE MEDIAL SESAMOID BONE

Place a digital grip on the plantar surface of the head of the first metatarsal bone and proceed with a transverse friction. This technique allows the perception under the finger of two "tubercles" separated by a depression.

In this picture, the index finger hooks up the medial sesamoid bone.

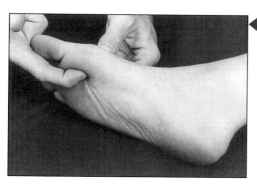

FIGURE 27-69
THE LATERAL SESAMOID BONE

The technique here is the same as that described in Fig. 27-68. The index finger is placed toward the lateral border of the foot to perceive (just beyond the depression mentioned) the lateral sesamoid bone.

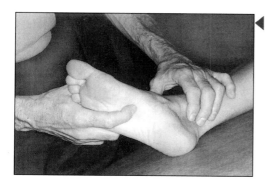

FIGURE 27-70
THE POSTEROLATERAL TUBERCLE OF THE FIRST METATARSAL BONE

After locating the base of the first metatarsal bone, move to the plantar surface of the foot toward the lateral border (this picture shows its position) (see also Fig. 27-34).

Comment: Since this structure is deeply located, the application of a reasonably firm pressure is recommended in order to have access to it. An approach using the thumb might prove more effective.

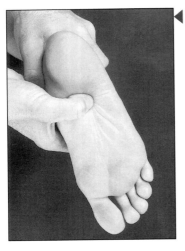

◀ FIGURE 27-71
THE ANTERIOR TUBERCLE OF THE INFERIOR SURFACE OF THE CALCANEUS

This figure presents a plantar view of the foot, which allows a more precise identification of the topographic position of the examined structure.

If the approach is carried from the medial border, the neck of the talus (Figs. 27-32 and 27-41) serves as a landmark when the thumb is placed at its level. Afterwards, the fingers move around the medial border of the foot in order to find the investigated structure.

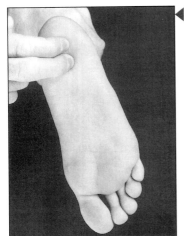

◀ FIGURE 27-72
THE POSTERIOR SEGMENT OF THE INFERIOR SURFACE OF THE CALCANEUS

Also designated as the posterior tuberosity, this structure occupies the posterior third of the bone and represents the part of the calcaneus lying on the ground (Fig. 27-7).

It presents two tubercles: the medial process (Fig. 27-73) and the lateral process (Fig. 27-74).

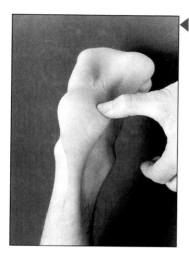

FIGURE 27-73
THE MEDIAL PROCESS

This is the largest of the two posterior tuberosities. It is the site of insertion of the flexor digitorum brevis and abductor hallucis muscles.

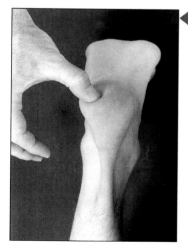

FIGURE 27-74
THE LATERAL PROCESS

This is the smallest of the two posterior tuberosities. It is the site of insertion of the abductor digiti minimi muscle.

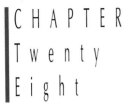
| CHAPTER
| Twenty
| Eight

ARTHROLOGY

THE ARTICULATIONS

THE ARTICULAR INTERSPACES AND THE LIGAMENTS

The articulations accessible during the surface investigation are (from the extremity of the toes to the ankle

- The interphalangeal joints (Figs. 28-2 and 28-3)
- The metatarsophalangeal joints (Figs. 28-4, 28-5 and 28-6)
- The tarsometatarsal joints (Lisfranc) (Figs. 28-7 through 28-11)
- The "medial tarsal" joint (Chopart's) (Figs. 28-12, 28-13, and 28-14), including the "Y" ligament (Fig. 28-13)
- The posterior calcaneotalar or subtalar joint and the anterior calcaneotalar joint (Figs. 28-15 and 28-16)

- The tibiotarsal joint (Figs. 28-17 through 28-22)
- The ligaments of the tibiotarsal joint (Figs. 28-23 through 28-28)
- The posteroinferior tibiofibular ligament (Fig. 28-29)
- The lateral annular ligament tarsi (Fig. 28-30)
- The anterosuperior and anteroinferior annular ligament tarsi (Fig. 28-31)
- The dorsal aponeurosis of the foot (Fig. 28-32)

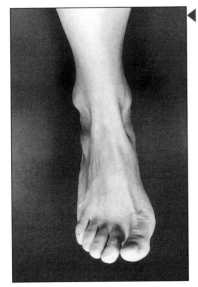

◀ **FIGURE 28-1**

ANTERIOR VIEW OF THE ANKLE AND DORSAL VIEW OF THE FOOT

Comment: The joint of Lisfranc (tarsometatarsal joints)

This structure joins the three cuneiform bones and the cuboid bone to the five metatarsal bones. It includes three tarsometatarsal joints:

- A medial joint between the medial cuneiform bone and the first metatarsal bone
- An intermediate joint, which joins the middle and lateral cuneiform bones to the second and third metatarsal bones
- A lateral joint between the cuboid bone and the fourth and fifth metatarsal bones

The articulation of Chopart (medial tarsal joint) joins the distal tarsum to the proximal tarsum. From a functional point of view, it is a single unit that includes the calcaneotalonavicular joint and the calcaneocuboid joint. The "Y" ligament of Chopart is the ligament shared by the two articulations mentioned above.

THE INTERPHALANGEAL JOINTS

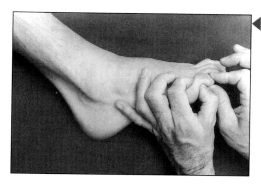

◀ FIGURE 28-2
THE INTERPHALANGEAL JOINTS OF THE FIFTH TOE

There are two of these and they can be identified without difficulty.

In this figure, the proximal grip immobilizes the proximal phalanx while the distal grip brings the distal phalanx into plantarflexion.

Comment: These are trochlear joints (ginglymus). The opposing surfaces are the articular surface of the anterior extremity of the more posterior phalanx, which has the shape of a pulley, and the articular surface of the posterior extremity of the more anterior phalanx, which has a minimally pronounced middle ridge.

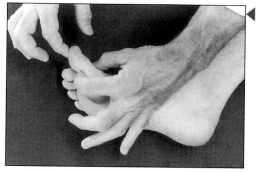

◀ FIGURE 28-3
THE INTERPHALANGEAL JOINT OF THE FIRST TOE IN DORSAL EXTENSION

At the level of the first toe there is only one interphalangeal joint. In this figure the proximal grip immobilizes the proximal phalanx while the distal grip brings the second phalanx into extension.

THE METATARSOPHALANGEAL JOINTS

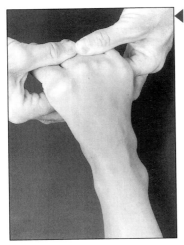

◄ **FIGURE 28-4**
THE METATARSOPHALANGEAL JOINTS — DORSAL VIEW

In this figure, the two hands grab the toes and bring them into plantarflexion, thereby uncovering the anterior and dorsal articular surfaces of the metatarsal heads.

Comment: The articular surface is perceived under the fingers as a smooth surface. The most accessible is obviously that of the first toe.

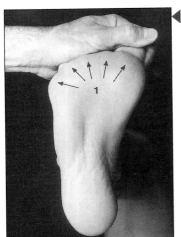

◄ **FIGURE 28-5**
THE METATARSOPHALANGEAL JOINTS — PLANTAR VIEW

In this picture, the hand grabs the toes and brings them into dorsiflexion, thereby uncovering the anterior and plantar articular surfaces of the metatarsal heads (1).

Comment: The articular surface of the head of each metatarsal bone extends widely on the plantar side.

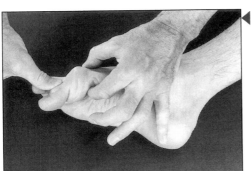

◄ **FIGURE 28-6**
THE METATARSOPHALANGEAL JOINT OF THE FIRST TOE

When this joint is examined, the sesamoid bones are palpated on its plantar portion (see Figs. 27-68 and 27-69).

THE ARTICULATION OF THE LISFRANC OR THE TARSOMETATARSAL JOINTS

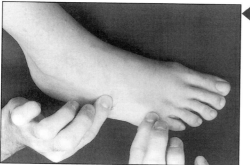

FIGURE 28-7
THE ARTICULAR INTERSPACE BETWEEN THE CUBOID BONE AND THE FIFTH METATARSAL BONE

The index finger of the distal hand is positioned on the anterior and lateral portion of the cuboid bone (Figs. 27-7, 27-9, 27-10 and 27-11) and the base of the fifth metatarsal bone (Figs. 27-7 and 27-8). To perceive the articular interspace, grab the head of the fifth metatarsal bone and mobilize it downward and then upward in a repetitive manner, allowing the index finger to perceive the investigated interspace clearly.

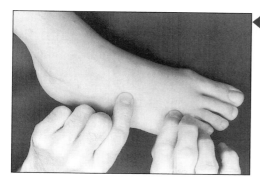

FIGURE 28-8
THE ARTIULAR INTERSPACE BETWEEN THE CUBOID BONE AND THE FOURTH METATARSAL BONE

While in contact with the base of the fourth metatarsal bone, move the index finger of the proximal hand slightly inward to face the anterior and medial portions of the cuboid bone.

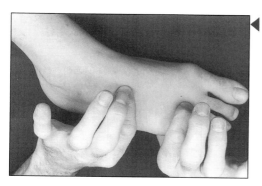

FIGURE 28-9
THE ARTICULAR INTERPACE BETWEEN THE LATERAL CUNEIFORM BONE AND THE THIRD METATARSAL BONE

From the grip described above, move the index finger approximately one fingerbreadth toward the medial aspect of the foot in order to contact both the anterior border of the lateral cuneiform bone and the base of the third metatarsal bone.

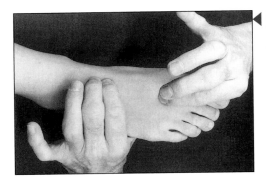

FIGURE 28-10
THE ARTICULAR INTERSPACE BETWEEN THE INTERMEDIATE CUNEIFORM BONE AND THE SECOND METATARSAL BONE

Using the previous grip (Fig. 28-9), move by approximately one fingerbreadth toward the medial aspect of the foot, keeping in mind that the anterior border of the middle cuneiform bone is withdrawn in relation to the anterior border of the two surrounding cuneiform bones. This will display the index finger toward the posterior aspect of the foot in order to be in contact with the middle cuneiform bone and the base of the second metatarsal bone.

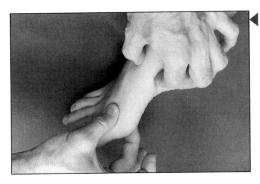

FIGURE 28-11
THE ARTICULAR INTERSPCE BETWEEN THE MEDIAL CUNEIFORM BONE AND THE FIRST METATARSAL BONE

In this picture, to locate the medial cuneiform bone (see Figs. 27-7 and 27-32) the proximal grip is positioned at the level of the investigated interspace. The distal grip mobilizes the head of the first metatarsal bone.

THE ARTICULATION OF CHOPART OR THE MEDIAL TARSAL JOINT

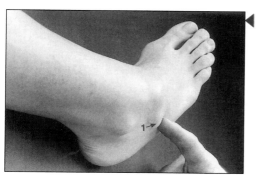

◀ FIGURE 28-12
THE LATERAL COMPONENT OF THE MEDIAL TARSAL JOINT ("LATERAL CHOPART")

The index finger is placed on the cuboid facet of the calcaneus. This facet corresponds to the anterior surface of the calcaneus. It articulates in front with the cuboid bone.

A foot inversion facilitates access to the lateral portion of this surface. (1) Greater process of the calcaneus.

See comment on page 258.

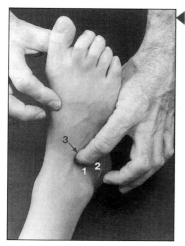

◀ FIGURE 28-13
THE "Y" LIGAMENT OF THE MEDIAL TARSAL JOINT

The ligament attaches posteriorly to the dorsal surface of the greater process of the calcaneus (1). It divides into two bundles:

• a lateral bundle, which inserts into the dorsal surface of the cuboid bone (2)
• a medial bundle, which inserts into the entire height of the lateral surface of the navicular bone (3)

Comment: It is considered the key ligament of this joint.

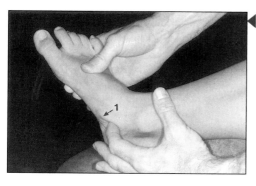

◀ FIGURE 28-14
THE MEDIAL ASPECT OF THE MEDIAL TARSAL JOINT ("MEDIAL CHOPART")

An eversion of the foot allows a clearing of the head of the talus, which articulates anteriorly with the navicular bone (1).

In this figure, the index finger faces the middle field of the head of the talus, which corresponds to the inferior calcaneonavicular ligament. This smooth surface is perceived beneath the index finger.

THE POSTERIOR CALCANEOTALAR OR SUBTALAR JOINT
AND THE ANTERIOR CALCANEOTALAR JOINT

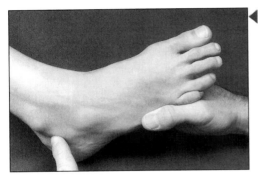

◄ FIGURE 28-15

THE POSTERIOR CALCANEOTALAR OR SUBTALAR JOINT —
LATERAL VIEW

The index finger indicates the lateral interspace of the subtalar joint. The bony prominence, facing the index finger, is
the lateral process of the talus, which supports the most lateral portion of the peroneal facet of the body of the talus.

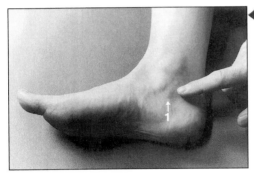

◄ FIGURE 28-16

THE ANTERIOR CALCANEOTALAR JOINT — MEDIAL VIEW

The index finger indicates the medial interspace of the subtalar joint. The bony prominence facing the index finger is
the lesser process of the calcaneus (1). It supports the
intermediate articular surface of the calcaneus and constitutes a combined articular body, since it is in continuity
with the anterior articular surface.

THE TIBOTARSAL JOINT

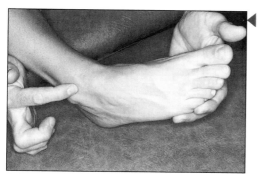

FIGURE 28-17
THE LATERAL BORDER OF THE LATERAL ASPECT OF THE TALAR TROCHLEA

The index finger of the distal hand is placed on the anterior border of the lower extremity of the peroneal shaft, while the foot is in neutral position. The foot may be slightly plantarflexed in order to perceive the investigated border under the finger.

The addition of a slight adduction of the foot may sharpen the perception.

Comment: Although smooth (since covered by cartilage), this border is perceived as sharp.

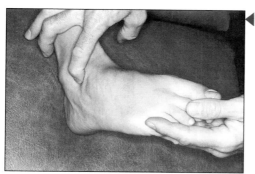

FIGURE 28-18
THE PERONEAL OR LATERAL MALLEOLAR FACET

With the subject's foot in neutral position, place the index finger of your proximal hand in front of the anterior border of the lower extremity of the fibula. With the distal hand, the foot is inverted and a slight plantarflexion is added. The articular facet is then perceived under the index finger as a smooth surface

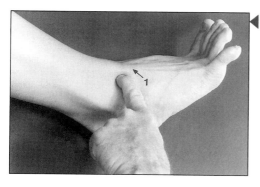

FIGURE 28-19
THE LATERAL ASPECT OF THE TALAR TROCHLEA

From the already located lateral border (Fig. 28-17), slide your finger behind the tendon of the extensor digitorum longus muscle (1) toward the medial border of the foot.

By inverting and plantarflexing the foot (projecting the talar trochlea toward the lateral aspect of the foot), access to this articular structure will be facilitated.

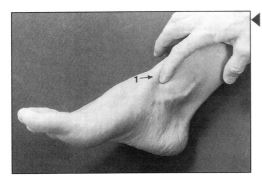

FIGURE 28-20

THE MEDIAL BORDER OF THE MEDIAL ASPECT OF THE TALAR TROCHLEA

With the subject's foot in neutral position, the index finger of your distal hand is positioned on the anterior border of the medial malleolus, at its junction with the anterior border of the lower extremity of the tibial shaft.

Slightly plantarflex the foot in order to perceive the investigated border under the finger. It is preferable to add a slight eversion of the foot so that the examination will not be hampered by the tendon of the anterior tibialis muscle (1).

Comment: This border, perceived as smooth structure beneath the finger, is much less pronounced on the medial side.

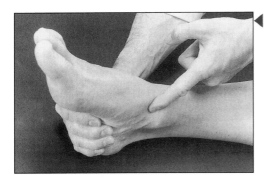

FIGURE 28-21

THE TIBIAL OR MEDIAL MALLEOLAR FACET

After placing the index finger of the distal hand in front of the anterior border of the medial malleolus, invert and slightly plantarflex the foot in order to expose the tibial facet optimally.

The investigated articular surface is perceived as a smooth surface beneath the finger.

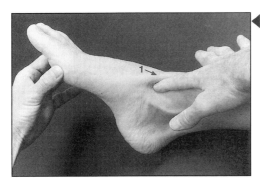

FIGURE 28-22

THE MEDIAL ASPECT OF THE TALAR TROCHLEA

From the already located medial border (Fig. 28-20), slide your fingers behind the tendon of the anterior tibialis muscle (1) toward the lateral border of the foot.

From this initial position, evert and plantarflex the foot in order to project the talar trochlea over the medial border of the foot. This will facilitate access to the investigated articular structure.

THE LIGAMENTS OF THE TIBITARSAL JOINT

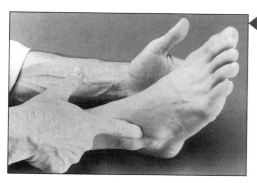

◀ FIGURE 28-23
THE ANTERIOR TALOFIBULAR LIGAMENT

To approach this ligament, remember its proximal insertion (into the middle aspect of the anterior border of the lateral malleolus) and its distal insertion (into the talus) just in front of the peroneal facet.

It is sometimes useful to bring the foot into adduction, supination, and slight plantarflexion in order to better access this ligamentous structure.

Comment: These three ligaments (Figs. 28-23, 28-24, and 28-25) are part of the lateral (collateral) ligament.

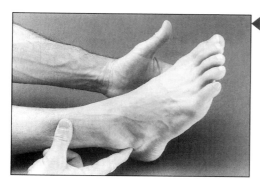

◀ FIGURE 28-24
THE CALCANEOFIBULAR LIGAMENT

To properly study this ligamentous structure, its course as well as its proximal insertion (into the anterior border of the lateral malleolus, under the ligament described in Fig. 28-23) and distal insertion (into the lateral surface of the calcaneus) must be well visualized.

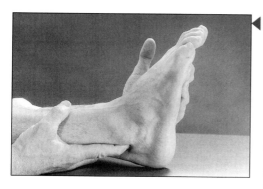

◀ FIGURE 28-25
THE POSTERIOR TALOFIBULAR LIGAMENT

To localize this structure, it is essential to remember its lateral insertion (into the medial surface of the lateral malleolus, below and behind its articular surface) as well as its medial insertion (into the lateral process of the posterior border of the talus).

Running between these two bony structures, its course is essentially horizontal.

Comment: It is located below the posterior inferior tibiofibular ligament of the inferior tibiofibular joint.

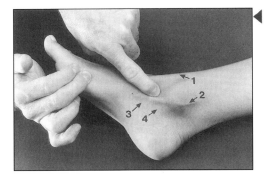

FIGURE 28-26
THE SUPERFICIAL LAYER OF THE DELTOID LIGAMENT —
THE TIBIONAVICULAR BUNDLE

To find this layer, remember the sites of proximal (anterior border and apex of the medial malleolus) and distal insertion (superior surface of the navicular bone; medial surface of the neck of the talus; inferior calcaneonavicular ligament (3), and lesser process of the calcaneus (4).

The simultaneous placement under tension of the tendons of the anterior tibialis muscle (1) and posterior tibialis muscle (2) (see figure) allows for localization of the most anterior part of this superficial layer, indicated by the index finger.

Comment: When the tibionavicular bundle of the medial laterial ligament is palpated, you are also in contact with the anterior talotibial bundle of the deep layer of this ligament.

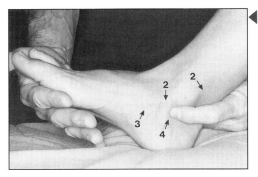

FIGURE 28-27
THE SUPERFICIAL LAYER OF THE DELTOID LIGAMENT —
THE CALCANEOTIBIAL BUNDLE

This part of the ligament, which attaches to the inferior calcaneonavicular ligament (3), is approached below the tendon of the posterior tibialis muscle (2).

In this figure, it is the most posterior part of the superficial layer of the approached ligament (the one inserting into the lesser process of the calcaneus) (4).

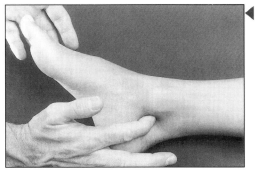

FIGURE 28-28
THE DEEP LAYER OF THE DELTOID LIGAMENT —
THE POSTERIOR TALOTIBIAL BUNDLE

It is important to remember its slightly withdrawn tibial insertion into the apex of the medial malleolus (closer to the talus than the insertions of the superficial layer) and its insertion into the talus on the medial process. The fibers of the deep layer are stretched between these two structures.

Comment: This region should be approached with care, since it is the site of passage of the posterior tibial artery and nerve.

THE POSTEROINFERIOR TIBIOFIBULAR LIGAMENT

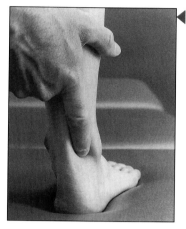

◀ FIGURE 28-29
THE POSTEROINFERIOR TIBIOFIBULAR LIGAMENT

When the index finger slides into the lateral retromalleolar groove, the first ligament perceived under the finger (moving inferiorly) is the posteroinferior tibiofibular ligament. Below this ligament, one finds a bundle of fibers reinforcing the articular capsule and, finally, lower down, one contacts the posterior talofibular ligament which is the posterior bundle of the lateral (collateral) ligament.

THE ANNULAR LIGAMENTS OF THE TARSUM AND THE DORSAL APONEUROSIS OF THE FOOT

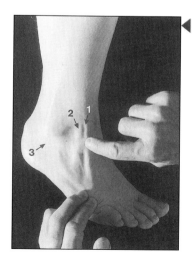

◀ FIGURE 28-30
THE LATERAL ANNULAR LIGAMENT OF THE TARSUM

In this figure, the index finger clearly indicates the visualized lateral portion of the anterior annular ligaments of the tarsum, which cover the tendons of the extensor digitorum longus (1) and the peroneus tertius muscles (2) and extend to the lateral border of the foot by the lateral annular ligament of the tarsum (3).

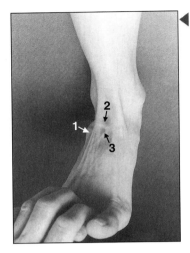

FIGURE 28-31
THE ANTEROSUPERIOR AND ANTEROINFERIOR ANNULAR LIGAMENTS OF THE TARSUM

At the point where they separate, just after covering the extensor digitorum longus muscle (1), you can clearly visualize the anterosuperior annular ligament of the tarsum (2) as well as the anteroinferior annular ligament of the tarsum (3).

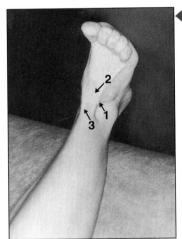

FIGURE 28-32
THE DORSAL APONEUROSIS OF THE FOOT

In this picture, you see clearly the dorsal aponeurosis of the foot (1), which covers the tendons of the extensor hallucis longus (2) and anterior tibialis muscles (3).

C H A P T E R
T w e n t y
N i n e

MYOLOGY

THE MUSCULOTENDINOUS STRUCTURES OF THE ANKLE AND THE FOOT

As you move around the ankle, you perceive

- The tendon of the anterior tibialis muscle (Fig. 29-2)
- The tendon of the extensor hallucis longus muscle (Fig. 29-3)
- The extensor hallucis brevis muscle, integral part of the extensor digitorum brevis muscle (Figs. 29-4 and 29-7)
- The tendon of the extensor digitorum longus muscle (Fig. 29-5)
- The tendon of the peroneus tertius muscle (Fig. 29-6)
- The muscular body of the extensor digitorum brevis muscle (Fig. 29-7)
- The tendon of the peroneus brevis muscle (Fig. 29-8)
- The tendon of the peroneus longus muscle (Fig. 29-9)
- The posterior part of the muscular body of the peroneus brevis muscle (Fig. 29-10)

- The Achilles tendon (Figs. 29-11 and 29-12)
- The tendon of the posterior tibialis muscle at the level of the medial malleolus (Fig. 29-13)
- The tendon of the posterior tibialis muscle over the medial border of the foot (Fig. 29-14)
- The tendon of the flexor digitorum longus muscle at the level of the medial malleolus (Fig. 29-15)
- The tendon of the flexor digitorum longus muscle over the medial border of the foot (Fig. 29-16)
- The tendon of the flexor hallucis longus muscle in the medial retromalleolar groove (Fig. 29-17)
- The tendon of the flexor hallucis longus muscle over the medial border of the foot (Fig. 29-18)

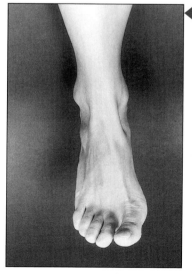

◀ **FIGURE 29-1**

ANTERIOR VIEW OF THE ANKLE AND DORSAL VIEW OF THE FOOT

Comment: The presentation of this topographic region should not be considered in its strict sense. It is only a didactic means of approaching structures that extend to the level of the foot.

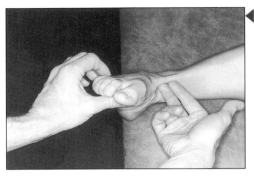

◀ **FIGURE 29-2**

THE TENDON OF THE ANTERIOR TIBIALIS MUSCLE

A large, powerful tendon, which has the shape of a cylindrical cord, appears in front of the medial malleolus, extending toward the medial border of the foot, where its principal site of insertion is the medial cuneiform bone. In this picture, the proximal hand positions the foot in inversion and dorsiflexion. The subject is asked to maintain this position.

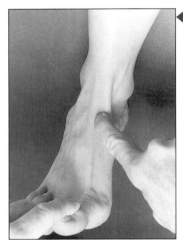

◀ **FIGURE 29-3**

THE TENDON OF THE EXTENSOR HALLUCIS LONGUS MUSCLE

Ask the subject to perform a double extension at the level of the interphalangeal and metatarsophalangeal joints of the first toe. A resistance may be applied by the thumb to the dorsal aspect of the first toe in order to sensitize the subject to the movement requested. The tendon appears just lateral to the tendon of the anterior tibialis muscle.

Comment: The tendon of this muscle also participates in the adduction, supination, and dorsiflexion of the ankle.

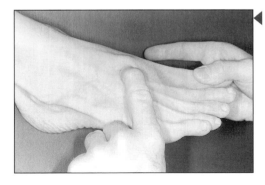

◀ **FIGURE 29-4**

THE MUSCULAR BODY OF THE EXTENSOR HALLUCIS BREVIS MUSCLE

Since it is the muscular head intended for the first toe, this body inconsistently constitutes the medialmost portion of the extensor digitorum brevis muscle.

Have the subject perform repeated extensions of the metatarsophalangeal joint of the first toe to assist in locating it on the dorsum of the foot, just lateral to the tendon of the extensor digitorum longus muscle, as located in Figure 29-3.

Comment: Its access is not easy and there are very few subjects in whom it is approached without difficulty (see also Fig. 29-23).

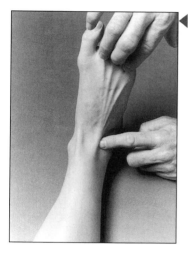

◀ FIGURE 29-5
THE TENDON OF THE EXTENSOR DIGITORUM LONGUS MUSCLE

This muscle participates in dorsiflexion of the ankle. The subject should therefore be asked to perform this muscular action in order to demonstrate the tendon at the level of the ankle, just lateral to the tendon of the extensor hallucis longus muscle (Fig. 29-4).

A resistance globally applied to the dorsal surface of the phalanges of the last four toes (against the extension of the interphalangeal and metatarsophalangeal joints of these toes) results in the demonstration of the tendons on the dorsum of the foot.

Comment: This muscle also participates in the abduction, pronation, and dorsiflexion of the foot.

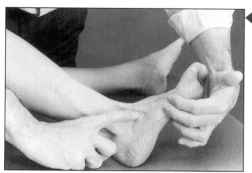

◀ FIGURE 29-6
THE TENDON OF THE PERONEUS TERTIUS MUSCLE

The subject is asked to abduct, pronate, and dorsiflex the foot against resistance as a grip is positioned on the lateral border of the foot, as shown in this picture.

The tendon appears lateral to the tendon of the extensor digitorum longus muscle, intended for the fifth toe. It extends toward the dorsal surface of the base of the fifth metatarsal bone, which is its site of distal insertion.

Comment: It is not constant.

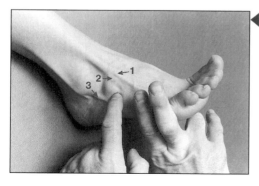

◀ FIGURE 29-7
THE MUSCULAR BODY OF THE EXTENSOR DIGITORUM BREVIS MUSCLE

The subject is asked to perform an extension of the interphalangeal and metatarsophalangeal joints of the toes in a global fashion (the fifth toe is not involved with this muscle).

The muscular body appears lateral to the tendons of the extensor digitorum longus muscle (1) and of the peroneus tertius muscle (2), in front of the lateral malleolus and medial to the tendon of the peroneus brevis muscle (3).

Comment: Resistance applied to the lateral border of the foot by the distal hand is intended to project the tendinous structures surrounding the investigated muscle, indicated by the index finger.

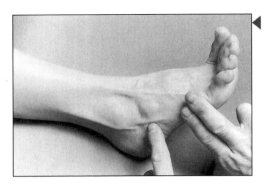

► **FIGURE 29-8**

THE TENDON OF THE PERONEUS BREVIS MUSCLE

With the foot in neutral position, the subject is asked to perform a pure abduction of the foot.

The distal hand may offer resistance on the lateral border of the foot.

The index finger of the proximal hand indicates the investigated structure.

Comment: This tendon passes in front of the peroneal tubercle.

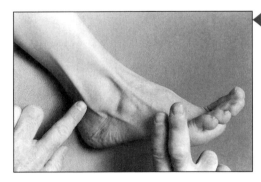

► **FIGURE 29-9**

THE TENDON OF THE PERONEUS LONGUS MUSCLE

The subject is asked to perform the same movement described above. This might be sufficient to demonstrate the tendon over the lateral border of the foot just before its entrance into the groove of the cuboid bone. A pronation and a plantarflexion may be added.

Comment: This tendon passes behind the peroneal trochlea.

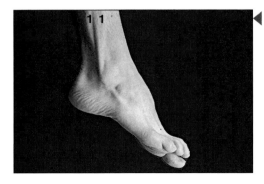

► **FIGURE 29-10**

THE POSTERIOR PORTION OF THE MUSCULAR BODY OF THE PERONEUS BREVIS MUSCLE

The muscular action requested from the subject is the same as that described in Figure 29-9.

The muscular body (1) is accessible slightly above the lateral malleolus and behind the tendon of the peroneus longus muscle.

In certain subjects (see figure), it may also be seen in front of this tendon.

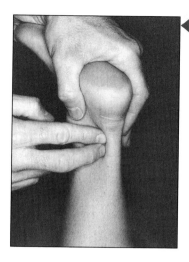

◀ **FIGURE 29-11**
LATERAL AND POSTERIOR APPROACH TO THE ACHILLES TENDON

This tendon, being superficial, does not present any difficulty of access.

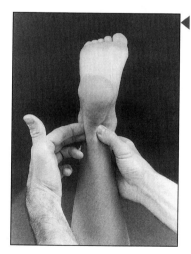

◀ **FIGURE 29-12**
THE ANTEROLATERAL AND ANTEROMEDIAL APPROACH
TO THE ACHILLES TENDON

Using the thumb, push the tendon laterally in order to gain access to its anterolateral portion, which may be investigated through sliding (back-and-forth) digital movements. Similarly, push the tendon medially with the thumb in order to gain access to its anteromedial portion.

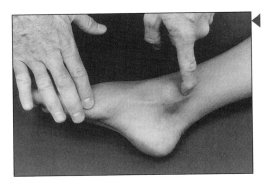

FIGURE 29-13

THE TENDON OF THE POSTERIOR TIBIALIS MUSCLE AT THE LEVEL OF THE MEDIAL MALLEOLUS

With the foot in plantarflexion, the subject is asked to adduct the foot against resistance over the medial border.

The tendon appears on the posterior border of the medial malleolus.

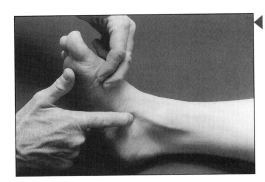

FIGURE 29-14

THE TENDON OF THE POSTERIOR TIBIALIS MUSCLE

The technique of placing this tendon under tension is the same as that described above.

After passing around the medial malleolus, the tendon follows the medial border of the foot, where it inserts, among other bony structures, into the tubercle of the navicular bone, indicated by the index finger.

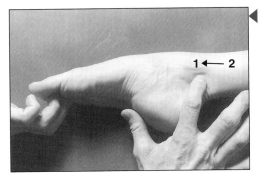

FIGURE 29-15

THE TENDON OF THE FLEXOR DIGITORUM LONGUS MUSCLE AT THE LEVEL OF THE MEDIAL MALLEOLUS

One hand is placed on the plantar surface of the last four toes in order to solicit repeated flexion of these toes. These repeated muscular actions are perceived by the other hand, which is positioned behind the posterior tibialis muscle (1). The index finger demonstrates the tendon of the flexor digitorum longus muscle (2), which is also situated behind the medial malleolus.

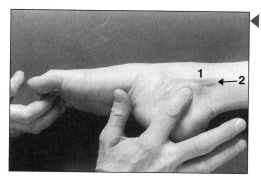

FIGURE 29-16
THE TENDON OF THE FLEXOR DIGITORUM LONGUS MUSCLE OVER THE MEDIAL BORDER OF THE FOOT

After passing around the medial malleolus in a special osteofibrous sheath, this tendon crosses the medial lateral ligament of the ankle joint and runs through its groove on the lesser process of the calcaneus. In this picture, the index finger is placed at the level of this groove. Beyond that, the tendon of the flexor digitorum longus muscle (2) extends into the plantar surface of the foot.

FIGURES 29-16, 29-17, AND 29-18

(1) Posterior tibialis muscle

(2) Flexor digitorum longus muscle

(3) Flexor hallucis longus muscle

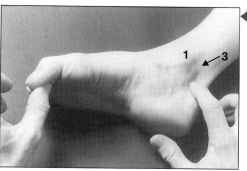

FIGURE 29-17
THE TENDON OF THE FLEXOR HALLUCIS LONGUS MUSCLE IN THE MEDIAL RETROMALLEOLAR GROOVE

One hand is positioned on the plantar surface of the first toe to solicit repeated flexions of the same toe.

These repeated muscular actions are perceived in the medial retromalleolar groove at some distance from the medial malleolus and very close to the Achilles tendon.

Comment: The tendon (3) of the investigated muscle, shown in this picture, is not visible in all patients.

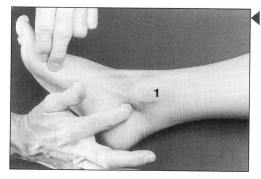

FIGURE 29-18
THE TENDON OF THE FLEXOR HALLUCIS LONGUS MUSCLE OVER THE MEDIAL BORDER OF THE FOOT

Beyond the tibiotarsal joint, the tendon slides into the groove of the posterior surface of the talus and positions itself under the tendon of the flexor digitorum longus muscle (Fig. 29-16) (2) in a special groove involving the medial surface of the calcaneus and located below the sustentaculum tali.

Comment: It may be interesting (as in this picture) to stress the tendon of the posterior tibialis muscle, since it is a landmark in the investigation of the examined tendon.

THE INTRINSIC MUSCLE OF THE FOOT

The muscular structures accessible by palpation are

- The extensor digitorum brevis and the extensor hallucis brevis muscles (Figs. 29-21 and 29-25)
- The abductor digiti minimi muscle (Fig. 29-26)
- The flexor digiti minimi brevis muscle (Fig. 29-27)
- The opponens digiti minimi muscle — visualization of its action (Fig. 29-28)
- The abductor hallucis muscle (Fig. 29-29)

- The flexor hallucis brevis muscle (Fig. 29-30)
- The adductor hallucis muscle (Fig. 29-31)
- The quadratus plantae muscle — visualization of its action (Fig. 13-32)
- The flexor digitorum brevis muscle — visualization of its action (Fig. 29-33)
- The dorsal and plantar interossei muscles — visualization of their actions (Figs. 29-34, 29-35, and 29-36).

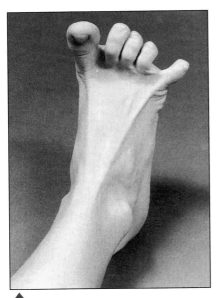

▲
FIGURE 29-19
DORSAL VIEW OF THE FOOT

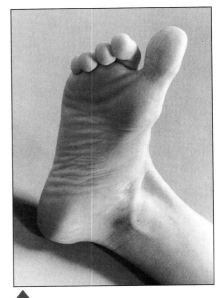

▲
FIGURE 29-20
PLANTAR VIEW OF THE FOOT

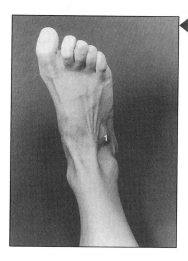

FIGURE 29-21
THE EXTENSOR DIGITORUM BREVIS MUSCLE — VISUALIZATION AND TOPOGRAPHY

This is the only muscle (1) in the dorsum of the foot.

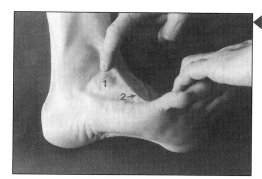

FIGURE 29-22
THE EXTENSOR DIGITORUM BREVIS MUSCLE

Ask the subject to perform an extension of the four proximal phalanges of the corresponding toes, with or without resistance, to perceive the muscular body (1), which is in front of the lateral malleolus and lateral to the tendon of the extensor digitorum longus muscle (2).

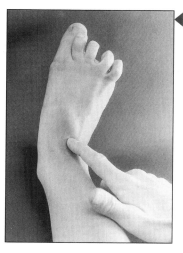

FIGURE 29-23
EXTENSOR HALLUCIS BREVIS MUSCLE

This is part of the extensor digitorum brevis muscle. The requested muscular action is the same as that described above. The muscular body is felt in front of the anterior annular ligament of the tarsum (Figs. 28-31 and 28-32), lateral to the tendon of the extensor hallucis longus muscle (Fig. 29-4) and medial to the tendon of the extensor digitorum longus muscle (Fig. 29-6).

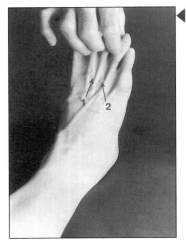

FIGURE 29-24

ENDING OF THE TENDONS OF THE EXTENSOR DIGITORUM BREVIS MUSCLE AT THE LEVEL OF THE SECOND AND THIRD TOES

The requested muscular action is the same as that described in Figure 29-22. A digital grip placed on the dorsal surface of the toes brings these toes into plantarflexion in order to demonstrate the two tendons, ending at the tendons of the extensor digitorum longus muscle serving the second (1) and third toes (2).

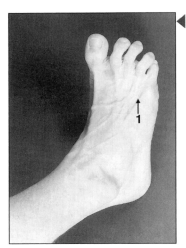

FIGURE 29-25

ENDING OF THE TENDON OF THE EXTENSOR DIGITORUM BREVIS MUSCLE AT THE LEVEL OF THE FOURTH TOE

This figure shows this tendon as it joins the tendon of the extensor digitorum longus muscle, serving the fourth toe (1).

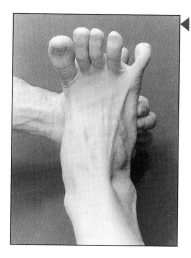

FIGURE 29-26

THE ABDUCTOR DIGITI MINIMI MUSCLE

Place a wide digital grip on the lateral border of the foot and the subject is asked for repeated abductions of the fifth toe. The muscular contraction is well perceived under the fingers.

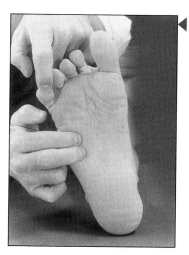

FIGURE 29-27

THE FLEXOR DIGITI MINIMI BREVIS MUSCLE

Position a bidigital grip on the plantar surface of the fifth metatarsal bone, moving slightly toward the medial border of the foot. Laterally, the muscular body is covered by the abductor digiti minimi muscle.

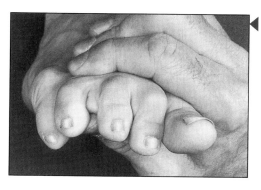

FIGURE 29-28

VISUALIZATION OF THE ACTION OF THE OPPONENS DIGITI MINIMI MUSCLE

Its action is to bring the fifth metatarsal bone medially.

Comment: Like the two muscles mentioned above, this one belongs to the lateral muscular group. It cannot be palpated individually.

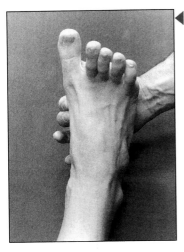

FIGURE 29-29
THE ABDUCTOR HALLUCIS MUSCLE

Place a wide digital grip on the medial border of the foot and the subject is asked to abduct the first toe on the first metatarsal bone.

If the subject cannot perform this type of muscular action, he or she should be asked to flex the first toe on the first metatarsal bone. The muscular contraction is well perceived on the medial border of the foot, more particularly on the plantar surface of the medial cuneiform bone and of the navicular bone.

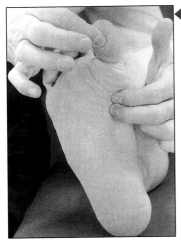

FIGURE 29-30
THE FLEXOR HALLUCIS BREVIS MUSCLE

Using a bidigital grip applied as widely as possible to the plantar surface of the first metatarsal bone behind the sesamoid bones, move slightly toward the medial border of the foot in order to perceive the medial bundle.

For the lateral bundle, the grip should be moved toward the lateral border of the foot, keeping in mind that this bundle is partially covered by the tendon of the flexor hallucis longus muscle. The requested action is a flexion of the first toe on the first metatarsal bone.

Comment: The superposition of the different muscular structures makes their individual palpation difficult.

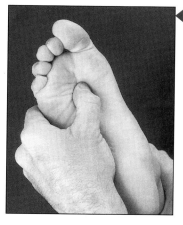

FIGURE 29-31

THE ADDUCTOR HALLUCIS MUSCLE

A wide grip using the thumb should be placed on the plantar surface of the first metatarsal interspace, with the hand placed on the lateral aspect of the foot. The subject is asked to flex the first toe at the first metatarsal bone in order to make the muscular contraction perceptible beneath the fingers. The contraction is perceived at the level of the oblique bundle and may be confused with the lateral bundle of the flexor hallucis brevis muscle. The perception of the contraction is difficult.

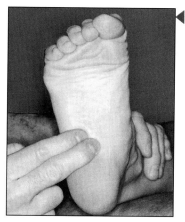

FIGURE 29-32

VISUALIZATION OF THE ACTION OF THE QUADRATUS PLANTAE MUSCLE

In this figure, the fingers are placed approximately at the junction of this muscle with the lateral border of the tendon of the flexor digitorum longus muscle.

Comment: Because of its oblique course, the tendon of the flexor digitorum longus muscle creates a certain deviation of the foot and toes. The purpose of the investigated muscle is to correct this tendency.

Therefore, it participates in the flexion of the last four toes.

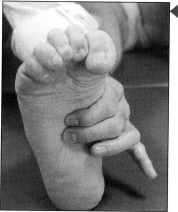

FIGURE 29-33

VISUALIZATION OF THE ACTION OF THE FLEXOR DIGITORUM BREVIS MUSCLE

A grip covering the foot through its medial or lateral border allows placement of a wide digital grip on the medial and plantar aspects of the foot. Next, the subject is asked to perform repeated flexions of the toes on the metatarsal bones in order to make the muscular contraction perceptible beneath the fingers.

Comment: The tendons described above are superposed on those of the flexor digitorum longus muscle.

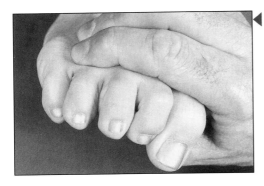

◀ **FIGURE 29-34**

VISUALIZATION OF THE ACTION OF THE PLANTAR INTEROSSEI MUSCLES AND OF THE LUMBRICALES MUSCLES

This figure visualizes the flexion of the proximal phalanges on the metatarsal bones of the lateral four toes. Contrary to what is shown in the figure, the first toe is not involved in this action. The plantar interossei muscles flex the proximal phalanx of the lateral four toes and draw the last three toes into the axis of the foot (which passes through the second toe). The lumbricales muscles flex the proximal phalanx of the lateral four toes and extend the two distal phalanges on the proximal phalanx.

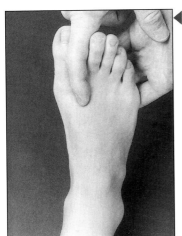

◀ **FIGURE 29-35**

THE FIRST DORSAL INTEROSSEUS MUSCLE

The dorsal interossei muscles can be approached in the four metatarsal interspaces.

They are directly accessible beneath the fingers when they are placed against the medial and lateral surfaces of the metatarsal bones.

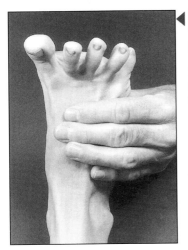

◀ **FIGURE 29-36**

VISUALIZATION OF ONE OF THE PRINCIPAL ACTIONS OF THE DORSAL INTEROSSEI MUSCLES

In this figure, the primary action is that of abduction of the second, third, and fourth toes in relation to the axis of the foot (which passes through the second toe).

Comment: These muscles also flex the proximal phalanx of the lateral four toes.

CHAPTER Thirty

NERVES AND VESSELS

The notable structures accessible by palpation are

- The superficial peroneal nerve (Figs. 30-3 and 30-4)
- The cutaneous lateral dorsal nerve and the anastomosis between the cutaneous intermediate dorsal nerve and the cutaneous lateral dorsal nerve (Fig. 30-4)
- The cutaneous intermediate dorsal nerve (Fig. 30-5)
- The posterior tibial nerve (Figs. 30-7 and 30-8)
- The posterior tibial artery (Figs. 30-7 and 30-8)
- The dorsalis pedis artery (Fig. 30-9)

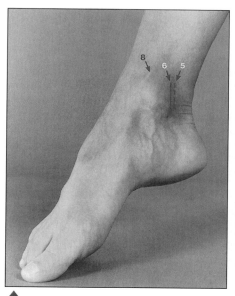

▲
FIGURE 30-1
MEDIAL VIEW OF THE ANKLE AND FOOT

(1) The superficial peroneal nerve
(2) The cutaneous intermediate dorsal nerve
(3) The cutaneous lateral dorsal nerve
(4) The anastomosis between the cutaneous intermediate dorsal nerve and the cutaneous lateral dorsal nerve

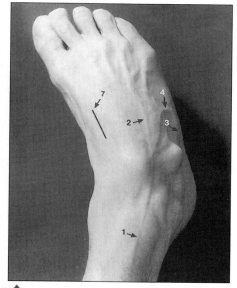

▲
FIGURE 30-2
ANTERIOR VIEW OF THE ANKLE AND DORSAL VIEW OF THE FOOT

(5) The tibial nerve
(6) The posterior tibial artery
(7) The dorsalis pedis artery
(8) The greater saphenous vein

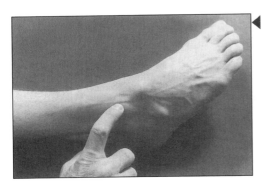

FIGURE 30-3
THE SUPERFICIAL PERONEAL NERVE

There are two possibilities for the investigation of this nerve:

- A relatively high search at the level of the inferior leg (at approximately the junction of the proximal two-thirds and of the distal third of the anterolateral aspect of the leg)
- A lower search at the level of the proximal foot

Comment: In either case, the nerve runs subcutaneously after perforating the aponeurosis of the leg.

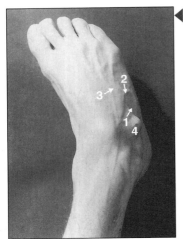

FIGURE 30-4
THE CUTANEOUS LATERAL DORSAL NERVE (1) AND THE ANASTOMOSIS (2) BETWEEN THE CUTANEOUS INTERMEDIATE DORSAL NERVE (3) AND THE CUTANEOUS LATERAL DORSAL NERVE (1)

In this figure, the musculocutaneous nerve is well visualized over the anterolateral and distal portion of the leg. At the level of the lateral malleolus, it extends through the cutaneous intermediate dorsal nerve (3), which travels along the third metatarsal interspace.

You can visualize the cutaneous lateral dorsal nerve (1), which is a prolongation of the sural nerve and travels along the lateral border of the foot. You can also see the anastomosis (2) between the two nerve structures described above, which passes just in front of the greater process of the calcaneus (4).

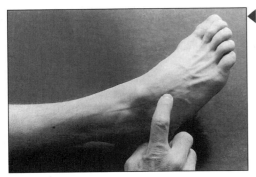

FIGURE 30-5
THE CUTANEOUS INTERMEDIATE DORSAL NERVE

Lateral view: Its topographic relationship with the other nerve elements of this region are described above for Figure 30-4.

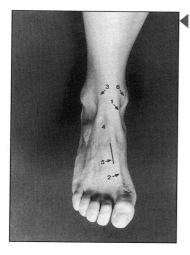

FIGURE 30-6
ANTERIOR VIEW OF THE ANKLE AND OF THE FOOT

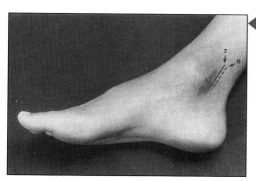

FIGURE 30-7
MEDIAL VIEW OF THE ANKLE AND OF THE FOOT

(1) The tendon of the anterior tibialis muscle

(2) The tendon of the extensor hallucis longus muscle

(3) The tendon of the extensor digitorum longus muscle

(4) The interior inferior annular ligament of the tarsum

(5) The dorsalis pedis artery

(6) The greater saphenous vein

(7) The posterior tibial artery

(8) The posterior tibial nerve

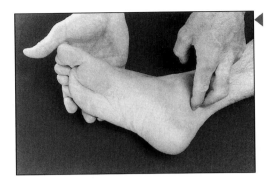

◀ FIGURE 30-8
THE POSTERIOR TIBIAL ARTERY AND THE POSTERIOR TIBIAL NERVE

The artery enters the medial retromalleolar groove between the flexor digitorum longus muscle located anteriorly and the flexor hallucis longus muscle located posteriorly.

The examination of the pulse and, therefore, its localization will be facilitated if the foot is first placed in slight inversion in order to relax the soft tissues of the region.
The posterior tibial nerve is palpated just behind the artery as a full cylindrical cord.

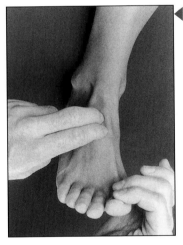

◀ FIGURE 30-9
THE DORSALIS PEDIS ARTERY

This is the name given to the anterior tibial artery at the level of the anterior annular ligament of the tarsum (Figs. 28-31 and 28-32).

The artery follows the dorsal surface of the foot down to the posterior extremity of the first interosseous space, where it crosses vertically to anastomose with the lateral plantar artery. The essential landmark is the tendon of the extensor hallucis longus muscle. Using a bidigital grip, look for the pulse of the dorsalis pedis artery on the dorsum of the foot just lateral to the tendon mentioned above and medial to the tendon of the extensor digitorum longus muscle serving the second toe.

INDEX

A

Abdomen
  anterior nerves in wall of, 32
  anterolateral muscles of, 64–65
  anterolateral view of, 62
Abdominal aorta
  palpation of, 67
  visualization of route of, 66
Abdominal oblique muscles, external, costal insertions of, 63, 64
Abductor digiti minimi muscle, 132, 162, 344, 401
  insertion of, 377
Abductor hallucis muscle, 345, 402
  insertion of, 377
Abductor pollicis brevis muscle, 132
Abductor pollicis brevis tendon, 162
Abductor pollicis longus muscle, 114, 130
  belly of, 147
Abductor pollicis longus tendon, 115, 130, 147, 162, 193, 194
  insertion of, 161
Abductor pollicis muscle, 132, 160
  fascia over, 160
Achilles tendon, 312, 313, 323, 328, 329, 333, 336, 344, 345, 372
  anterolateral and anteromedial approach to, 395
  attachment of, 371
  lateral and posterior approach to, 395
Acromial angle, 78
  posterior inferior border of acromion medial to, 79
Acromion, 31, 70, 78, 101
  apex of, 79
  lateral view of, 5
  medial border of, 80
  posterior inferior border of, 79
Adam's apple, 8
  anterior view of, 13
  lateral view of, 12
Adductor brevis muscle, 241, 255
Adductor hallucis muscle, 403
Adductor longus muscle, 218, 221, 222, 240, 241, 245, 254, 255, 256
  sartorius muscle and, 246
Adductor magnus muscle, 209, 241, 242
  distal tendon insertion of, 245, 254, 257
    sartorius muscle and, 246
  distal tendon of vertical bundle of, 299
  inferior bundle of, 299
  ischial tuberosity insertion of, 256
  lateral portion of, 256
  median portion of, 256
Adductor magnus tendon, 256, 269, 295
  vertical, 278
Adductor minimus muscle, 241
Adductor muscles, thigh, 247
Adductor tubercle, 278, 299

Anatomical snuffbox, 130
  location of, 176
  presentation of, 169
  radial artery in, 161, 162
Anconeus muscle, 101, 114, 130, 140, 146
Ankle
  anterior surface of, 366–369
  anterior view of, 320, 378, 391, 405, 407
    muscles of, 343
  anterolateral view of, 346
  anteromedial view of, 346
  articulations of, 378–389
  lateral border of, 347–355
  lateral lateral ligament of, 364
  medial border of, 356–365
  medial lateral ligament of, 365
  medial view of, 405, 407
  musculotendinous structures of, 391–397
  myology of, 343, 391–404
  nerves and vessels of, 405–408
  osteology of, 347–377
  posterior surface of, 370–372
  posterior tibialis tendon at, 335
  medial, 345
Annular ligaments
  of radius, 117
  of tarsus, 389
  interior inferior, 407
Anserine bursa, 266, 269
Aponeurosis, internal oblique, 32
Aponeurosis, plantar, 345
Aponeurotic expansions, extensor digitorum tendon for, 143
Aponeurotic extension, extensor digitorum muscle, 145
Arcuate artery, 311, 342
Arm
  brachial artery of, 100
  deep artery of, 100, 101
    middle collateral branch of, 114
  inferior lateral cutaneous nerve of, 101
  medial cutaneous nerve of, 32, 100
  medial view of, 111
  myology of, 103–110
    anterior view of, 103–107
    posterior view of, 101, 108–110
  nerves and vessels of, 111–112
  posterior cutaneous nerve of, 101
  posterolateral view of, 102
  superior lateral cutaneous nerve of, 101
  topographic presentation of, 102
Arthrology, knee, 285–290
Articular cartilage, elbow, 117
Articular interspaces
  between cuneiform bone and metatarsals, 381–382
  of foot, 368